A Practical Guide to Basic Laboratory Andrology

Lars Björndahl
Karolinska Institutet

David Mortimer
Oozoa Biomedical Inc., Vancouver

Christopher L. R. Barratt
University of Dundee

Jose Antonio Castilla
Hospital Virgen de las Nieves

Roelof Menkveld
University of Stellenbosch

Ulrik Kvist
Karolinska Institutet

Juan G. Alvarez
Institut Marques

Trine B. Haugen
Oslo University College

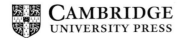

CAMBRIDGE
UNIVERSITY PRESS

CAMBRIDGE UNIVERSITY PRESS
Cambridge, New York, Melbourne, Madrid, Cape Town,
Singapore, São Paulo, Delhi

Cambridge University Press
The Edinburgh Building, Cambridge CB2 8RU, UK

Published in the United States of America by
Cambridge University Press, New York

www.cambridge.org
Information on this title: www.cambridge.org/9780521735902

© Cambridge University Press 2010

First published 2010

Printed in the United Kingdom at the University Press,
Cambridge

*A catalog record for this publication is available from the
British Library*

ISBN 978-0-521-73590-2 Paperback

Contents

List of authors   *page* vi
List of abbreviations   vii

1   **Introduction**   1
2   **Basic physiology**   5
3   **Basic semen analysis**   33
4   **Extended semen analysis**   77
5   **Sperm function tests**   113
6   **Tests of sperm–cervical mucus interaction**   147
7   **Sperm preparation**   167
8   **Sperm cryobanking**   189
9   **Preparation of surgically retrieved spermatozoa**   219
10 **Quality management and accreditation**   227
11 **Risk management**   249
12 **Reproductive toxicology**   257

Appendices
1   *Reference values*   261
2   *Equipment required for a basic andrology laboratory*   277
3   *Supply companies*   287
4   *Recommendations on the application of CASA technology in the analysis
    of spermatozoa*   291
5   *Home testing*   295
6   *Example laboratory and report forms*   297
7   *Comparison of replicate counts*   305
8   *Safety*   313
    Index   323

The color plates are to be found between pages 148 and 149.

Authors

Lars Björndahl
Centre for Andrology and Sexual Medicine,
Department of Medicine, Karolinska
University Hospital, Huddinge, S-141 86
Stockholm, Sweden

David Mortimer
Oozoa Biomedical Inc., Box 93012,
Caufeild Village RPO,
West Vancouver BC V7W 3G4, Canada

Christopher L.R. Barratt
Reproductive and Developmental
Biology Group, Centre for Oncology
and Molecular Medicine, Division of
Medical Sciences, Ninewells Hospital,
University of Dundee, Dundee,
Scotland, DD1 9SY

Jose Antonio Castilla
Hospital Virgen de las Nieves, Ribera del
Beiro, Avda. de las Fuerzas Armadas,
Granada, Andalucia, 18005, Spain

Roelof Menkveld
Andrology Laboratory E3,
Tygerberg Academic Hospital and
University of Stellenbosch,
Tygerberg, 7505, South Africa

Ulrik Kvist
Centre for Andrology and Sexual Medicine,
Department of Medicine, Karolinska
University Hospital, Huddinge,
S-141 86 Stockholm, Sweden

Juan G. Alvarez
Instituto Marques, Manuel Girona,
33, 08034 Barcelona, Spain

Trine B. Haugen
Oslo University College,
Pb 4 St. Olavs plass, 0130 Oslo,
Norway

Abbreviations

A list of common abbreviations and acronyms used in andrology and assisted conception laboratories, which may be used in this book without further definition, is provided below. Standard SI units and chemical formulae are not defined here, nor are many abbreviations that are in general English usage.

A23187	a calcium ionophore
AATB	American Association of Tissue Banks (USA)
AI	artificial insemination (unspecified source of spermatozoa)
AID	artificial insemination by donor (no longer used since the advent of AIDS, see DI and TDI)
AIDS	acquired immunodeficiency syndrome, caused by HIV infection
AIH	artificial insemination homologous *or* artificial insemination by husband
ALH	amplitude of lateral head displacement, a sperm kinematic measure (μm)
APAAP	alkaline phosphatase:anti-alkaline phosphatase complex
AR	acrosome reaction
ARIC	acrosome reaction following ionophore challenge
ART	assisted reproductive technology
ASAB(s)	antisperm antibody(ies)
ASRM	American Society for Reproductive Medicine (USA)
ATP	adenosine triphosphate
AZF	azoospermia factor, a region on the Y-chromosome
BBT	basal body temperature
BCF	beat cross frequency, a sperm kinematic measure (Hz)
BSA	bovine serum albumin (Cohn fraction V)
CAP	College of American Pathologists (USA)
CASA	computer-aided sperm analysis (*not* computer-automated semen analysis)
CBS	Cryo Bio System (Paris, France), the manufacturer of High Security Straws for cryobanking spermatozoa
CD (-ROM)	compact disk (read-only memory)
CD45	the "pan-leukocyte" antigen
C.I.	Color Index number (for stains)
CJD	Creutzfeldt–Jakob disease
CLIA	Clinical Laboratory Improvement Amendments (USA)
CMV	cytomegalovirus
COLA	Commission on Laboratory Accreditation (USA)
CPA	cryoprotective agent *or* Clinical Pathology Accreditation (UK)

CPM	cryoprotectant *or* cryopreservation medium
Cryo	cryopreservation *or* cryopreserved
CSF	cryosurvival factor, the proportion of motile spermatozoa post-thaw expressed as a percentage of the motile spermatozoa pre-freeze
CV	coefficient of variation
CZBT	competitive (sperm–)zona binding test
–D	sometimes added to acronyms such as IVF to denote the use of donor spermatozoa
DGC	density gradient centrifugation (sperm preparation method)
DHA	docosahexaenoic acid
DI	donor insemination
DMSO	dimethyl sulfoxide (a cryoprotectant and also a carrier molecule for A23187)
DNA	deoxyribonucleic acid
DPX	a microscopy mountant
DSUS	direct swim-up from semen (sperm preparation method)
DTT	dithiothreitol
DVD	digital versatile disk
EBV	Epstein–Barr virus
ECA	European Cooperation for Accreditation
EDTA	ethylenediamine tetraacetic acid, a chelator of divalent cations
EFQM	European Foundation for Quality Management
EGTA	ethyleneglycol tetraacetic acid, a chelating agent with a high affinity for calcium ions
EQA	external quality assurance
EQAP	external quality assessment program
EQAS	external quality assessment scheme
EQC	external quality control
ESHRE	European Society of Human Reproduction and Embryology
EtOH	ethyl alcohol or ethanol
EU	European Union (*not* enzyme unit)
FITC	fluorescein isothiocyanate, a fluorochrome
FMEA	failure modes and effects analysis
FMLP	formyl-methionyl-leucyl-phenylalanine, a purportedly leukocyte-specific probe to induce the generation of ROS
FNA	fine needle aspirate (a technique for performing TESA)
FSH	follicle-stimulating hormone
GAT	Kibrick's gelatin agglutination test for spermagglutinating antisperm antibodies
GEYC	glycerol-egg yolk-citrate, a modified Ackerman's CPM for human spermatozoa
GLP	Good Laboratory Practice
GMP	Good Manufacturing Practice
H33258	Hoechst dye 33258, a DNA fluorochome that can be used as a vital stain
HA	hyaluronic acid *or* hyperactivation/hyperactivated
HBV	hepatitis B virus

hCG	human chorionic gonadotrophin
HCV	hepatitis C virus
HEPES	N-(2-hydroxyethyl)piperazine-N'-(2-ethanesulfonic) acid, a zwitterionic pH buffer, pKa at 25°C = 7.5, useful pH range = 6.8–8.2
HEPT	(zona-free) hamster egg penetration test
HFEA	Human Fertilisation and Embryology Authority (UK)
hFF	human follicular fluid
H-H	head-to-head spermagglutination
HIV	human immunodeficiency virus, types-1 and -2 (causes AIDS)
H-MP	head-to-midpiece spermagglutination
HMT	hyaluronate migration test
HOS test	hypo-osmotic swelling test
HPF	high power field (40× objective)
HPM	high power magnification (40× objective)
HPV	human papillomavirus
HSA	human serum albumin (Cohn fraction V)
HSPM	human sperm preservation medium, a particular CPM formulation for human spermatozoa
HSV	herpes simplex virus
H-T	head-to-tail spermagglutination
HTF	human tubal fluid culture medium
HTLV	human T-cell lymphotropic virus, types-I and -II (HTLV-III was renamed HIV-1)
HZA	hemizona assay
IAAC	InterAmerican Accreditation Cooperation (USA)
IBT	immunobead test
ICI	intracervical insemination
ICSI	intracytoplasmic sperm injection
ID	identification
Ig	immunoglobulin
ILAC	International Laboratory Accreditation Cooperation
IMV	Instruments de Medecine Veterinaire (L'Aigle, France), the original manufacturer of semen straws
IPA	isopropyl alcohol
IQA	internal quality assurance (scheme)
IQC	internal quality control (scheme)
ISO	International Organization for Standardization (Geneva, Switzerland)
IU	International Unit (IU for enzymes refers to the conversion of 1 μmol of substrate/minute at 37°C)
IUI	intrauterine insemination
IVF (–ET)	in-vitro fertilization (and embryo transfer)
JCAHO	Joint Commission on Accreditation of Healthcare Organizations (USA)
LCR	ligase chain reaction
LH	luteinizing hormone
LIN	linearity, a sperm kinematic measure calculated as VSL/VCL × 100 (%)
LN2	or as LN_2, liquid nitrogen

LPF	low power field (10× objective)
LPM	low power magnification (10× objective)
MAR	mixed antiglobulin reaction
MESA	micro-(surgical) epididymal sperm aspiration
MI	(sperm) motility index
MOPS	3-(N-morpholino)propanesulfonic acid, a zwitterionic pH buffer, pKa at 25°C = 7.2, useful pH range = 6.5–7.9
MSDS	material safety data sheet
mtDNA	mitochondrial DNA
NA	numerical aperture (of a microscope objective)
NADH	β-nicotinamide adenine dinucleotide, reduced form
NAFA	Nordic Association for Andrology
NATA	National Association of Testing Authorities (Australia)
NCD	nuclear chromatin decondensation
NH	negative high phase contrast microscope optics
NPM	non-progressively motile (spermatozoa)
OI	oil immersion
PBS	phosphate buffered saline
PCR	polymerase chain reaction
PCT	post-coital test
PDCA	the Plan-Do-Check-Act quality cycle or Deming wheel
PESA	percutaneous epididymal sperm aspiration
PETG	polyethylene terephthalate glycol
PL	positive low phase contrast microscope optics
PMA	phorbol 12-myristate 13-acetate, an agent that provokes the generation of ROS by leukocytes and spermatozoa
PNA	peanut agglutinin, a lectin from *Arachis hypogea* that binds to the outer acrosomal membrane
PNP	p-nitrophenol
PNPG	p-nitrophenyl α-D-glucopyranoside
PR	(sperm motility) progression rating
PSA	prostate-specific antigen *or Pisum sativum* (pea) agglutinin, a lectin that binds to the acrosomal contents
PT	proficiency testing
PVA	polyvinyl alcohol
PVC	polyvinyl chloride
PVP	polyvinylpyrrolidone
QA	quality assurance
QC	quality control
QI	quality improvement
QMS	quality management system
RBC	red blood cell (erythrocyte)
RCA	root cause analysis
RFID	radiofrequency identification (device)
ROS	reactive oxygen species (a type of free radical)
RPLND	retroperitoneal lymph node dissection

SCD test	sperm chromatin dispersion test
SCMC test	sperm–cervical mucus contact test
SCSA	sperm chromatin structure assay
SD	standard deviation
SDS	sodium dodecyl (lauryl) sulfate
SEM	standard error of the mean *or* scanning electron microscopy
SIT	Isojima's sperm immobilization test for complement-dependent cytotoxic antisperm antibodies
SMIT	sperm–mucus interaction test
SOP	standard operating procedure
SPA	sperm penetration assay (North American term for the HEPT)
STD	sexually transmissible disease
STR	straightness, a sperm kinematic measure calculated as VSL/VAP × 100 (%)
TAT	Friberg's tray agglutination test for spermagglutinating antisperm antibodies
TBS	TRIS-buffered saline
TEM	transmission electron microscopy
TDI	therapeutic donor insemination (an alternative to DI)
TES	N-[Tris(hydroxymethyl)methly]-2-aminoethanesulfonic acid, a zwitterionic pH buffer, pKa at 25°C = 7.5, useful pH range = 6.8–8.2
TESA	testicular sperm aspiration
TESE	testicular sperm extraction, usually by surgical testicular biopsy
TEST	or TES-TRIS, a buffer combination of TES and TRIS
TQM	total quality management
TRIS	tris(hydroxymethyl)aminomethane, pKa at 25°C = 8.1, useful pH range = 7–9
TRITC	tetramethyl rhodamine isothiocyanate, also known simply as rhodamine, a fluorochrome
Tt	tail-tip (of the spermatozoon)
T-T	tail-to-tail spermagglutination
TUNEL	terminal deoxynucleotidyl transferase
TUR	trans-urethral resection, of the prostate
TYG	TEST-yolk-glycerol, a particular CPM formulation for human spermatozoa
TZI	teratozoospermia index
U	(International) Unit; see IU
UPS	uninterruptible power supply
u.v.	ultra violet
VAP	average path velocity, a sperm kinematic measure (μm/s)
vCJD	variant Creutzfeldt–Jakob disease
VCL	curvilinear velocity, a sperm kinematic measure (μm/s)
VCR	videocassette recorder
VHS	the most common standard for domestic and commercial videocassettes
VOC	volatile organic compound
VSL	straight-line velocity, a sperm kinematic measure (μm/s)
WBC	white blood cell (leukocyte)
WHMIS	Workplace Hazardous Material Information Scheme

WHO	World Health Organization (Geneva, Switzerland)
WOB	wobble, a sperm kinematic measure calculated as VAP/VCL × 100 (%)
XHT	crossed hostility test
ZBT	(sperm–)zona binding test
ZP	zona pellucida
ZP3	zona pellucida glycoprotein 3

Introduction

Male subfertility is a very significant global problem. Epidemiological data show that approximately 1-in-7 couples are classed as subfertile [1]. Sperm dysfunction is the single most common cause of male subfertility. Indeed, studies using semen assessment criteria for male subfertility (sperm concentration $<20 \times 10^6$/ml) illustrate that 20% of 18-year-olds are classed as subfertile [2]. Although it is too simplistic to base a classification as subfertile solely on sperm concentration, the reported frequency of male subfertility points to a high proportion of the population being affected, compared with other prevalent diseases such as diabetes. Moreover, what is more worrying is the possibility that the prevalence of male subfertility is increasing [3]. Andrology is therefore a pivotal discipline in modern medicine, and it is against this background that we have assembled this handbook.

Semen analysis provides a comprehensive view of the reproductive functioning of the male partner of the subfertile couple. It includes assessments of sperm count (which examine sperm production, transport through the male genital tract and ejaculatory function), sperm motility (a basic functional marker of likely sperm competence), sperm vitality (to distinguish between dead spermatozoa and live, immotile spermatozoa), sperm form (aspects of sperm production and maturation), and the physical appearance of the ejaculate (semen production). In addition to this basic semen assessment there are further tests that can be performed – what we have termed extended semen analysis – permitting further analyses that assess more functional aspects of the semen sample. Such tests include biochemical examinations to evaluate the secretions from the auxiliary sex glands, the detection of antisperm antibodies, and the use of computer-aided sperm analysis (CASA) to examine sperm motility patterns (kinematics).

A high quality, comprehensive semen assessment is not just the cornerstone of the diagnosis of male subfertility; it is also the starting point for providing prognostic information. While the basic semen assessment has been performed for over 60 years, there have been a number of studies questioning the value of the traditional semen characteristics (sperm concentration, motility, and morphology) in the diagnosis and prognosis of male subfertility [4]. Partly, this is the result of an incomplete understanding of what clinical information a semen assessment can provide (see below), but primarily it is because the basic assessments are usually performed using inadequate methods with limited understanding of the technical requirements, and poor quality assurance. An example of this is the UK survey of laboratories performing andrology tests, which showed dramatic variation from World Health Organization (WHO) standardized procedures leading to uncritical reporting of results [5]. In this handbook we provide a detailed, step-by-step guide using robust methods for examining human semen. We have also included comprehensive documentation for training of staff and sections on quality control (QC), quality assurance (QA), and quality improvement (QI). Adoption of such methods and procedures will lead to a significant improvement in the quality of the data produced by the andrology laboratory, and therefore more robust clinical information.

One matter that has been discussed in relation to semen analysis is the number of samples that must be analyzed from each individual. Quite often, at least two samples are said to be required to get a representative result for the individual [6,7]. However, when based on laboratory data, a considerable portion of the variability in results could be ascribed to technical variability due to substandard laboratory methods. Thus, with poor technical quality (including low numbers of spermatozoa assessed) investigations of multiple samples from the same man can, at least in part, compensate – but it is cost-efficient for neither the patient and his partner, nor the laboratory. The reason why, in epidemiological studies, men investigated for possible reproductive toxicological effects only need to produce one sample is most likely that the variability in individual samples will "disappear" when the average is used and differences in averages between groups can be analyzed [8]. Although there is a considerable biological variability in semen analysis results (see Chapter 2), especially concerning sperm concentration, the clinical evaluation of the man does not always require analyses of several repeated samples. For the primary investigation of the man in a subfertile couple, information from the very first semen sample can be enough to direct the continued investigation – either a very poor result indicating the need for direct clinical andrological investigations, or a very good result indicating that further basic semen analyses will not reveal any more information [9,10]. In the group of men with intermediate results, valuable information can be gained from repeated semen analysis. The methods described in this handbook have been developed to minimize the varia-bility due to technical factors, to optimize the evaluation of the man as well as the laboratory work.

For the proper use of semen analysis results, appropriate interpretation is fundamental. With a few clear exceptions (e.g. azoospermia), the data cannot provide unambiguous information about the chances of future conception, either *in vivo* or *in vitro*. Currently, there is a clear tendency to overemphasize the value of a single parameter, e.g. sperm morphology with strict cut-offs as used for assisted reproductive technology (ART). However, as there is a considerable overlap between the semen characteristics of fertile and subfertile men, no single parameter can be used to provide prognostic information about the fertility potential of the couple. A combination of several variables (motility, morphology, and concentration) does give more accurate diagnostic and prognostic information, although there will always be overlaps between what is considered fertile and subfertile [11,12]. Irrespective of the low predictive value for the reproductive success of the couple, a comprehensive semen analysis provides information about the status of the male reproduc-tive organs, and this is important in the well-being of the man. The results of a semen analysis are often used as a sentinel marker for the potential treatment pathway for patients. For example, a primary question in ART clinics remains: is the semen of this man suitable for intrauterine insemination (IUI), or is in-vitro fertilization (IVF), or even intracytoplasmic sperm injection (ICSI) needed? Primarily, what the clinic is trying to do is determine whether there are indications that the man will have a high likelihood of *failure* using a particular treatment modality, i.e. the man's spermatozoa are unsuitable for insemination by IUI, and IVF is indicated. However, despite the plethora of literature surrounding this area, there are still no simple answers. For example, a meta-analysis of the literature trying to ascertain the number of spermatozoa that have been (can be) used as a cut-off for IUI success concluded that there was no such cut-off, and that the data available were of insufficient quality to provide a robust answer [13]. Of course, the quality of the sperm preparation methodology (and also the products used) will also impact on treatment outcome, confounding any simple relationship between pre-treatment semen characteristics and treatment outcome.

For the comprehensive investigation of a man's fertility potential it is essential not only to perform a semen analysis, but also that a physical examination be performed, a complete medical carried out, and a history taken [14]. Accurate interpretation of a semen analysis cannot be made without knowing the patient's history, and having information from a physical examination and other laboratory investigations, e.g. hormone analysis. Reduced fertility potential can be secondary to other diseases that should be properly investigated and treated. It is thus irresponsible and unethical to embark upon an infertility work-up without a complete physical examination and history.

A common source for misunderstandings and misinterpretations is the use of qualitative terms such as oligozoospermia and asthenozoospermia. Originally, these terms were used to characterize laboratory findings before the quantitative measures had become usable and reliable. Subsequently, these terms have been given precise limits on quantitative scales, creating the false impression of dichotomy (two clearly separated outcomes, such as subfertile and fertile) based on semen characteristics – as opposed to the true situation of a sliding scale between severely infertile (but not sterile) and fertile. In an effort to reduce such confusion in the future, we have abandoned the use of all such qualitative terms and urge everyone working in the field to do likewise: just describe what you see, as objectively and quantitatively as possible, and interpret the test results within the holistic medical context for the man, especially the particular circumstances that exist within the reproductive unit of which he is part, i.e. with his partner, since (sub)fertility is always a feature of the couple.

References

1. Hull MG, Glazener CM, Kelly NJ, et al. Population study of causes, treatment, and outcome of infertility. Br Med J (Clin Res Ed) 1985; 291: 1693–7.

2. Andersen AG, Jensen TK, Carlsen E, et al. High frequency of sub-optimal semen quality in an unselected population of young men. Hum Reprod 2000; 15: 366–72.

3. Sharpe RM, Irvine DS. How strong is the evidence of a link between environmental chemicals and adverse effects on human reproductive health? BMJ 2004; 328: 447–51.

4. Björndahl L, Barratt CL. Semen analysis: setting standards for the measurement of sperm numbers. J Androl 2005; 26: 11.

5. Riddell D, Pacey A, Whittington K. Lack of compliance by UK andrology laboratories with World Health Organization recommendations for sperm morphology assessment. Hum Reprod 2005; 20: 3441–5.

6. Keel BA. Within- and between-subject variation in semen parameters in infertile men and normal semen donors. Fertil Steril 2006; 85: 128–34.

7. Castilla JA, Alvarez C, Aguilar J, et al. Influence of analytical and biological variation on the clinical interpretation of seminal parameters. Hum Reprod 2006; 21: 847–51.

8. Stokes-Riner A, Thurston SW, Brazil C, et al. One semen sample or 2? Insights from a study of fertile men. J Androl 2007; 28: 638–43.

9. Hirsh A. Male subfertility. BMJ 2003; 327: 669–72.

10. Mishail A, Marshall S, Schulsinger D, Sheynkin Y. Impact of a second semen analysis on a treatment decision making in the infertile man with varicocele. Fertil Steril 2009; 91: 1809–11.

11. Guzick DS, Overstreet JW, Factor-Litvak P, et al. National Cooperative Reproductive Medicine Network. Sperm morphology, motility, and concentration in fertile and

infertile men. *N Engl J Med* 2001; **345**: 1388–93.

12. Jedrzejczak P, Taszarek-Hauke G, Hauke J, *et al*. Prediction of spontaneous conception based on semen parameters. *Int J Androl* 2008; **31**: 499–507.

13. van Weert JM, Repping S, Van Voorhis BJ, *et al*. Performance of the postwash total motile sperm count as a predictor of pregnancy at the time of intrauterine insemination: a meta-analysis. *Fertil Steril* 2004; **82**: 612–20.

14. Jequier AM. The importance of diagnosis in the clinical management of infertility in the male. *Reprod Biomed Online* 2006; **13**: 331–5.

Chapter 2

Basic physiology

What are gametes good for? Protection against microorganisms

One prerequisite for multi-cellular organisms to survive is to be able to repulse attacks by microorganisms; attacks by their deoxyribonucleic acid (DNA), ribonucleic acid (RNA), and proteins and prions. Every individual multi-cellular organism has developed an immunological defense system that is directed towards everything but itself. However, to discriminate *foreign* cells and microorganisms from cells belonging to itself it is essential to be unique. The problem of becoming unique was solved some 600 million years ago with the evolution of a new type of cell division, meiosis, which enabled the formation of genetically unique gametes. Coupled with this, the fusion (fertilization) of two genetically unique gametes (the spermatozoon and the oocyte), results in a genetically unique, new individual. Due to meiotic recombination, every gamete is supplied with one out of four unique DNA molecules for every chromosome pair. In human beings there are 23 pairs of chromosomes, so the number of possible DNA combinations in any gamete is 4^{23}, i.e. any gamete achieves 1 out of 70×10^{12} combinations (one out of seventy million million) of genetic material. At fertilization, gametes from two different individuals fuse and form one new individual; the genetic composition of the child is thus one combination out of 4900×10^{24} possible combinations. A man produces some 100 million unique genetic lots per day. A woman produces one mature oocyte a month; and again, each oocyte is genetically unique.

Thus, the evolution of meiosis and unique gametes was a prerequisite for an individual immune defense, which in turn was a prerequisite for the evolution and survival of multi-cellular organisms exposed to endless attacks by microorganisms [1].

Outside the body the laboratory staff must protect the gametes

Outside the body there is no immune system or reproductive tract to protect the gametes. The laboratory must therefore fulfill these functions to protect gametes and embryos. Assisted reproduction *in vitro* would be impossible if microorganisms were not actively combated. Laminar-air-flow benches, UV-light protected airlocks, sterile and controlled handling and culture media, rooms with controlled air purity and special clothing for the involved staff are some precautions regulatory bodies seek. Sometimes chemical weapons such as antibiotics are necessary, yet microorganisms with foreign DNA and RNA may still manage to invade our culture media and become incorporated into embryos and thereby future generations [1].

Every man is a unique experiment of nature

Most multi-cellular organisms have both testes and ovaries, usually (but not always) in different individuals, of the male and female genders, respectively. Since oocytes are immobile these organisms exchange spermatozoa either while they are in direct contact or with the aid of wind, water or other vectors.

In mammals, some 300 million years ago the genes controlling sperm production were transferred from one of the two ancient X-chromosomes onto a "shortened X-chromosome", today called the Y-chromosome. The Y-bearing organism developed into a mobile, sperm-producing individual. In order for the "species" to survive, the sperm producer must succeed in finding signs of ovulation and be able to deliver spermatozoa for fertilization of the oocytes. In mammals, the default development (phenotype) is the female development. The development of a fertile man able to react to signs of ovulation requires the selection of a handful of specific male development routes during embryonic, fetal, and early childhood development [2,3]. Many of these traits are known to be dependent on testosterone. The traits result in the development of (a) the testes, (b) inner male genitalia, (c) outer male genitalia, (d) male sexual identity and (e) "oocyte-bearing" women as a sexual preference.

Production of the male gamete or spermatozoon

Spermatogenesis is the process by which spermatozoa are produced from spermatogonia in the testis. The light microscopic examination performed during semen analysis aims to give information about the success of spermatogenesis including the number of spermatozoa, their morphology and motility. A more thorough evaluation of the ejaculate can reveal a variety of disturbances originating in the different steps of spermatogenesis, and might shed light on disturbed testicular function, or even disclose the presence of early testis cancer [3,4].

Spermatogenesis preparations occur in the embryo

Already during the embryonic and fetal stage, preparations for spermatogenesis are being made. Immature germ cells from the epiblast migrate from the yolk sac and invade the seminiferous cords (which will become tubules at puberty) in both testes, and start to proliferate up to week 18 in the fetus. The other cells inside the seminiferous cords, the Sertoli cells, also multiply. The somatic Sertoli cell and its spermatogonia could be regarded as a unit for future sperm production. If the migration of germ cells is disturbed, or if the germ cells degenerate, few or no spermatogonia will be left for sperm production, and the only cells left would be the Sertoli cells (known clinically as the "Sertoli cell-only" syndrome).

Spermatogenesis is comprised of five different processes
Renewal of stem cells

There are two types of spermatogonia type A: dark and pale (Figure 2.1). Both belong to the stem cell population and are continuously renewed by mitotic divisions. It is estimated that spermatogonia undergo some 20 mitotic cell divisions a year, so at 35 years of age the spermatogonia have undergone some 400 mitotic cell divisions, whereas the female oocyte rests from embryonic week 10 until ovulation. Thus, hazards linked to cell division events (mutations in DNA, aneuploidy, mutations and deletions in mitochondrial DNA) are more likely to affect spermatogenesis than oogenesis.

Human spermatogenesis

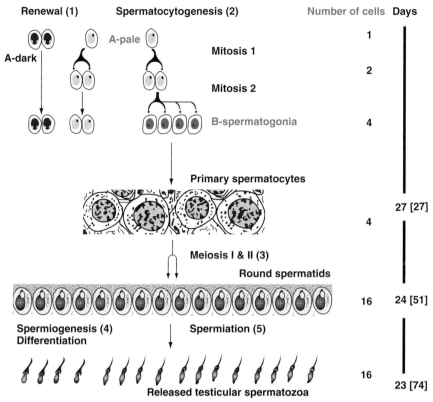

Figure 2.1 A schematic drawing of human spermatogenesis compiled from data given by references [4] and [5]: (1) shows that A-pale spermatogonia renew by mitosis and that A-dark spermatogonia mainly rest; (2) outlines that another A-pale spermatogonium is chosen to undergo two mitotic cleavages into four B-spermatogonia and that B-spermatogonia differentiate into primary spermatocytes (spermatocytogenesis); (3) shows the two meiotic divisions of each of the primary spermatocytes into four round spermatids, and finally (4) the differentiation of round spermatids into elongated spermatids (spermiogenesis) that through (5) spermiation are released as testicular spermatozoa in the lumen of the seminiferous tubule. Number of cells refers to the number of daughter cells (finally spermatozoa) resulting from one spermatogonium. Days mark the duration of each step and, in brackets, the accumulated duration.

Spermatocytogenesis

An important process is an exponential increase in number of spermatozoa; in the human testis two consecutive mitotic divisions prepare for the meiotic cell division. One spermatogonium A pale is recruited for sperm production and undergoes two mitotic cell divisions, resulting in a clone of four spermatogonia B. Each of these then differentiates into four primary spermatocytes. The latter two mitotic cell divisions increase the possible number of spermatozoa by a factor of four. If one mitotic division does not occur then only half the number of spermatozoa can be produced. It means that missing mitotic divisions could be one cause of low sperm numbers. In rodents there may be 11 mitotic divisions before the meiotic divisions begin, and in the rhesus monkey there may be five mitotic divisions. Thus, in those species, one A-spermatogonium will theoretically result in 8192 and 128 spermatozoa, respectively, whereas the number of resulting spermatozoa in man is 16 [5].

Meiosis

The purpose of this process is to ensure that every spermatozoon achieves (a) a unique combination of DNA, and (b) a haploid genome in which the original 23 pairs of chromosomes are reduced to 23 single copies of the DNA. Each of the four primary spermatocytes in a clone undergoes the two meiotic divisions. The eight secondary spermatocytes finally result in the formation of 16 round spermatids.

Spermiogenesis

This is the process where the round spermatid transforms (differentiates) into a functional messenger cell called the testicular spermatid, which is still attached to the Sertoli cell (Figure 2.2).

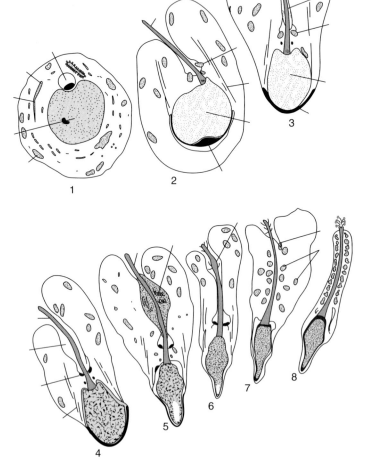

Figure 2.2 The steps of spermiogenesis. (1) Immature spermatid with round shaped nucleus. The acrosome vesicle is attached to the nucleus; the tail anlage still fails contact to the nucleus. (2) The acrosome vesicle is increased and flattened over the nucleus. The tail establishes contact with the nucleus. (3–8) Acrosome formation, nuclear condensation, and development of tail structures take place. The mature spermatid (8) is delivered from the germinal epithelium. Semi-schematic drawing on the basis of electron micrographs by AF Holstein [4].

Spermiation

Initiated by the Sertoli cell, testicular spermatozoa are released from the Sertoli cells, which take up the surplus cytoplasm and membrane from the sperm midpiece (the residual body).

Spermatogenesis takes place in the seminiferous tubules

A normal tubule has a diameter of about 180 μm, and the diameter is decreased when spermatogenesis is impaired (Figure 2.3). The tubule walls are composed of five layers of myofibroblasts in connective tissue, which cause peristaltic waves of contraction to transport the immotile testicular spermatozoa to the rete testis for further transportation, via the efferent ducts, to the caput of the epididymis. The thickness of the peritubular tissue is 8 μm, corresponding to the size of the neighboring spermatogonia. A thickened wall is associated with impaired spermatogenesis [4].

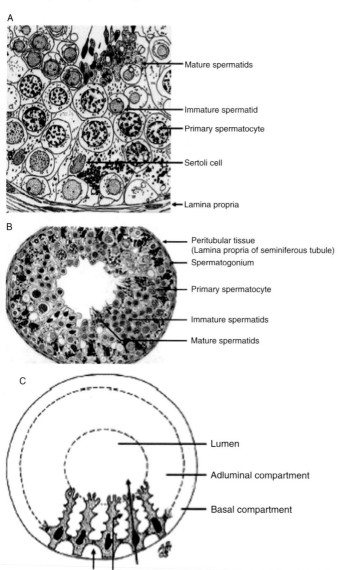

A

— Mature spermatids

— Immature spermatid

— Primary spermatocyte

— Sertoli cell

← Lamina propria

B

— Peritubular tissue
(Lamina propria of seminiferous tubule)

— Spermatogonium

— Primary spermatocyte

— Immature spermatids

— Mature spermatids

C

— Lumen

— Adluminal compartment

— Basal compartment

Figure 2.3 (A) Cross-section of a seminiferous tubule of a fertile man 32 years of age. Drawing of a semithin section ×300. (B) A sector of the germinal epithelium in the seminiferous tubule. Drawing on the basis of a semithin section ×900. (C) Sertoli cells divide the germinal epithelium in a basal and adluminal compartment. Arrows indicate that the passage of substances from the outside stops at the tight junctions in the basal compartment, and that the adluminal compartment and the lumen can only be reached by transport through the Sertoli cells. Drawings by AF Holstein [4].

The Sertoli cell

The Sertoli cell is the dominating cell in the seminiferous cords and tubuli. It is a supporting cell that provides nutrition and mediates paracrine signals for spermatogenesis, as well as protection of the developing germs cells from the immune system. The Sertoli cell communicates, via factors and testosterone, with the Leydig cells in the interstitium between the seminiferous tubules. It produces inhibin-B, which exerts a negative feedback on the follicle-stimulating hormone (FSH) secretion from the pituitary gland. In about half of men with azoospermia, the Sertoli cells produce low levels of inhibin-B, resulting in elevated FSH levels in blood. However, low levels of inhibin-B and high levels of FSH do not exclude that focal spermatogenesis can be found at testicular biopsy, making sperm retrieval and ICSI a possible treatment [6,7]. Protection from the immune system is mediated by neighboring Sertoli cells forming tight junctions between them, thereby dividing the seminiferous tubules into two compartments (Figure 2.3C): (a) the basal compartment facing the *inside* where the immune system can act against *foreign* objects, and (b) the one facing the *outside world* – the adluminal compartment, from which the spermatozoa are released and transported out of the man. At meiosis, the primary spermatocytes, which soon are going to give rise to spermatids with unique DNA (and therefore will appear as *foreign* to the immune system), are transferred from the basal to the adluminal (outside) compartment, thus escaping the risk of being attacked by the immune system. The so-called blood-testis barrier consists of a combination of these inter-Sertoli cell connections, the peritubular tissue in the walls of the tubules, and the endothelium of the testicular capillaries in the interstitium between the tubules [4].

The testicular interstitium and the Leydig cells

Besides spermatogenesis the testis has another vital physiological role: testosterone production by the Leydig cells which surround the capillaries in the interstitium.

The embryonic male

In response to human chorionic gonadotrophin (hCG) from the placenta anlagen (chorion cells) and thereafter the developing placenta of the embryo, Leydig cells produce testosterone necessary for the differentiation and development of a fertile man. Disturbed function of the placenta during critical time intervals of the embryonic development can jeopardize the specific male development and hence future male fertility.

The adult man

At puberty, gonadotrophin-releasing hormone (GnRH) is secreted from the hypothalamus in isolated peaks (once every 90 minutes), which stimulates the pituitary to secrete FSH and LH (named luteinizing hormone from its effect in females). LH stimulates the Leydig cells to produce testosterone. No less than 90% of the testosterone is taken up by the Sertoli cells in the tubules and is used for spermatogenesis and by luminal flow for the androgen-specific functions of the excurrent duct system up to the corpus of the epididymis. Some 10% is delivered to the capillary blood and exerts systemic androgen effects on the man, including male secondary sex characteristics such as body and face hair, deep voice, increased muscle mass, decreased body fat, increased male hemoglobin, and reinforced skeleton, as well as brain function resulting in "male temper" [3].

The human spermatozoon

The messenger cell

The morphology of the human spermatozoon is depicted in Figure 2.4, drawn by the German scientist Adolph Holstein, based on electron microscopic studies [4].

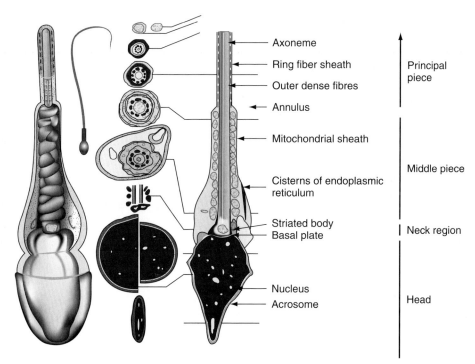

Axoneme

Ring fiber sheath

Outer dense fibres

Annulus

Mitochondrial sheath

Cisterns of endoplasmic reticulum

Striated body
Basal plate

Nucleus

Acrosome

Principal piece

Middle piece

Neck region

Head

Figure 2.4 The human spermatozoon. Left: Virtual preparation of the spermatozoon showing the acrosome, the nucleus and nuclear envelopes, and the mitochondrial sheath of the main piece of the flagellum. Middle: Cross-sections of the human spermatozoon of different levels indicated on the right: longitudinal section of the human spermatozoon. Semi-schematic drawing by AF Holstein [4] on the basis of electron micrographs.

The spermatozoon is a messenger cell – a conveyer of information – carrying the unique paternal messages needed to create a healthy child and grandchildren. As a messenger it needs special properties, such as being motile in order to reach the immotile oocyte and deliver its information after fusion with the oocyte membrane. The motility of the spermatozoon depends on the axoneme structures (e.g. microtubule doublets, dynein arms, spokes), the presence of functional mitochondria and functional outer dense fibers, both providing energy (ATP), functional centriole (tail insertion) and fibrous tail sheath (rigid tail movements).

The sperm chromatin, DNA, protamines and zinc

The DNA of the spermatozoon is temporarily well-protected in a semi-crystalline structure stabilized by zinc (Figure 2.5). This unique, dense packaging of sperm chromatin offers protection and could compensate for the lack of DNA repair systems. The sperm chromatin is primarily arranged like a "rope" with three intermingled strands: the two DNA strands constitute two strands while the third strand is constituted of protamines. There is one zinc ion for every protamine molecule and turn of the DNA helix, i.e. for every 10 base-pairs of DNA. Zinc withdrawal enables a quick unwrapping of the chromatin into separate DNA threads (double-stranded helices), when studied almost immediately after ejaculation. This ability promptly declines among spermatozoa left in the liquefying ejaculate *in vitro* [1,8,9,10].

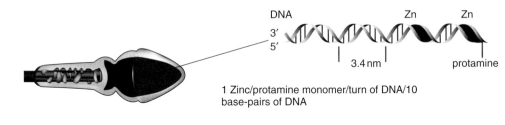

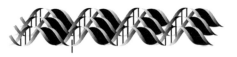

Figure 2.5 Outline of a model for human sperm chromatin stabilization. Chromatin string arranged by three threads: the two DNA strands and the protamine string composed of protamine monomers. One zinc is present for every protamine monomer for every turn of the DNA helix, i.e. for every 10 base-pairs. Chromatin fibers arranged condensed, side by side, when the negative charges of DNA have been neutralized by positive charges of the protamines.

This unique, dense packaging of the sperm genome is due to exchange of DNA-binding histones in the nucleus. During the late phases of spermiogenesis somatic histones are replaced first by temporary proteins and then by protamines. At the same time zinc is incorporated into the sperm nucleus. The positive amino groups ($-NH_3^+$) of arginine in the protamines *neutralize* the negative phosphate groups ($-PO_4^{3-}$) of the DNA backbone, which is the basis for the tight packing of the DNA-protamine complex. In human sperm chromatin there are mainly two types of protamines: protamine 1 and protamine 2. Besides arginine, these protamines contain the amino acids cysteine and histidine that can form stable temporary salt-bridges with zinc. The NH group of the imidazole ring of histidine, and the reduced SH group of the cysteine, have high affinity for zinc (cf. zinc-fingers). Moreover, the presence of zinc facilitates the binding of DNA to protamine [11,12,13]. Sperm nuclear zinc deficiency induced *in vitro* provokes liberated sulfhydryl groups to form disulfide-bridges and thereby changes the type of chromatin stability from zinc-dependent to non-zinc-dependent chromatin stability, caused by disulfide-bridges leading to an abnormal (covalently bonded) and less easily reversible stabilization of the chromatin. This is likely to hinder or at least delay sperm chromatin decondensation in the ooplasm, and could therefore be an important cause for male factor infertility.

Sperm mitochondrial DNA and impaired spermatogenesis

Mutagenic destruction of mitochondrial DNA (mtDNA) is a condition that limits the lifespan of each individual. By regeneration of mitochondria with undamaged native mtDNA in the oocyte a new individual is provided with fully functional mitochondria from the one-cell stage of the zygote. This appears to be the evolutionary mechanism for family eternity, by which every new generation can start off with fresh mitochondria.

Mutagenic deletions of mitochondrial DNA are likely to propagate relatively rapidly in cells with frequent cell divisions. For a 35-year-old man, his spermatogonia have undergone some 400 mitotic divisions. This means that a deletion of the mtDNA in his spermatogonia would lead to a metabolic exhaustion of the processes involved in spermatogenesis and could therefore be manifested by, for example, severely reduced sperm concentration, motility, and morphology. Thus, genetic characterization of germ cell mtDNA or sperm mtDNA could be a future tool to estimate whether disorders in spermatogenesis are due to inadequate mitochondrial functions.

Efficiency of the spermatogenesis

Spermatogenesis in man appears to be a process of redundancy. Developing germ cells and spermatozoa are lost during and after spermatogenesis, and only some 25% of spermatozoa formed reach the ejaculate [4]; among them, the proportion of malformed spermatozoa is extremely high. One can argue that if the man has *some* "typical" spermatozoa (i.e. appearance as spermatozoa able to pass through cervical mucus and bind to the zona pellucida), then the genetic "blueprints" for a typical spermatozoon are present. But, the control of the process is apparently of very low priority for fertility, and is therefore not given high efficiency in terms of quality management. This type of pleiomorphism (a large range of sperm forms in the ejaculate) is almost never seen in laboratory animals or inbred farming animals where spermatozoa have excellent morphology. This may be due to natural selection when males compete for the oocytes at the sperm level, or man-made selection of animals with good sperm morphology. Besides man, gorillas and some mice species have pleiomorphic spermatozoa. A plausible explanation for this could be that the performance (and thereby the structure and function) of spermatozoa is not critical when the competition for reproduction is between males (the female only receives spermatozoa from one male), rather than between their spermatozoa (the female receives spermatozoa from several males during an ovulatory cycle) [14]. It should be emphasized that if a man has only 1% of spermatozoa with morphology typical for those spermatozoa that reach the site for fertilization, an ejaculate of 100 million spermatozoa still contains 1 million spermatozoa with "typical" morphology.

Note that pleiomorphism means that many different types of morphological variants exist in an ejaculate. This must be distinguished from conditions where most spermatozoa have the same type of atypical morphology. In such cases a genetic reason could be suspected and a chromosomal analysis (karyotyping) can rule out chromosomal translocations and inversions. In fact, morphology screening in mice is used as a method to monitor exposures inducing chromosomal translocations.

Sperm transport – from testis to urethra

Testicular spermatozoa are transported from the seminiferous tubules in the testis by the flow of fluid to the rete testis, and then by the 15–20 efferent ducts to the convoluted, approximately six-meter-long, epididymal duct on each side (Figure 2.6). The epididymis is anatomically divided into the caput, corpus, and cauda regions (Figure 2.7). There is

13

also a more functional subdivision of the epididymal duct into the initial, middle, and terminal segments. The epididymal duct, and its continuation into the vas deferens and the seminal vesicles, is developed from the embryonic Wolffian duct. In the vas deferens, spermatozoa are transported from the distal cauda to the urethra. Before passing through the prostate the vas deferens is widened, forming the ampulla of the vas deferens, from which the seminal vesicles are developed. The ampulla and the seminal vesicle on each side have a common excurrent duct named the ejaculatory duct, which opens into the urethra [2,3].

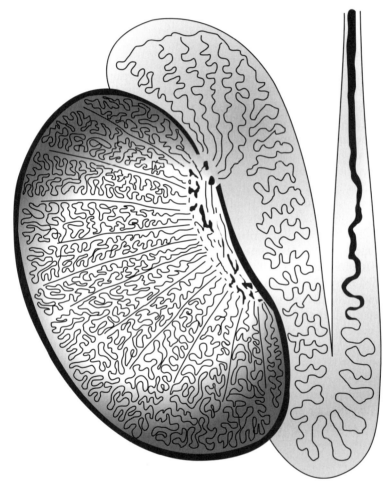

Figure 2.6 A semi-schematic drawing by AF Holstein [4] showing the arrangement of the seminiferous tubules in the human testis, the efferent ductules (6 of 10–15 shown) connecting the rete testis to the epididymal duct, and the continuation of the epididymal duct into the vas deferens.

The differentiation, development and secretory function of these organs are dependent on androgens. From the testes to the corpus of the epididymis, most androgens are provided by the local fluid transportation from the testis (luminal fluid, lymphatic fluid, and local venous plexa), while the systemic circulation provides androgens to the cauda, the vas deferens, the seminal vesicles and the prostate. The prostate has developed from the embryonic genitourinary sinus.

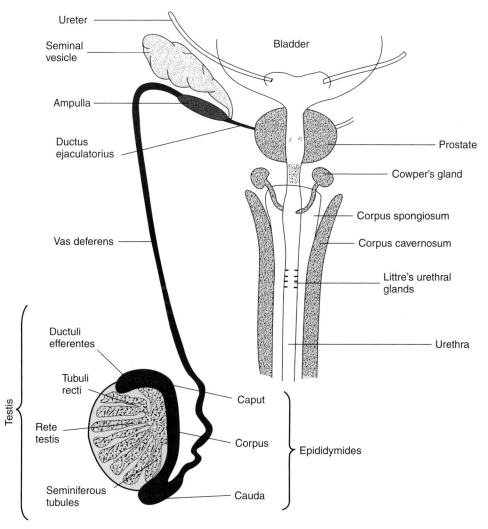

Figure 2.7 Outline of the male genital tract in man.

The epididymis and sperm transport

In most mammals the epididymal transit time has been reported to be 7–10 days. However, the transit time is dependent on the amount of spermatozoa to be transported (i.e. daily sperm production). Men with high sperm output (>200 × 10^6 spermatozoa per day) had an average transit time of 2 days, whereas men with lower output (mean approximately 70 × 10^6 per day) reached 6 days of transit time [15]. The luminal transport from corpus to cauda seems independent of nervous regulation, but involves local spontaneous waves of contraction of seven to nine waves per minute. In the distal cauda and vas deferens the spontaneous contractility is only one to two waves per minute, resulting in an accumulation of spermatozoa in the distal cauda (i.e. it is a region of sperm storage).

Transit time through the caput, corpus and proximal cauda is independent of ejaculatory frequency. The transport of spermatozoa from the distal cauda to the urethra is dependent on neurogenic activity, and frequent ejaculation results in a decline in sperm numbers there, while sexual abstinence results in increased numbers stored. One ejaculation a day for 2 days seems enough to normalize and equalize an increased or depleted sperm storage to the level of the daily sperm output [16].

The epididymis, sperm maturation and sperm fertilization capacity

During epididymal transit the spermatozoon undergoes a maturation process by which it acquires capabilities as a messenger cell to traverse and survive the female genital tract, and eventually deliver its genetic information to the embryo-to-be. Among these properties are progressive motility, the ability to fuse with and fertilize the oocyte, and the ability to sustain embryonic development into a viable offspring. The maturation process appears not to be restricted to particular parts of the epididymis, but occurs as a function of time. Thus, spermatozoa withheld in the caput by occlusion of the duct in the corpus develop fertilizing capacity. Normal development and function of the caput and corpus epididymides is dependent on luminal flow of testosterone, which is locally transformed to the active dihydrotestosterone by the converting enzyme 5-α-reductase type 1 (5-αR1).

Epididymis and sperm storage

The cauda epididymis has evolved as the sperm storage organ in animals forced to wait for female ovulation. It seems that when reaching the proximal cauda, the spermatozoa have achieved "conservation factors" enabling prolonged storage. Two major factors contribute to this sperm storage: (a) a low temperature (34°C), and (b) an androgen-dependent environment, including secretory products, created in the cauda epididymis. The androgen acting in the cauda epididymis is testosterone, transported by the systemic circulation and taken up by the epididymal epithelial cells and locally converted to dihydrotestosterone by 5-α-reductase type 2 (5-αR2). Factors jeopardizing the scrotal temperature and the testosterone effects (e.g. compounds interacting with 5-αR2) would decrease the functional storage time.

Conservation and capacitation

The conservation processes involve inactivation of motility and metabolism, and the stabilization of various sperm structures and membranes. At ejaculation, the mixing of spermatozoa with the prostatic fluid restores motility, and it is plausible that the capacitation process needed to activate mammalian spermatozoa for fertilization involves restoration of conserved mechanisms [17].

The size of the sperm storage

Man is a mammal with relatively low sperm production, a mere $100–500 \times 10^6$ per day. Sperm production is continuous, and similar to the ram the man can have several ejaculations a day with fertile spermatozoa. Ejaculation every 4th hour after 3 days of abstinence can give results such as 1000×10^6 (first sample after 3 days of abstinence), 125×10^6 (4 h later), and 20×10^6 (another 4 h later). It is worth noting that a decline from 1000×10^6 to 20×10^6 fresh spermatozoa due to sexual activity has no negative impact on the man's fertility. In this respect, the evaluation of sperm number is totally different from the evaluation of red and white cells in blood. Therefore, when evaluating sperm counts, the ejaculatory frequency (i.e. sexual behavior) is of critical importance: not only the time interval between the preceding ejaculation to that collected for investigation, but also the frequency of ejaculations preceding collection for investigation. Of all the spermatozoa in the epididymis, 50–80% are localized in the cauda, and half of them are available for ejaculation.

DNA damage upon sperm storage

Experiments show that spermatozoa aged within the epididymis (or in the laboratory or within the female genital tract) first lose their potential to contribute to a normal embryonic development (probably due to the fact that prolonged sperm storage results in sperm DNA strand breaks and chromosomal aberrations of the embryos [11]). Thereafter they lose the ability to fully decondense their nuclear chromatin within the oocyte; followed by the loss of their ability to fertilize the oocyte and, long thereafter, they have a reduction in motility.

Animal studies have shown that if the transport of fresh spermatozoa from the testis to the cauda epididymis is hindered, those spermatozoa remaining in the cauda more frequently cause aneuploidies in resulting embryos after only six days in the epididymis. The question arises, therefore, as to how those spermatozoa that, upon aging in the epididymis, have damaged DNA are eliminated and "hindered" in reaching the site of fertilization. Possible explanations include:

1. That old spermatozoa are mixed with fresh ones in the cauda, and these fresh gametes with undamaged DNA are more likely to reach the oocyte. There is so far no evidence that the female genital tract can select spermatozoa based upon their genomes, and about 0.5–1% of newborns have chromosomal aberrations. Moreover, DNA damage occurs before the ability to fertilize is decreased.

2. Male sexual drive could result in nocturnal emissions, masturbation and non-ovulation-related intercourse, which in turn would eliminate old spermatozoa, making way for fresh ones.

3. Local muscle contractions of the cauda–vas deferens can emit spermatozoa to the urethra, where they are voided with the urine. Spermatozoa in morning urine are diagnostic for spermarche [15,18].

4. An as yet unexplored possibility might be that there is an intrinsic system for eliminating aged spermatozoa in men.

Vas deferens

The vas deferens can be palpated as a 3- to 5-mm-thick "string" in both sides of the scrotum. The vas has three robust layers of smooth muscle, one outer longitudinal, one circular, and one inner longitudinal layer, and facing the lumen is a convoluted mucosal layer. The epithelium has one layer with secretory cells. Stimulation of sympathetic neurons releases noradrenaline which stimulates adrenergic α_1-receptors on the smooth muscles leading to a mass-contraction that, within a second, transports spermatozoa from the distal cauda to the urethra.

Seminal vesicles, ampullae and ejaculatory ducts

The seminal vesicles and the ampullae have one layer of secretory epithelium of common origin that is highly convoluted. The secretory cells are stimulated by sympathetic neurons using acetylcholine as the transmitter; acetylcholine stimulates the formation of androgen-specific secretory products like fructose. The smooth muscles of the walls are stimulated to contract by the sympathetic adrenergic neurons; noradrenaline stimulates adrenergic α_1-receptors, which initiates contraction whereby the contents are emitted to the urethra. The ejaculatory ducts open in the prostatic part of the urethra. In cases of agenesis of the Wolffian duct system (epididymis, vas deferens, seminal vesicles, and ejaculatory ducts), either parts of the system, or the whole system are missing. The ejaculate then lacks secretory markers for the missing parts (neutral α-glucosidase for the epididymis; fructose for the seminal vesicles and ampullae).

The physiological role of the seminal vesicles in humans is unknown

Human spermatozoa ejaculated in, or incubated in seminal vesicular fluid show decreased motility, vitality, chromatin zinc content, and profound changes in chromatin stability.

The importance of fructose and prostaglandins is unknown

In many textbooks fructose is mentioned as a substrate for sperm metabolism. However, considering the negative effects that seminal vesicular fluid has on spermatozoa (decrease in vitality, motility and affected chromatin packaging) and that spermatozoa normally do not come into contact with seminal vesicular fluid, the paradigm of seminal fructose being a substrate for human spermatozoa should be challenged [19]. Another role for fructose, and other "unusual" sugar-types in semen of other animals, could be to normalize the osmotic pressure to 290 mosmol/l. The seminal vesicles contain 40 million times higher concentrations of prostaglandins than the blood, and their physiological role also remains to be clearly determined.

The prostate

The prostate is composed of 20–30 different glands that open into the urethra. These glands evolved as branching buds from the sinus urogenitalis (i.e. an origin similar to the lower parts of the vagina). Testosterone from the systemic circulation is locally transformed to 5-α dehydro-testosterone by the type-2 testosterone dehydrogenase. Sympathetic cholinergic nerves stimulate the accumulation of androgen-specific secretory products such as zinc, magnesium, calcium, citrate, acid phosphates and prostate-specific antigen (PSA) [20]. Anti-cholinergic compounds thus counteract the formation of prostatic secretion, as do inhibitors to testosterone-dehydrogenase type 2. At emission, smooth muscle cells surrounding the glands are contracted and the fluid from the 20–30 glands is expelled and mixed with spermatozoa in the urethra. Emission is mediated by the adrenergic α_1-receptors on the smooth muscle cells, stimulated by noradrenaline released from sympathetic adrenergic neurons.

Prostatic fluid also contains many substances that are normally present in blood plasma and are transudated from the blood plasma to the prostatic fluid. An acute inflammatory reaction in the prostate increases the transudated part, resulting in higher semen volume with lower concentration of androgen-specific compounds.

The bladder neck and emission

Emission involves emptying of spermatozoa and the various fluids into the urethra. The sympathetic neurons also release noradrenaline on the smooth muscles surrounding the urinary bladder neck, which results in a closure of the urethra, preventing the emitted spermatozoa and fluid from passing up into the urinary bladder.

Diseases or surgery affecting the sympathetic neurons, e.g. diabetes, trans-urethral resection of the prostate (TUR), or retroperitoneal lymph node dissection (RPLND), can result in disturbed emission. Either there is no or decreased emptying of spermatozoa and fluid into the urethra, or fluid is expelled up into the urinary bladder. This condition results in lower or no volume expelled at ejaculation, with little or no antegrade ejaculation. Presence of many spermatozoa in urine collected after orgasm means that there has been a retrograde ejaculation.

Often, low or no antegrade ejaculation is associated with impaired emission from the epididymis and the glands and no or few spermatozoa are found in the urine. In some cases α_1-stimulators can stimulate emission, bladder neck closure and result in antegrade ejaculation.

Innervations of the smooth muscles of the emission organs

The ductuli efferentis, the Wolffian duct system, the prostate and the bladder neck constitute a functional transport system of smooth muscles. In the efferent ducts, caput, corpus, and proximal cauda the smooth muscles are rich in intercellular tight junctions. The consequence is that spontaneous electrical depolarizations can be spread, and induce waves of spontaneous contractions transporting spermatozoa and fluids without regulation by nerves. In contrast, the smooth muscles of the distal cauda, the vas deferens, the seminal vesicles, the ejaculatory ducts, the prostate and the bladder neck have fewer junctions and are therefore dependent on neurogenic stimulation to induce waves of contraction [21].

The post-synaptic nerves stimulating the smooth muscles are specific to the genital tract and are called short adrenergic neurons. The pre-synaptic sympatic neurons emanate from the lateral horns of the thoracic and lumbar regions of the spinal cord. They reach the genitalia through the hypogastric plexus and the hypogastric nerves running lateral to the rectum. Inside the genital organs they are connected to the post-synaptic, short neurons. Ejaculation induced by vibrators uses, as does masturbation or coitus, the whole emission reflex. Electric stimulation of the hypogastric plexus or hypogastric nerves results in contractions in the distal cauda, vas deferens, the seminal vesicles, the ejaculatory ducts, the prostate, and the bladder neck. By rectal electro-stimulation, various parts of the system can be activated to cause emission without the normal ejaculatory sequence.

The smooth muscles in the whole system respond to noradrenergic α_1-stimulation. Emission is blocked by α_1-receptor blockers (e.g. phentolamine, and some anti-depressive agents) and is augmented by α_1-agonists (e.g. phenylpropanolamine, as used against oedema in the nasal mucosa). The adrenergic neurons are inhibited by the cholinergic neurons that stimulate secretion. Thus, during formation of fluid during sexual arousal, emission is partly inhibited.

Innervations of secretory cells

The secretory cells in the epididymis, the vas deferens, the ampulla, the seminal vesicles, and the prostate are innervated by short, sympathetic, cholinergic neurons releasing acetylcholine. The secretory neurons are inhibited by the adrenergic neurons. Thus, secretory stimulation decreases upon emission.

Ejaculation

At orgasm, spermatozoa in the cauda of the epididymis are emitted into the urethra and suspended in prostatic fluid. Striated muscles in the pelvis contract and increase the pressure in the urethra so that its contents are expelled. Later expelled fractions are mainly composed of a fluid from the seminal vesicles, which form a gel. Spermatozoa in the zinc-rich prostatic fluid preserve motility, vitality and a zinc-dependent stabilization of their nuclear chromatin. Spermatozoa that meet seminal vesicular fluid lose motility, vitality and zinc and lose the normal stabilization of the nuclear chromatin [1,10].

Ejaculatory muscles

The urethral walls are extended by prostatic fluid with spermatozoa. This extension evokes somatic reflexes of rhythmic contractions in the bulbo- and ischio-cavernosus muscles and also in the muscles of the pelvic floor. The bulbo-cavernosus muscle surrounds the corpus spongiosum of the penis and inserts into the corpus cavernosum on both sides. The ischio-cavernosus muscle inserts into the crus of the penis on both sides. These striated muscles of the perineum are innervated by the pudendal nerve. Note that whereas emission is controlled by autonomic nerves, ejaculation is governed by striated muscles under *voluntary* control. However, men seldom practice training these muscles, as is done with the striated muscles controlling the bladder and the rectum, so ejaculation is experienced as an involuntary process once orgasm is reached.

Intra-urethral pressure and ejaculatory flow speed

The contractions create an increase in intra-urethral pressure which forces the urethral contents outwards through the penis (when the bladder neck is closed). The flow speed of the ejaculate portions is dependent on how effectively the contraction force is transduced to increased pressure in the urethral lumen. The more powerful the erection, the more the force is transferred to pressure, giving a high-flow velocity and a good separation of the ejaculate fractions. In contrast, a poor erection means more penile plasticity and less separation of ejaculatory fractions.

The high ejaculatory flow-speed is physiological, but also one reason why the sperm-containing first fraction of an ejaculate is often lost at semen collection. Such ejaculates, where many of the spermatozoa have escaped collection, should not, of course, be used to evaluate sperm production.

The sequence of ejaculation

Our knowledge of the normal ejaculatory sequence comes from studies using split-ejaculates [10,19,22]. At ejaculation, each fraction is collected and characterized by counting the spermatozoa and measuring secretory markers for the prostate (zinc) and the seminal vesicles (fructose). Such studies revealed that spermatozoa from the distal cauda are suspended in the simultaneously emitted fluid from the prostatic glands and expelled in a first ejaculatory portion: thus, the physiological ejaculate that is deposited onto the cervical mucus comprises spermatozoa in prostatic fluid. Shortly thereafter, fluid from the seminal vesicles is expelled. A specific sequence of ejaculation is also true for several animals; for example, in the boar, where the sperm-rich fraction is collected for assisted reproduction.

Abnormal ejaculatory sequence

As early as 1965, Amelar and Hotchkiss [22] instructed men to withdraw after expulsion of the first portion of the ejaculate, and they also used the first half of the ejaculate for insemination. A common disorder is delayed emptying of the prostatic fluid, seen especially in men with an inflammatory reaction of the prostate [23,24,25]. The spermatozoa are then primarily expelled mixed with the seminal vesicular fluid, which has the potential to affect sperm motility, vitality, and chromatin packaging. Amelar and Hotchkiss also noted that some 6% of infertile men had a delayed expulsion of spermatozoa.

Redistribution of zinc at ejaculation

Zinc is secreted as both free ions and ions bound to citrate in the prostatic fluid. Seminal vesicular fluid contains powerful zinc-binding, high-molecular-weight proteins which can extract zinc from spermatozoa and redistribute the citrate-bound and free zinc to the proteins of vesicular origin during and after liquefaction [23,26]. The proportion of zinc bound to high-molecular-weight proteins shows huge variations between men and ejaculates (2–67%) [27]. Although a semen sample may have high zinc concentration, compounds in the liquefied ejaculate can act as zinc-chelators, thereby affecting the sperm chromatin.

The ejaculatory sequence, ejaculate composition, and sperm chromatin stability

Forces that normally stabilize the sperm chromatin seem essential for a safe transfer of the genetic material to the oocyte. Fertile donors have been shown to have higher sperm chromatin zinc content than infertile men, and some 25% of infertile men can have altered chromatin stability. Zinc withdrawal enables a quick unwrapping of the whole nucleus into separate threads, when studied within minutes after ejaculation. This ability promptly declines when spermatozoa are stored *in vitro* [8,9]. Compounds from the seminal vesicles can deprive the sperm chromatin of zinc, affecting the normal protective packaging of the sperm DNA. The chance for pregnancy at IVF is severely reduced among men with low seminal zinc concentration.

The "standardized" methods for semen analysis and sperm handling

In reality, the standardized semen sample only exists in the laboratory, when the entire ejaculate is collected and mixed in one vessel. From a physiological perspective, the standard semen sample is therefore an artifact that forces spermatozoa in the prostatic fluid to be trapped by the expanding vesicular gel for up to 20 minutes. PSA from the prostate degrades the gel-forming seminogelins of vesicular origin. Due to this process, and to the general conditions during the in-vitro procedures, the spermatozoa are exposed to increasing osmolarity, increased oxygen tension and elevated levels of free radicals [1,10].

A change in semen osmolarity *in vitro* affects sperm selection *in vitro*

In vivo, spermatozoa are expelled in the isotonic prostatic fluid onto the isotonic cervical mucus extruding from the cervical opening into the vagina. *In vitro*, enzymatic digestion of macromolecules starts at ejaculation, resulting in a rapid increase of the semen osmolarity from 290 up to 450 mosmol/l three hours later [10]. There are two implications of this. One is the possible direct effect of the increasing osmolarity on spermatozoa, while the other is the risk and effects of hypo-osmotic stress, when spermatozoa in hypertonic seminal plasma are exposed to isotonic culture media. This occurs during both the ordinary swim-up procedure and in sperm selection by density gradient centrifugation (DGC). The actual level and the rate of increase in osmolarity is an individual property that varies between samples. The increment in osmolarity is strongly associated with the concentration of prostatic fluid, and increases exponentially with increased temperature. One approach to eliminate the effects of increasing osmolarity would be to apply the selection provided by nature – i.e. to select spermatozoa at ejaculation, for instance by using the first, non-coagulated, ejaculated, split-ejaculate fraction for DGC within minutes after ejaculation [10].

The importance of sperm number is overestimated

Just 10 to 200 spermatozoa normally reach the ampullar parts of the oviducts, of which only one will fertilize [28,29]. Fatherhood has been proven among vasectomized men without any detectable spermatozoa in the ejaculate. No spermatozoa, assessed in one 10-μm-deep chamber, only tell us that the probability is 95% that the sample has less than 720 000 spermatozoa. No spermatozoa observed in a centrifuged sample after examination by microscopy of 400 fields tell us, with the same probability, that there are fewer than 200 spermatozoa in the sample. Thus, if no spermatozoa are found under the microscope it does not exclude the possibility that there were spermatozoa present in the ejaculate.

In a study from Norway, men contributing to pregnancy within one month had higher total sperm number (mean 410×10^6 per ejaculate) compared to men needing up to 12 months to contribute to a pregnancy (mean 254×10^6 per ejaculate). Of all men contributing to a pregnancy within one year, 95% had $\geq 22 \times 10^6$ sperm per ejaculate [24]. Among infertile couples in France, studied after a period of at least six months of infertility, those with $<5 \times 10^6$ spermatozoa/ml, i.e. approximately corresponding to a total number of 22×10^6 per ejaculate in the study above, had a low (11%) chance of achieving a pregnancy within the next year, whereas men with $>5 \times 10^6$/ml had a 62% probability of contributing to a pregnancy during the same time frame [25]. A cut-off of 5×10^6/ml was also found in one Danish study [26], while another Danish study advocates a cut-off concentration of 40×10^6 per ml (corresponding to $\sim 170 \times 10^6$ spermatozoa per ejaculate). However, the confidence interval for this chosen level was zero to infinity, and the data given allowed the reader to recalculate a cut-off level close to 10×10^6/ml. Moreover, some 20% of the men included in this study failed to collect the first, sperm-rich fraction, biasing the results and conclusions [27]. Thus, a clinical cut-off for the chance to achieve pregnancy within one year seems close to approximately 20×10^6 spermatozoa per ejaculate.

The risk for damaged sperm DNA is increased among men with low sperm number

Studies of the integrity of sperm DNA show that men with few spermatozoa have spermatozoa with more chromosomal aberrations and more DNA strand breaks.

The spermatozoon is the only cell in the body that lacks DNA repair systems. This means that damage to the DNA during sperm formation, maturation, storage, ejaculation, *in vitro* handling, and transfer to the oocyte cannot be repaired by the spermatozoon itself. DNA damage does occur and can be repaired by the oocyte, although this repair could be complete, wrong or incomplete. Faulty repair might result in *de novo* translocations (genes are wrongly transferred onto other chromosomes) or inversions (genes are inserted onto the right chromosome but in the opposite direction). If all genetic material is present, the translocation or inversion is called balanced, but if not, it is unbalanced. If DNA strand breaks are left unrepaired, genes are lost and the condition is called chromosome deletion. Deletions and unbalanced aberrations often result in miscarriage or malformations, and can also affect psychomotor development after birth. A balanced translocation results in a healthy child with normal psychomotor development and normal puberty. However, its own fertility could be reduced and it has higher risk of contributing to miscarriage, fetal death, malformations and affected psychomotor development in the subsequent generation. This is because individuals with balanced translocation produce gametes with variable genomes: some gametes have too much DNA, some too little, some have normal DNA, and some have the same balanced translocation as the individual himself.

A spermatozoon used for fertilization that has acquired DNA damage might therefore not only affect the child-to-be but also, or only, affect the generation thereafter. Consequently, the full safety of any assisted reproduction method can only be judged in a two-generation perspective [1].

Female physiology from a sperm perspective

Sperm invasion threatens the human oocyte: hundreds of millions against one

With the evolution from external to internal fertilization, and internal embryonic and fetal development, the numbers of embryos and fetuses must be limited. Women who ovulated multiple oocytes were at an evolutionary disadvantage. Men are, in this evolutionary aspect, still at primitive invertebrate level, i.e. 100s of millions of genetic lots are produced a day and released in vast numbers. Human females are unsuited for multiple pregnancies. The increased prevalence of obstetrical problems, and adverse outcomes in spontaneous twin pregnancies are eloquent expressions of humans being an essentially monotocous species.

However, in some 1% of families there is a hereditary propensity for spontaneous twin pregnancies. In these cases, the survival of females and fetuses has been less incompatible with twin pregnancies. This is, however, not the case for the twin pregnancies produced by ART [1].

The evolution of the female resulting in the ovulation of a single oocyte created another problem for nature. The single oocyte is threatened by an invasion; 100×10^6 spermatozoa against one single oocyte. Evolutionary biologists discuss the need for the female to protect her oocyte from this invasion. The cervical mucus, the isthmus of the Fallopian tubes, and the barriers protecting the oocyte can be viewed as central components of this defense.

Passage through the cervical mucus, the uterus, and the Fallopian tubes

From a physiological point of view the cervical mucus is where the man deposits the first expelled population of spermatozoa suspended in prostatic fluid. Thereafter, the gel-forming, seminal vesicular fluid is expelled – and there is no evidence that these two secretions are mixed in the vagina as they are mixed in a semen collection vessel. Rather, it seems that *in vivo*, the freely swimming spermatozoa in the prostatic fluid, some of which enter the cervical mucus, and the gel-formed vesicular secretion form two separate compartments.

The cervix, its mostly impermeable mucus, and the low pH of the vagina are barriers in the female between microorganisms in the outer world and the interior of the female reproductive tract and the peritoneal compartment.

To enable fertilization, these barriers must allow penetration of motile male gametes at ovulation. FSH leading to follicular development also results in increased levels of estradiol (E2), which stimulate the cervical glands to produce mucus that (a) does not kill the spermatozoa, and (b) allows them to penetrate using their own power (motility). At ovulation, the cervical mucus has conditions optimal for sperm passage, the highest anti-bacterial activity and, at the same time, the pH of the vagina is the lowest. Soon after ovulation, increased levels of progesterone affect the cervical glands and make the mucus impermeable to spermatozoa.

The textbook picture of the vagina as an open tube with cervical mucus restricted to the cervical canal must also be challenged. Close to ovulation, the narrow, collapsed lumen of the vagina contains the "sperm-catching" cervical mucus protruding from the external cervical os into the vagina – unless it has been interfered with by, for instance, hygiene procedures. Using natural family planning procedures, samples of cervical mucus are collected at the vulva. Clinical protocols for vaginal examination prescribe that this expression of physiology – protruding cervical mucus – should be removed to give the examiner a clear view of the cervix. However, the procedure can give the examiner the wrong impression – that cervical mucus is restricted to the cervix only.

It has been suggested that the cervix functions as a sperm reservoir. However, the major evidence is that spermatozoa can survive deep up in the crypts of cervical mucus, but this does not prove that spermatozoa temporarily surviving in the crypts actually constitute a reservoir since there is no evidence that these spermatozoa ever re-emerge from the crypts into the cervical canal.

The progressive motility of the spermatozoon is essential for it to pass through cervical mucus, and hence spermatozoa with poor motility are filtered out during their passage through it. Concomitantly, spermatozoa with abnormal morphology are also removed, resulting in only a minority of ejaculated spermatozoa actually entering the cervix. Some hours after ejaculation the uterus is invaded by leukocytes that attack the spermatozoa. It is therefore reasonable to assume that the fertilizing spermatozoon has to traverse the uterus and reach the immune-privileged oviductal epithelium in the isthmus of the oviduct ahead of this elimination of spermatozoa in the uterus. In the uterus, muscular contractions may enhance passage of sperm through the uterine cavity to the uterotubal junctions since radio-labeled spheres placed in the vagina can be translocated to the isthmus during the late follicular phase [30].

The uterotubal junction and the isthmus sperm reservoir

The anatomy of the uterotubal junction, the folded mucosa and contracted smooth muscle layer, along with a mucus secretion that flows towards the uterus, together constitute a functional barrier for the spermatozoa to pass, as well as a barrier that can prevent a fertilized oocyte reaching the uterine cavity too soon. Short, adrenergic neurons release noradrenaline that triggers the smooth muscles of the isthmus to contract when dominated by estradiol during the follicular phase before ovulation. Following ovulation, increased levels of progesterone hyperpolarize the smooth muscles, thus counteracting the adrenergic action, and the muscles relax allowing the zygote to pass at day 3 to 4 after fertilization. There is some evidence indicating that more than good sperm morphology and progressive motility are needed for spermatozoa to pass into the isthmus of the Fallopian tubes. A few thousand spermatozoa may swim through the uterotubal junctions to reach the isthmus part of the oviducts. Whereas other mammals reveal a distinct sperm reservoir, the human isthmus constitutes at least a functional reservoir that could prolong the availability of spermatozoa maintained in a fertile state, as the spermatozoa interact with the oviductal epithelium. Subpopulations of a few spermatozoa become capacitated and hyperactivated, which enables them to proceed towards the tubal ampulla. At any time, only some 10 to 200 spermatozoa could be flushed from normal human oviducts, while some thousands could be recovered in distally obstructed oviducts [22,30,31].

Which are the few spermatozoa that reach the oviductal ampulla?

These spermatozoa constitute a subpopulation of those few thousands that traversed the uterotubal junction and connected to the oviductal epithelium in the isthmus. Then, which are they?

Are they: (a) spermatozoa reaching the tubes before the invasion defense-system in the uterus reacts and hinders spermatozoa arriving later? Or is it (b) a subpopulation of spermatozoa that reaches the isthmus and in addition has a special competence to pass? Or is it (c) a subpopulation that is *invisible* to an invasion defense system? If it is the former groups (a + b), spermatozoa in the first, expelled ejaculate fraction would be more representative for these than spermatozoa residing in the liquefied, whole ejaculate. If it is the latter groups (b + c), these spermatozoa would be true subpopulations we need to be able to identify. In the future we might be able to identify and select spermatozoa that can reach the tubes from the first expelled fraction. However, we can never truly predict whether a man will become a father or not, regardless of the sophistication of methods we use, as long as we only assess the *messenger* functions of the spermatozoa. The messages would only be possible to study in some spermatozoa representative for selected subpopulations, since it is doubtful whether we will ever be able to study the messages of a given spermatozoon without affecting its integrity [1].

When will competent spermatozoa reach the place of fertilization?

There is no valid support for a rapid (minutes) transport, although some early observations indicated that e.g. human and rabbit spermatozoa could reach the ampulla minutes after insemination. However, these spermatozoa were mostly dead and did not contribute to fertilization [30,31]. Experimental studies to clarify the physiological situation, especially in humans, are lacking.

Allowing speculation: a sperm linear velocity of 25–50 μm/s would correspond to 1.5–3.0 mm/min. Considering that the distance from the cervical os to the oviductal ampulla is some 150 mm, theoretically a spermatozoon would need some 50–100 min to swim the distance by itself. Adding a delay (minutes to days) in transport through the isthmus, it being a functional barrier and reservoir that also is influenced by the female hormonal status and ovulation, competent spermatozoa might arrive in the ampulla from 1 hour to days after ejaculation. During assisted reproduction using selected spermatozoa from a liquefied ejaculate, additional time (30–60 min) is needed for the spermatozoa to adjust from hypertonic semen to the isotonic cervical mucus [10].

Sperm responses to signals from the female genital tract

Capacitation

At ejaculation, the mammalian spermatozoon has not yet acquired full fertilizing capacity. The biochemical, molecular and physiological changes that the spermatozoon experiences in the female genital tract are collectively referred to as capacitation and result finally in a spermatozoon fully competent for fertilization. During capacitation, changes occur in membrane properties, enzyme activities, and motility which make spermatozoa responsive to stimuli that induce hyperactivated motility, and later on the acrosome reaction, and thereby prepare the spermatozoon for penetration of the egg investments prior to fertilization. These changes are accompanied by the activation of cell-signaling cascades *in vivo*, or in defined media *in vitro* [32,33]. At present the nature of these signaling complexes, their temporal and spatial activations, remains to be elucidated.

Hyperactivated motility

Hyperactivation is usually considered a part and an expression of the capacitation process seen in all Eutherian mammals studied. However, the regulatory pathway that finally gives rise to an increase in flagellar Ca^{2+} and triggers hyperactivation can operate independently from capacitation [34,35].

Hyperactivation is characterized by high-amplitude, asymmetrical flagellar bending, and assessment of hyperactivation needs parameters measured by CASA. Besides promoting the passage through the zona pellucida, hyperactivation may also facilitate release of sperm from the oviductal storage reservoir at the isthmus and may propel sperm through mucus in the oviductal lumen and the matrix of the cumulus oophorus.

The acrosome reaction

The acrosome reaction is a "metamorphosis event" that must be completed by the spermatozoa of many animal species prior to fusion with eggs. In Eutherian mammals it follows capacitation and is triggered by the spermatozoon binding to the zona pellucida. It involves multiple fusions between the sperm plasma membrane and the underlying outer acrosomal membrane resulting in many small vesicles allowing release of the acrosomal content. In the mouse, this exocytosis is triggered by one of the three zona pellucida glycoproteins, ZP3. Following binding of the spermatozoon to the zona, ZP3 promotes a sustained influx of Ca^{2+} into the spermatozoon that is necessary for the acrosome reaction [36]. Among substances released during the acrosome reaction are hyaluronidase and acrosin. These are enzymes capable of degrading the cumulus mass and the zona pellucida, respectively. However, the hyaluronidase is apparently released at the zona pellucida, i.e. after the cumulus mass has already been traversed, and interestingly spermatozoa lacking acrosin can still fertilize although they are less efficient [37]. In a sea-snail, acrosin helps the spermatozoon open the oocyte-surrounding gel without acting as an enzyme. Thus the presence of a molecule that can act as an enzyme does not mean that it actually has a physiologically important enzymatic effect.

The barriers of the oocyte allow the passage of competent spermatozoa

The mammalian oocyte is surrounded by a thick glycoprotein layer, the zona pellucida, which the spermatozoon takes some 3–4 min to penetrate. Furthermore, around the zona pellucida is the huge cumulus mass, which is composed of about 50 cell layers of cumulus cells, surrounded by the matrix produced by the cells. Hyaluronic acid is the predominant matrix macromolecule. The cumulus mass contains progesterone and nitric oxide, both of which induce calcium signaling within the sperm. Most spermatozoa fail to pass through, and become stuck in the cumulus. The specific reasons why some sperm do not pass remain to be elucidated.

One factor could be lack of hyperactivated motility. Sperm penetration through the cumulus matrix, as well as through the zona pellucida, is dependent on hyperactivated motility, which is a type of motility characterized by high-amplitude flagellar waves that generate powerful propulsive force, capable even of breaking covalent bonds [38]. After passage through the cumulus the fertilizing spermatozoon must bind to the zona pellucida (a largely species-specific process), undergo the acrosome reaction, and then penetrate through the matrix of the zona. Thus, the zona pellucida constitutes a barrier which, in most mammals, admits only spermatozoa of the same species. Following the acrosome reaction new ligands are exposed on the equatorial segment of the sperm head, by which the spermatozoon can bind to the oocyte plasma membrane after passing through the zona.

In conclusion, the spermatozoon that finally fuses with the oocyte is one that underwent capacitation, developed hyperactivated motility, had the competence to pass the cumulus mass, showed the right code to bind to the zona pellucida, underwent the acrosome reaction, traversed the zona, and finally showed the right code for binding to the oocyte membrane and was able to fuse with it.

The spermatozoon does not penetrate – it fuses with the oocyte

Fertilization by fusion of the gametes is a fundamental mechanism, and was the first evolutionary step towards sexual reproduction some 600 million years ago. After fusion the sperm membrane and the oocyte membrane are contiguous. The internal parts of the sperm cell are then automatically inside and surrounded by the ooplasm. The contaminated outside of the sperm membrane remains on the outside surface of the fertilized oocyte.

ICSI penetrates and bypasses fusion

ICSI (intracytoplasmic sperm injection) is a new biological concept. From an evolutionary perspective, injection of spermatozoa (with membranes and some suspending medium) means that the barriers of the oocyte are breached, raising the possibility for bypassing the natural barriers without physiological control, potentially exposing the zygote and the future generations to the entrance of compounds or organisms that otherwise would not have had access to the inside of the oocyte. This new evolutionary concept requires that we use controlled conditions, especially not using culture media that contains biological material from other species [1].

After fusion – sperm messages

As far as is known at present, the spermatozoon brings four messages to the zygote:

1. Factors for oocyte activation;

2. An intact haploid genome;

3. A centrosome (needed for mitotic divisions in the new individual); and

4. Factors necessary for the initiation of placental development.

Besides DNA, the spermatozoon also brings proteins and mRNA to the oocyte, but the specific functions of these compounds still remain to be elucidated.

1. Activation of the oocyte

The exact signals are unknown, but electrical events in the oocyte membrane, and a rise in calcium in the ooplasm must occur. There is also the release of the cortical granules, which induce changes in the oocyte membrane so that it cannot fuse with other spermatozoa. Only if two spermatozoa are fusing with the oocyte almost simultaneously should polyzoospermic fertilization occur. Fertilization by two spermatozoa usually results in three pronuclei and a diandric, triploid zygote, which can develop to term (although human triploids always die within hours of birth).

The oocyte also completes its second meiotic division, which is then followed by the fusion of the male and female pronuclei and, some hours later, the first mitosis. However, the oocyte can also be activated spontaneously, or by chemicals such as ethanol or even by physical manipulation with a glass pipette. This capacity for parthenogenetic development means that even if an oocyte divides into two cells there is no guarantee that it was fertilized by a spermatozoon.

2. An intact haploid genome

Immediately upon sperm–egg fusion the nuclear envelope surrounding the sperm nucleus dissolves and the tightly condensed nucleus rapidly decondenses to form the male pronucleus.

3. Male centriole is needed for mitoses of the zygote

The centrosome is a self-replicating organelle. In humans and most mammals it is derived from a centriole in the sperm and pericentriolar material (PCM) from the oocyte. It serves as the main microtubular organizing center and a regulator of cell-cycle progression. It can initiate the aggregation, orientation and function of certain intracytoplasmic threads or tubules. It can also reproduce and is claimed to carry its own RNA-genome. The centrosome contains a pair of perpendicularly oriented cylindrical centrioles and a protein matrix named pericentriolar material (PCM). One specialized expression of the centrosome is the centriole. A centriole can in turn give rise to a cilium or a flagellum. In some cells the centrosome forms many centrioles (basal bodies), each giving rise to a cilium, as in ciliated cells in e.g. the Fallopian tubes and in the respiratory epithelium. The spermatozoon carries one centrosome, which has given rise to two centrioles. One of the centrioles gave rise to the sperm flagellum, the basic element of the tail, and can still be seen posterior to the connecting piece by transmission electron microscopy (TEM). The other may have helped in the organization of the chromosomes in the nucleus, but cannot be detected within the connecting piece of the sperm flagellum.

Immediately upon sperm–egg fusion the sperm proximal centriole duplicates and forms a centrosome together with the oocyte pericentriolar material. The centrosome organizes gamma-tubulin molecules in the ooplasm into long tubular threads starting at the centrosome, which grow rapidly and radiate like a "sperm aster" all over the ooplasm. They anchor to the female pronucleus containing the maternal chromosomes. By contraction of the threads the sperm centrosome drags the female genome down to the male genome. From here on, the centrosome duplicates and then sustains the first, and all future, mitoses of the new individual. If it fails, the oocyte centrosome can take over but this development will apparently only last for a few cell divisions and the blastocyst will die. This knowledge has many implications. A sperm centriole that has been seriously damaged during sperm transfer will fail to sustain embryonic development. Fertilized oocytes that do not divide, or divide only slowly, could have a damaged sperm centriole. Even dividing fertilized oocytes chosen for embryo transfer could be destined to die due to sperm centriolar failure. The anti-cough drug noskapin and also diazepam interfere with sperm aster formation, but the extent to which drugs that interfere with centrosome function might have affected human fertility is not known.

Interestingly, in mice and other rodents, the zygote does not receive a centriole from the spermatozoon, but the whole centrosome (two centrioles and the PCM) from the oocyte, a fundamental difference in mammalian evolution [39].

4. Factors necessary for initiation of placental development

In placental mammals like humans, the nutrition in the oocyte lasts for a few days only. Chorionic villi grow out from the surface in all directions and when meeting the endometrium, these villi actively transform the endometrium into the maternal part of the placenta-to-be. Thus, the embryo plays the active role. The acceptance of a foreign individual intermingling with the tissue (here the endometrium) of the host was a step taken by evolution and its full consequences for e.g. acceptance of cancer growth is being explored at present.

Two sperm nuclei in a frog oocyte will result in a frog. Two oocyte nuclei in a frog oocyte also will result in a frog. In a placental mammal the situation is different: two sperm nuclei in a mouse oocyte will result in mainly placental tissue. The human equivalent has been known for several years, although its implications were not understood. Two sperm nuclei in an oocyte result in a hydatid mole. In contrast, two oocyte nuclei in an oocyte result in mainly embryonic tissue without initiation of proper placental tissue. The embryo will die. The mechanism by which the spermatozoon initiates placental growth is not understood. Genomic imprinting, i.e. different inactivation of genes by epigenetic control within the male or female gonad, is a favorable candidate for this mechanism.

Evolution of placental animals thus has given the spermatozoon a "new" important function. Paternal factors thus secure a passage of nutrients and other vital substances to the fetus while the block for placental formation within the oocyte genome protects the female from offspring achieved through parthenogenesis.

A consequence of this is that research on factors contributing to subfertility must also consider the possibility that damage to the sperm and its messages might disturb placental formation and function and therefore might also be involved in problems related to growth and development a long time after fertilization.

Sperm mitochondria and their DNA are targeted to be destroyed by the oocyte

Each mitochondrion in the body contains several copies of circular mitochondrial DNA (mtDNA). At fertilization, the spermatozoon brings some 100 copies of mitochondrial DNA, whereas the oocyte has some 100 000 copies. Sperm mtDNA has passed up to 400 cell divisions and is more likely to be mutated than the mtDNA in the oocyte that has been selected, multiplied and then kept resting since the 10th fetal week. Sperm mitochondrial DNA is already ubiquitin-targeted in the testis to be destroyed upon entrance into the oocyte.

Thus, the mitochondria are inherited through the female germ cell line. There are reports suggesting that mutated sperm mitochondrial DNA may escape destruction and cause mitochondrial disease in the offspring. If so, it seems to be an extremely rare event.

References

1. Kvist U. Genetics, ethics and the gametes – on reproductive biology, multiple pregnancies and ICSI. *Acta Obstet Gynecol Scand* 2000; **79**: 913–20.
2. Neill JD, ed. *Knobil and Neill's Physiology of Reproduction.* 3rd edn. Amsterdam: Elsevier Academic Press 2005.
3. Nieschlag E, Behre HM, Nieschlag S, eds. *Andrology: Male Reproductive Health and Dysfunction.* 2nd edn. Berlin and Heidelberg: Springer-Verlag 2001.
4. Holstein AF, Schulze W, Davidoff M. Understanding spermatogenesis is a prerequisite for treatment. *Reprod Biol Endocrinol* 2003; **1**: 107.
5. Ehmcke J, Schlatt S. A revised model for spermatogonial expansion in man: lessons from non-human primates. *Reproduction* 2006; **132**: 673–80.
6. Westlander G, Ekerhovd E, Bergh C. Low levels of serum inhibin B do not exclude successful sperm recovery in men with nonmosaic Klinefelter syndrome. *Fertil Steril* 2003; **79** Suppl 3: 1680–2.
7. Rosenlund B, Kvist U, Ploen L, *et al.* Percutaneous cutting needle biopsies for histopathological assessment and sperm retrieval in men with azoospermia. *Hum Reprod* 2001; **16**: 2154–9.
8. Kvist U, Björndahl L, Kjellberg S. Sperm nuclear zinc, chromatin stability, and male fertility. *Scanning Microsc* 1987; **1**: 1241–7.
9. Björndahl L, Kvist U. Loss of an intrinsic capacity for human sperm chromatin decondensation. *Acta Physiol Scand* 1985; **124**: 189–94.
10. Björndahl L, Kvist U. Sequence of ejaculation affects the spermatozoon as a carrier and its message. *Reprod Biomed Online* 2003; 7: 440–8.
11. Kjellberg S. *Zinc and human sperm chromatin.* PhD thesis, Department of Gynecology and Obstetrics, University of Linköping, 1993.
12. Bal W, Dyba M, Szewczuk Z, *et al.* Differential zinc and DNA binding by partial peptides of human protamine HP2. *Mol Cell Biochem* 2001; **222**: 97–106.
13. Brewer L, Corzett M, Balhorn R. Condensation of DNA by spermatid basic nuclear proteins. *J Biol Chem* 2002; **277**: 38895–900.

14. Birkhead TR, Immler S. Making sperm: design, quality control and sperm competition. *Soc Reprod Fertil Suppl* 2007; **65**: 175–81.

15. Johnson L, Varner DD. Effect of daily spermatozoan production but not age on transit time of spermatozoa through the human epididymis. *Biol Reprod* 1988; **39**: 812–7.

16. Johnson L. A re-evaluation of daily sperm output of men. *Fertil Steril* 1982; **37**: 811–6.

17. Bedford JM. Enigmas of mammalian gamete form and function. *Biol Rev Camb Philos Soc* 2004; **79**: 429–60.

18. Richardson DW, Short RV. Time of onset of sperm production in boys. *J Biosoc Sci Suppl* 1978; **5**: 15–25.

19. Mann T, Lutwak-Mann C. *Male Reproductive Function and Semen*. Berlin and Heidelberg: Springer-Verlag 1981.

20. Eggert-Kruse W, Reimann-Andersen J, Rohr G, et al. Clinical relevance of sperm morphology assessment using strict criteria and relationship with sperm-mucus interaction in vivo and in vitro. *Fertil Steril* 1995; **63**: 612–24.

21. Wagner G, Sjöstrand NO. Autonomic pharmacology and sexual function. In: Sjösten A, ed. *The Pharmacology and Endocrinology of Sexual function*. Amsterdam: Elsevier Science Publishers 1988.

22. Amelar RD, Hotchkiss RS. The split ejaculate: its use in the management of male infertility. *Fertil Steril* 1965; **16**: 46–60.

23. Björndahl L, Kjellberg S, Kvist U. Ejaculatory sequence in men with low sperm chromatin-zinc. *Int J Androl* 1991; **14**: 174–8.

24. Kvist U. Sperm nuclear chromatin decondensation ability. An in vitro study on ejaculated human spermatozoa. *Acta Physiol Scand Suppl* 1980; **486**: 1–24.

25. Kvist U. Can disturbances of the ejaculatory sequence contribute to male infertility? *Int J Androl* 1991; **14**: 389–93.

26. Arver S. Studies on zinc and calcium in human seminal plasma. *Acta Physiol Scand Suppl* 1982; **507**: 1–21.

27. Kjellberg S, Björndahl L, Kvist U. Sperm chromatin stability and zinc binding properties in semen from men in barren unions. *Int J Androl* 1992; **15**: 103–13.

28. Ahlgren M. Sperm transport to and survival in the human fallopian tube. *Gynecol Invest* 1975; **6**: 206–14.

29. Mortimer D, Templeton AA. Sperm transport in the human female reproductive tract in relation to semen analysis characteristics and time of ovulation. *J Reprod Fertil* 1982; **64**: 401–8.

30. Suarez SS, Pacey AA. Sperm transport in the female reproductive tract. *Hum Reprod Update* 2006; **12**: 23–37.

31. Mortimer D. Sperm transport in the female genital tract. In: Grudzinskas JG, Yovish JL, eds. *Gametes – The Spermatozoa*. Cambridge: Cambridge University Press 1995.

32. Salicioni AM, Platt MD, Wertheimer EV, et al. Signalling pathways involved in sperm capacitation. *Soc Reprod Fertil Suppl* 2007; **65**: 245–59.

33. Gadella BM, Tsai PS, Boerke A, Brewis IA. Sperm head membrane reorganisation during capacitation. *Int J Dev Biol* 2008; **52**: 473–80.

34. Suarez SS. Control of hyperactivation in sperm. *Hum Reprod Update* 2008; **14**: 647–57.

35. Publicover S, Harper CV, Barratt C. [Ca2+]i signalling in sperm – making the most of what you've got. *Nat Cell Biol* 2007; **9**: 235–42.

36. Florman HM, Jungnickel MK, Sutton KA. Regulating the acrosome reaction. *Int J Dev Biol* 2008; **52**: 503–10.

37. Raterman D, Springer MS. The molecular evolution of acrosin in placental mammals. *Mol Reprod Dev* 2008; **75**: 1196–207.

38. Mortimer ST. A critical review of the physiological importance and analysis of sperm movement in mammals. *Hum Reprod Update* 1997; **3**: 403–39.

39. Schatten G. The centrosome and its mode of inheritance: the reduction of the centrosome during gametogenesis and its restoration during fertilization. *Dev Biol* 1994; **165**: 299–335.

Chapter 3

Basic semen analysis

This chapter describes the steps involved in performing a basic semen analysis. Table 3.1 shows an overview of the entire recommended working process for basic semen analysis: following the recommended order for the different component procedures will provide a basis for efficient and high quality working [1].

Table 3.1 The component analytical procedures of a complete semen analysis are a sequence optimized for efficiency and quality in the laboratory work. Details of the individual procedures are given in this, and following chapters. Some steps can be considered optional.

Time from ejaculation	Procedure
Immediately	Weigh the sample container with the semen sample, ascertain correct labeling, and place it in 37°C incubator.
	Register and label the corresponding laboratory documents.
25–30 min	Assess semen liquefaction, visual appearance, and smell.
30–60 min	Semen viscosity assessment.
	Examination of the wet preparations (motility; selection of dilution; assessment of other cells, debris, aggregates and agglutination).
	Antisperm antibody test(s).
	Make smears for sperm vitality testing if sperm motility is <40%.
	Make dilutions for sperm concentration determination.
	Make smears for sperm morphology assessment.
	Take a 100-µl aliquot of semen for assessment of inflammatory cells.
	Centrifuge and freeze semen for any requested biochemical analyses.
Later	Counting of spermatozoa in the hemocytometer.
	If there are >1 × 10^6/ml round cells, perform an assessment of inflammatory cells.
	Biochemical analyses of the secretory contributions from the prostate (e.g. zinc), seminal vesicles (e.g. fructose), and epididymis (e.g. α-glucosidase).
	Stain the smears for sperm morphology assessment.
	Perform the sperm morphology assessments.

Sample collection and delivery

Principles

The circumstances under which a semen sample is collected and delivered to the laboratory can influence the results of the analysis. Since the time that spermatozoa are held in semen can reduce their survival, motility and fertilizing ability, it is essential that the start of diagnostic investigations is standardized to 30 minutes after ejaculation (in order to allow most ejaculates to liquefy properly) [1,2]. If the sample can be collected in a special room adjacent to the laboratory there is a significant reduction of the risk for delays during transportation, and for cooling of the sample with concomitant loss of motility. This situation calls for proper design and equipping of the semen collection room, and for situations that might cause stress for the men, such as long waiting times, embarrassing encounters, and disturbing noise from outside the room, to be avoided. Duration of stimulation can be important for the outcome, and men should be allowed ample time so as not to feel rushed to produce their samples [3].

In general, patients are expected to collect a semen sample for investigation after between 2 and 7 days of ejaculatory abstinence. However, if the abstinence time can be held to 3–5 days the variability due to abstinence duration can be kept reasonably low [1].

Equipment and materials

- Waiting area with patient flow minimizing embarrassing contact between patients
- Secluded semen collection room
- Semen sample collection container – non-toxic plastic (Figure 3.1)
- Self-adhesive labels for secure identification of the sample collection vial
- Special condoms (non-toxic, non-spermicidal)

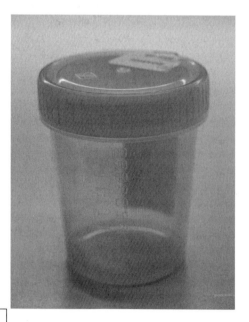

Figure 3.1 Example of a sample collection container with a tight-fitting lid and ample space for at least two separate, unique identifiers, as well as space to write the container weight and the time of ejaculation.

Notes

1. If a man has difficulties collecting a sample at the laboratory, he might be allowed to produce a first sample at home and transport it (protected from cooling by keeping the sample close to the body) to the laboratory for investigation, preferably within 30 min after ejaculation, but at most within 1 h. In cases where the main problem is to produce a sample by masturbation, a special, non-spermicidal condom can be used to collect a sample at intercourse [4].

2. Retrograde ejaculation can be suspected if no ejaculate is expelled at orgasm. In some cases, antegrade ejaculation can be achieved if the man ejaculates with a full bladder. Other men might be helped by intake of drugs that counteract parasympathetic activity (e.g. imipramine 50 mg; in most countries patients must be prescribed such drugs by a clinician). In other cases it will probably be necessary to alkalinize the urine in order to be able to retrieve live spermatozoa in urine after ejaculation [5].

3. If a lubricant must be used then it must *not* show any toxicity to spermatozoa. Currently, the only suitable commercial product for this particular purpose is *Pre'*, an external use version of the *Pre~Seed* vaginal lubricant (INGfertility, Valleyford, WA, USA; see www.preseed.com/MedicalProfessionals/People_Products.php). It is also available in bulk to physicians/laboratories as *Pre' MD*.

Patient instructions

Principles

Written information for the layman about the purpose of the investigation, and circumstances that could interfere with the analysis and with the interpretation of the results should be supplied either directly from the referring clinician or by letter to the patient when an appointment for the semen analysis is made with the laboratory. This information should also include a short explanation of the male reproductive organs and their functions. Special attention should be given to the relevance of correct abstinence time and the importance of collecting the entire ejaculate [1,6]. Further oral information should be given when the patient comes to the laboratory to deliver the sample. On the day of sample collection, relevant information about sample collection and abstinence time should be recorded, and other pertinent questions regarding, for instance, recent periods of high fever or inflammatory diseases should be asked and the man's responses noted [7].

Equipment and disposable materials

- Information sheet on the purpose of semen analysis (written for laymen)
- Information sheet about the male reproductive organs and their functions (written for laymen)
- Checklist for laboratory staff regarding the verbal information to be given to patients when the appointment is made
- Checklist for laboratory staff regarding the verbal information to be given to, and obtained from, patients when the sample is collected
- Questionnaire for the patient at the time of sample collection and delivery

35

Semen volume and handling of the sample container

Background

The first part of the investigation of a semen sample is its physical examination, which includes measurement of semen volume as well as assessment of viscosity, general visual appearance and smell (odor).

Assessments that follow measurement of the ejaculate volume are best done after full liquefaction of the sample, followed by the microscopic investigations. For an efficient flow of procedures optimizing the quality of the analytical steps (to reduce variability and any negative influence of post-ejaculatory factors), it is recommended that the component investigations are performed in the order shown in Table 3.1 (above).

Principle

Even before the coagulated sample has liquefied, the volume can be determined by weighing, provided that the sample collection container has been weighed before the sample was collected. If at least 30 different containers from a batch have been weighed, and the variation in weight between containers is less than 0.1 g, then all containers can be assumed to have the same weight and then it is not necessary to weigh each one before use. For every new batch of containers, a set of 30 should be tested to establish the consistency of their weight for that specific batch. The specific gravity of semen can be assumed to be 1.0 g/ml, and weighing is preferred to using measuring pipettes since no semen is lost by the weighing procedure [8].

The sample container should be uniquely labeled in accordance with all laboratory documentation. It is recommended that the container be given two independent but unique identifiers (one of which must be a number), for example patient identity and laboratory sample number. To facilitate the proper work sequence in the laboratory, the time of sample collection should be clearly marked on the container and also recorded in the sample record form.

The sample should be placed in a temperature-controlled (37°C) incubator, if possible on an orbital mixer. The sample is left in the incubator until 25–30 min after ejaculation, so that examination can be initiated at 30 min after ejaculation. The mixing of the sample is checked by "swirling" the sample around the bottom of the container for 15–20 s. When the sample has been transported to the laboratory after collection at another location, it must be allowed to warm up to 37°C in the incubator (e.g. for 5–10 min) before examination.

Specimen
- Freshly ejaculated human semen

Equipment and disposable materials (see also Appendix 2)
- Top-load balance
- Air incubator at 37°C
- Marker pen for laboratory use, and labels for secure identification
- Calculator to calculate sample weight

Calibration and quality control

The balance should be serviced by the manufacturer/supplier or other specialist at least annually. Balance accuracy should be tested (QC) at least monthly to ensure that it delivers reliable results. If deviating results are found, servicing and recalibration of the balance must be carried out as soon as possible. Procedures for balance service and testing should be described in the laboratory's Quality Manual.

Procedure

1. After the sample has been collected the container is weighed and the result recorded together with the batch vial weight (tare weight) on the sample record form.
2. Time of ejaculation is clearly written on the vial.
3. Immediately place the collection vial in the incubator and record the time on the form; leave in the incubator until 25–30 min after ejaculation.
4. Calculate the sample volume by subtracting the tare weight from the result of weighing after sample collection and record the value on the form.

Calculations and results

The initial vial weight is subtracted from the total weight measured after sample collection. Weight in grams (g) is recorded as volume (ml) on the sample record form to one decimal place (i.e. 0.1 g accuracy).

Interpretation guidelines

A low volume (<2 ml) could have different explanations:

- Incomplete sample collection
- Secretory dysfunction of accessory sex glands (infections, agenesis of seminal vesicles)
- Stress during sample collection

A high ejaculate volume (>6 ml) could be due to different causes, although no general, direct relationship has been shown between high semen volume and male infertility. A high volume can cause a relatively high dilution of the spermatozoa, causing a relatively low sperm concentration. High semen volume has also been associated with a high risk for semen loss from the vagina. Causes for increased semen volume can be:

- Inflammatory exudate from, for instance, an infected prostate during the acute (exudative) phase of inflammation
- Extensive sexual stimulation, possibly combined with long abstinence time

Semen liquefaction

Principles

The ejaculate coagulates due to macro-proteins originating from the seminal vesicles. In the laboratory the entire ejaculate is brought together in one collection container, including the first sperm-rich fraction, and all fractions are involved in the coagulum. Most samples are fully liquefied within 15–20 min, at least when stored at 37°C, due to enzymes (proteases) originating from the prostate.

The physiological importance of ejaculate liquefaction in humans is not known and it has been suggested that the formation of a coagulum does not represent the normal physiology for the human spermatozoa [9,10]. Disturbances of the process are most probably markers for pathological processes in the male accessory sex glands, which could also result in a negative effect on sperm functions.

Specimen

- Ejaculated semen, ideally 25 min after ejaculation, stored for at least 15 min in an incubator at 37°C

Equipment and disposable materials (see also Appendix 2)

- Air incubator at 37°C

Procedure

1. Take the sample collection container from the incubator 25–30 min after ejaculation.
2. Swirl the sample around the bottom of the container for 15–20 s to ensure that mixing is complete.
3. Inspect the specimen for signs of incomplete liquefaction, e.g. gel clumps or streaks.
4. In case considerable parts of the specimen are still not liquefied, the sample should be returned to the incubator and re-inspected 15 and 30 min later.
5. Samples still not liquefied 60 min after ejaculation are evaluated to the best extent possible. Lack of liquefaction is noted in the laboratory report, as well as a note that further investigations have been done on any material available outside the coagulum.

Results

Results are reported as "normal," "delayed" (fully liquefied at 60 min, but not at 30 min), "incomplete" (still not completed at 60 min), or "not liquefied" (intact coagulum at 60 min). Comments should describe whether solitary gel clumps and/or streaks are visible in the otherwise liquefied sample.

Interpretation guidelines

Since the end result of coagulation and liquefaction mainly depends on the actions of compounds secreted from two different glands, both general and localized infections and inflammatory reactions in the male reproductive tract are likely to interfere and possibly cause changes in the process.

It is therefore advisable that a man with disturbed liquefaction is given a full clinical examination by a clinical andrologist or a urologist.

Visual appearance

Principle

A normal semen sample is usually grayish-white and opalescent. Unusual coloration or translucence of an ejaculate can provide diagnostic information regarding the man.

Specimen

- As for the assessment of semen liquefaction

Equipment and disposable materials

- None required

Procedure

While examining the extent of liquefaction, the color and opalescence (clear appearance) of the sample are also assessed.

Results

A normal semen sample is usually grayish-white and opalescent; lack of opalescence should be recorded. Any change in color (red, brownish or yellowish) should be recorded.

Interpretation guidelines

1. It is not uncommon that a very clear or translucent sample is azoospermic or has a very low sperm concentration (severely oligozoospermic).

2. Human semen can have a pale yellow coloration that is not necessarily abnormal. A yellowish color can be due to an increased concentration of flavoproteins of seminal vesicular origin, often related to long abstinence time. A combination of very low volume and yellow color can appear in acute infections with high concentration of inflammatory cells in semen. On rare occasions yellow semen can be due to jaundice, which should be properly investigated medically.

3. The presence of erythrocytes or hemoglobin (red or brownish appearance) as a solitary finding is not considered to reflect any pathological condition. Red staining of semen is an indication of blood and can be due to a skin injury while producing the sample or the blood might originate from one of the accessory glands, and hence might be a sign of infection. If the finding is consistent, the patient should be investigated further to establish the source for the blood.

Semen odor

Principle

Perception of the smell of normal semen is generally quite variable, but samples with a strong smell can usually be perceived by most laboratory staff members.

Specimen

- As for the assessment of semen liquefaction

Equipment and disposable materials

- None required

Procedure

When the sample is inspected for liquefaction, the lid of the container is removed and the smell of the sample evaluated.

Results

If present, a strong, disgusting smell (putrescent), or a urine smell is recorded in the sample form.

Interpretation guidelines

A strong and repugnant smell can be caused, for instance, by a bacterial infection. The patient should be examined by a clinician to decide whether medical treatment of an infection is indicated.

Semen viscosity

Principle

A viscous semen sample forms long threads instead of discrete drops when it is allowed to run out of a pipette. This is not the same phenomenon as coagulation and liquefaction, but abnormalities can have the same cause – disturbed accessory gland function causing both viscosity problems and problems with coagulation and liquefaction.

Specimen

- As for the assessment of semen liquefaction

Equipment and disposable materials

- Wide-bore serological pipette or glass or plastic rod validated for being in contact with fresh semen
- Measuring scale (e.g. ruler) of 2 cm to facilitate assessment

Procedure

1. Aspirate the semen into (for example) a 5-ml plastic, volumetric pipette.
2. Let the semen run out of the pipette back into the sample collection container.
3. Estimate the length of the threads formed between the droplets.

Results

If threads >2 cm long are formed when the sample drops from the pipette the sample is considered to have an abnormal viscosity, and this finding should be recorded on the report form.

Interpretation guidelines

The main problem with a highly viscous semen sample is the difficulty it creates for performing proper assessments of sperm motility, concentration, and antisperm antibodies, as well as for the preparation of good smears for sperm morphology assessment.

Notes

Addition of a known volume of saline or suitable culture medium followed by careful mixing can often give a sufficiently homogeneous dilution to allow proper investigations. The original volume should be used to give the true original sperm concentration in the undiluted semen. Since the motility characteristics will change due to the dilution (an effect of reduced viscosity), it is essential that it is clearly stated on the sample record form that the motility assessment was performed on a diluted sample. For samples intended for treatment (assisted reproductive techniques) the risk for contamination should be minimized by using the same culture medium as will be used for clinical sperm preparation.

Semen pH

Principle

Semen pH is the result of hydrogen ion content in prostatic secretion (acidic), seminal vesicular secretion (alkaline), carbon dioxide evaporation after ejaculation, and effects of chemical reactions occurring from ejaculation until the time of pH assessment. In contrast to the situation in for instance blood, there are no specific homeostatic control systems in the ejaculate. It is therefore extremely difficult to standardize measurements. Due to the lack of homeostatic control and difficulties in standardizing measurements there are no reliable and useful reference ranges. Therefore, measurement of pH does not provide any further information to the basic semen analysis.

There is, however, one situation when measurement of pH can contribute significantly to the investigation: in cases with no sperm in the ejaculate and a relatively low volume a low pH (7 or lower) points to lack of the alkaline secretions from the seminal vesicles, indicating agenesis of the Wolffian duct system (including the seminal vesicles) as a cause for the azoospermia. Biochemical analysis (zinc and fructose as markers for prostatic and seminal vesicular fluid, respectively) will strengthen this diagnosis (see Chapter 4).

Specimen

- As for the assessment of semen viscosity

Equipment and disposable materials

- Merck/EM Science *ColorpHast* pH test strips; range 6.5–10.0. These have been found to be the most accurate pH test strips; they comprise a plastic strip with a single piece of indicator paper attached to one side at one end

Procedure

1. Using an air-displacement pipette, transfer a small droplet of semen onto the test strip.
2. Allow the color to develop.
3. Compare the color of the test strip with the appropriate color scale to read the pH.

Interpretation guidelines

Azoospermia, low volume (usually <1.0 ml), and pH <7.0 is often indicative of obstructive azoospermia due to agenesis of the Wolffian duct system, provided the semen sample was completely collected. A pH above 7.5 indicates a significant contribution of seminal vesicular fluid, which indicates that at least the seminal vesicles (at least in part) can contribute to the ejaculate, but does not rule out agenesis of other parts of the Wolffian duct system.

Making a wet preparation

Background

A wet preparation is used for direct observation of spermatozoa, along with the other cells and particles in the native semen sample. The primary methods of investigation are observation, classification and counting.

Principle

For proper evaluation of sperm motility it is essential that the depth of the preparation is about 20 μm. The depth of a preparation can be calculated by dividing the aliquot volume by the coverslip size (area). Using an 18 × 18 mm coverslip requires a semen aliquot of 6 μl, while a 22 × 22 mm coverslip requires a volume of 10 μl.

It is essential that the coverslip is applied immediately after the semen droplet is placed on the slide – if delayed there is a considerable risk for errors due to desiccation, resulting in a ring of dead sperm and debris around the periphery of the preparation.

Specimen

- As for the assessment of semen liquefaction

Equipment (see also Appendix 2)

- Air-displacement pipetter, 0–20 μl

Disposable materials

- Glass microscope slides
- Coverslips, 18 × 18 or 22 × 22 mm, #1½ or #2 thickness (heavy enough to spread the semen)
- Disposable tips for the automatic pipetter (sterile if the sample is for treatment purposes)
- Gloves

Procedure

1. Use a clean microscope slide that has been pre-warmed to 37°C; store the slide warm during the making of the preparation and ideally keep it at 37°C during the entire investigation of the preparation.
2. Make sure the sample is well mixed by swirling the sample before taking the aliquot for the wet preparation.
3. Aspirate the appropriate volume with an air-displacement pipette and deposit it as a droplet on the microscope slide.
4. Apply the coverslip to the droplet immediately.

Results

No results are recorded at this stage.

Notes

If air bubbles appear centrally under the coverslip it must be discarded and a new preparation made.

Hint: If the pipette plunger is depressed past the first stop before releasing it to take the sample aliquot, the volume in the pipette tip will be slightly larger than the desired volume. Then, when the aliquot is dispensed onto the slide by depressing the pipette plunger only to the first stop, the extra material will stay in the pipette tip, greatly reducing air bubble formation.

Initial investigation of a wet preparation

Principle

Observation under the microscope of spermatozoa, cells and other particulate material (Figure 3.2).

Specimen

- A freshly prepared wet preparation from the semen specimen being analyzed

Equipment (see also Appendix 2)

- Microscope, 10×, 20×, and 40× phase contrast objectives, ideally equipped with a heated stage set at 37°C

Procedure and results

1. The examination of the wet preparation should begin as soon as the flow has ceased, which should happen within 1 min after placing the coverslip on the semen droplet; if not, then the preparation should be discarded and a new one prepared.
2. Count the number of spermatozoa visible in randomly chosen microscope fields. If less than one spermatozoon is observed per field of vision (40× objective with wide-field

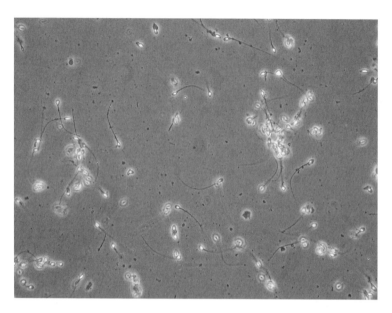

Figure 3.2 Typical appearance of normal semen under phase contrast optics (positive low phase contrast). Note the presence of small and larger particulate debris, as well as a few aggregates of debris and dead (immotile) spermatozoa.

eyepieces) the sample should be treated as an azoospermic or severely oligozoospermic sample (see Notes).

3. If spermatozoa are observed, sperm motility is assessed (for details, see below).

4. *Assess the presence of sperm aggregation and agglutination*: The degree of sperm aggregation or agglutination is determined in 10 randomly chosen microscope fields not adjacent to the coverslip edges. The proportion of spermatozoa trapped in clumps is estimated to the nearest 5%.

   - Agglutination is defined as at least some motile spermatozoa adhering without other cells and debris, most likely due to the presence of multivalent antisperm antibodies. If the agglutinates are very large, it may be difficult to assess whether the spermatozoa are specifically (e.g. head-to-head or tail-to-tail), or more randomly bound to each other.

   - Clumps comprising immotile (dead) spermatozoa and debris are described as aggregation. Small aggregates are common in normal samples, while large aggregates, which can contain hundreds of spermatozoa each, are considered as abnormal.

   - In samples where the proportion of spermatozoa involved in clumping is estimated to be 25% or more, motility is assessed on the free spermatozoa only. The proportion of spermatozoa involved in clumping, and that motility was assessed on the free sperm only, must be recorded on the sample form.

5. *Assess the presence of other cells and debris*: It is common to find other cells and debris in semen samples. Therefore the increased presence of such material should only be reported if seen in multiple fields. Such abnormalities should be commented upon in the report form using a few different, standardized expressions:

   "Round cells" are common in semen samples. "Leukocytes" must be differentiated from immature germinal epithelium cells *or* precursors or large cell bodies (often without nuclei) consisting of cytoplasm that has become exfoliated from the seminiferous epithelium of the testis. Other round cells can be of prostatic origin. There are two equally valid methods to assess the number of round cells present in semen. Round cells can be counted in the Neubauer hemocytometer chamber (at the same time as the assessment of sperm concentration). Alternatively the number of round cells can be counted in the same fields used for motility assessments. The separately determined sperm concentration, the number of spermatozoa counted in the motility assessment fields, and the number of round cells in the same fields, are used to calculate the concentration of round cells (see Note 1). If more than 1 million round cells per milliliter are found, a method for the specific determination of leukocytes should be used (see below) to assess the concentration of inflammatory cells in semen.

"Debris" (differentiate between particulate debris and motile bacteria):

No debris at all is quite rare

Some debris is very common

Moderate contamination with debris is not considered abnormal

Large amounts of debris should be regarded as abnormal

"Erythrocytes" (red blood cells) should not be found in semen, although the presence of a few does not indicate pathology.

"Epithelial cells" (squamous, cubic and transitional) can often be found in low numbers in semen samples; their increased presence has not been linked to any specific pathology.

"Bacteria" and "protozoa" should not be found in normal semen when examined under a phase contrast light microscope. However, if small motile particles are seen in a fresh sample (not to be confused with debris showing Brownian motion), high contamination with bacteria should be suspected and reported. Any observation of characteristic *Trichomonas* protozoa should also be reported (Figure 3.3).

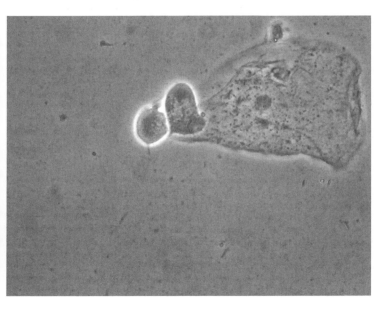

Figure 3.3 Protozoon (to the left) adjacent to a squamous epithelium cell (to the right); note the shade of the beating flagellum at the top of the *Trichomonas* organism.

Notes

1. *Handling of azoospermic and severely oligozoospermic samples*: When no or only very few spermatozoa have been observed in multiple microscope fields of the wet preparation, the sperm concentration cannot be determined using the quality-controlled quantitative technique (see below), and it is recommended that this be recorded on the report form and that the observed numbers of motile and immotile spermatozoa are given as free text comments.

   A sample with very few spermatozoa could be centrifuged (at least 1000 *g* for 15 min) and the pellet examined under the microscope (phase contrast optics, 40× objective). The presence of motile or immotile spermatozoa is assessed by scanning the whole area of the coverslip (corresponding to about 400 fields under a 22 × 22 mm coverslip) and the numbers of motile and immotile spermatozoa are recorded on the sample report form.

2. To calculate the concentration of round cells/ml semen, the numbers of sperm and round cells in the wet fields, respectively, and the separately determined sperm concentration are used:

$$\text{Round cell concentration} = \frac{\text{sperm concentration} \times \text{round cells}}{\text{\# spermatozoa in the field}}.$$

Sperm motility assessment

Background

Manual sperm motility assessment is performed on duplicate wet preparations as soon as possible after the presence of spermatozoa has been confirmed. Preparations should always be made and assessed in sequence, so that the second preparation is fresh when its motility assessment is started.

Sperm motility assessment – motility categories

Principle

If possible, it is recommended that motility assessments are made using a video monitor, in order to minimize the difference between daily routine and quality control assessment. If video equipment is not available, then assessments are done under phase contrast microscopy using a 20× or 40× objective.

It is essential that the motility assessment be commenced as soon as possible after the wet preparation has been made (see above) in order to minimize any negative influence of temperature decrease or dehydration.

Sperm motility is assessed by classifying each spermatozoon into one of three classes of motile spermatozoa, or as immotile, in at least five randomly chosen fields from each wet preparation; at least 200 spermatozoa should be classified in each preparation. Rapidly progressive spermatozoa (WHO class *a*) move forward with a speed of at least 25 µm/s (half a tail length or 5 head lengths), slowly progressive ones (WHO class *b*) move forward more than 5 µm/s (one head length) but less than 25 µm/s, non-progressive spermatozoa (WHO class *c*) move less than 5 µm/s, and immotile spermatozoa (WHO class *d*) have no active tail movements [1,11,12].

If at least 25% of the spermatozoa are estimated to be involved in clumps, then the motility assessment is made only on the free spermatozoa, and a comment is recorded on the sample report form. Only complete spermatozoa (head with tail) are included in the counts. However, spermatozoa with no or extremely small sperm heads should be commented upon if estimated to correspond to at least 20% of the intact spermatozoa.

In order to minimize the influence of random errors, motility assessments should always be done in duplicate. If comparison of the duplicate results does not show sufficient similarity, the assessments are discarded and new preparations made and assessed.

Specimen

- Freshly made wet preparations on warm microscope slides (see above)

Equipment (see also Appendix 2)

- Microscope, 10×, 20×, and 40× phase contrast objectives, ideally equipped with a heated stage set at 37°C
- Tally counter with at least 4 channels

Quality control

- Comparison of duplicate assessments for each sample
- For novices: Repeated training with experienced staff and using archived material with known results
- For all staff members: Internal quality control (IQC) monitoring of the variation between staff members and over time (imprecision)
- For the laboratory as a unit: External quality assurance (EQA) monitoring of the laboratory's performance in relation to other laboratories (accuracy)

Procedure

1. A wet preparation is prepared as described earlier.
2. Assessment is started as soon as any flow in the preparation has ceased.
3. First, count the rapid and slow progressive spermatozoa. Thereafter, count the non-progressive and immotile spermatozoa in the same field. If the concentration of spermatozoa is very high, it is advisable to only count spermatozoa in a smaller field, e.g. in the area of four central squares in an eyepiece grid (graticule or reticle).
4. Assess at least five different fields. At least 200 spermatozoa should be counted in each preparation.
5. Repeat the assessment of the motility of at least 200 spermatozoa in a second wet preparation from the same semen sample.

Calculations and results

First calculate the proportions for the four categories (WHO a,b,c,d) for each of the two preparations: the total number of spermatozoa in each motility group is divided by the total of number of spermatozoa assessed in that preparation. Then take the results for the dominant (largest) group, and calculate the average proportion for the two duplicates, and the difference between the duplicates. Refer to the table in Appendix 7 (Table A7.1) to establish whether the difference is small enough to accept the assessments. If the difference between the duplicates is less than the limit value in the table the assessments can be accepted, otherwise the data are discarded and two new preparations are made and assessed.

When duplicate counts are accepted, all the category proportions (i.e. proportions of WHO *a*, *b*, *c*, and *d*, respectively) are calculated from the duplicate results, as well as the proportions of motile (*a* + *b* + *c*), and progressively motile (*a* + *b*) spermatozoa.

All motility results are presented as integer percentage values. The sum of the four motility categories (*a*,*b*,*c*,*d*) in a sample should be 100. If, due to rounding errors, the sum is 99 or 101, adjust the dominant group to get a sum of 100.

Interpretation guidelines

- Decreased motility (poor progression, reduced overall motility) can be due to disorders such as infections with inflammatory processes in the excretory glands (prostate and seminal vesicles).

- The presence of some types of antisperm antibodies (especially spermotoxic antibodies) can reduce sperm motility.

- Complete absence of sperm motility can be seen in men with cytotoxic antisperm antibodies, but also among men with ciliary dyskinesia (immotile cilia syndrome or Kartagener's syndrome).

Notes

The proportion of rapid progressive spermatozoa (category *a*) at 37°C is an important, functional sperm property related to fertility and fertilization success [13,14]. It is possible to do repeatable, manual assessments of the proportion of rapid, progressive spermatozoa provided staff members are trained using a visual scale for the 25 μm/s rate. Although there is no need to record all specimens, there is a major advantage in using a video screen for motility assessments. Furthermore, the use of video recordings for training and QC/QA is of additional value.

Sperm motility on video monitor

Principle

The use of a video monitor for assessing sperm motility has many advantages. Training in small groups assessing the same screen simultaneously is more efficient than individual training. The use of video monitors for routine analysis also eliminates the difference between assessments of *live* samples and QC assessments of recorded samples, which increases the validity of all recorded samples used for training and QC (Figure 3.4).

To obtain the same help to estimate sperm velocity that a grid in a microscope ocular gives, a black acetate with a central, circular, transparent field with a grid with squares corresponding to 25 × 25 μm could be attached in front of the screen.

To avoid sperm swimming in and out of focus in the 20-μm-deep preparation, it is best to use a 10× phase contrast objective to avoid sperm swimming in and out of focus, and then additional magnification in the camera tube to obtain a suitable magnification.

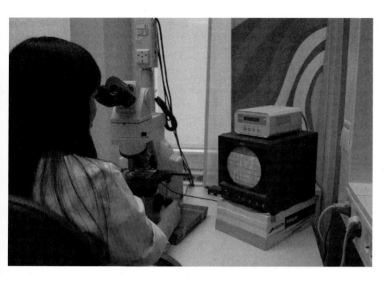

Figure 3.4 Illustration of a video setup for the routine assessment of sperm motility.

Specimen

- The same preparation as for the basic sperm motility assessment

Equipment (see also Appendix 2)

- Videomicrography system
- Stage micrometer

Disposable materials

- As for the basic sperm motility assessment

Calibration

Ideally, the total magnification on the video monitor screen should be adjusted so that 100 μm in the sample equals 70–90 mm on the screen (total magnification is adjusted by choosing appropriate intermediate magnification in the photo tube). Check the overall on-screen magnification using a micrometer scale in the microscope, and a ruler for the screen.

Quality control

- Duplicate assessments with comparisons are used to reduce the risk for random errors

Procedure

1. Adjust the microscope for optimal function (correct settings for phase contrast optics and Köhler illumination).
2. Adjust the focus through the oculars of the microscope, and then adjust the focus while looking at the image on the video monitor.
3. Chose a microscope field at random.

4. First, count the rapid and slow progressive spermatozoa. Thereafter, count the non-progressive and immotile spermatozoa in the same field; if the concentration of spermatozoa is very high, it is advisable to only count spermatozoa in a smaller field (e.g. in the area of four squares of the on-screen grid).

5. Assess at least five different fields. At least 200 spermatozoa should be counted in each preparation.

6. Repeat the motility assessment in a second preparation from the same semen sample.

Calculations and results

Calculations are done in the same way as for a basic motility assessment, and the same results are reported.

Interpretation guidelines

The same interpretation guidelines as for basic motility assessment.

Notes

The monitor should not be too large, since it is being viewed close-up; a screen size of about 13 cm is sufficient.

Video recording of sperm motility

Principle

Recording samples for motility assessments gives extra value for the laboratory by generating training material for novices and other staff members requiring qualitative training, as well as an archive of material that can be used for IQC and for exchange with other laboratories for EQA.

Specimen

- As for a basic sperm motility assessment

Equipment (see also Appendix 2)

In addition to the equipment needed for motility assessment on a video screen the following capabilities are needed:

- Recording facilities (VHS video recorder, DVD recorder, computer with video clip facilities) with the ability to view recordings frame-by-frame.
- Text generator connected to a video recorder or computer software, in order to add identifying text to the video recordings.

Disposable materials

- As for a basic sperm motility assessment
- Recording medium for video clips (video tapes, recordable CD-ROMs or DVD disks)

Calibration

- As for motility assessment using a video monitor

Quality control

- Recorded samples should be examined by all members of staff and the average results from experienced members used as target (or "true") values
- In recorded semen samples the velocity of individual spermatozoa can be measured frame-by-frame to classify spermatozoa objectively into the four groups (WHO *a–d*)
- Recorded samples can also be used for training and QC exchange with other laboratories
- When copies are made of the master recording, especially when converted to other formats, it is important to check that the copy gives the same results. This should be done by comparing results from blinded assessments of original and transferred versions of the recording. This problem is minimal with digital recordings, but a significant issue with analog video recordings

Procedure

1. Turn on the video camera, video monitor and video clip capture unit (video recorder and text generator or computer with appropriate software).

2. First record, for about 10 s, an image of a micrometer scale as the calibration image.

3. Then record a 5- to 10-s-long "scene" without the microscope image, preferably with an identifying text (e.g. "Andrology Laboratory, Xxxxxx Hospital, Quality Control").

4. Make a fresh wet preparation using pre-warmed microscope slide and coverslip (37°C) and make sure that there is no flow in the preparation.

5. Prepare the text function and create a unique identification (ID) for the recorded sample that cannot be used to reveal the identity of the patient (recorded samples for these purposes should be irreversibly anonymized). Either record the ID for 5 s before the first sample clip, or align the text so that it does not interfere with the central field of the view for the sample.

6. Make recordings.

7. Check the focus.

8. Record for 15–20 s and then add 5 s with a blank screen.

9. Estimate the number of spermatozoa that could be counted in that field. At least 200 "valid" spermatozoa must be recorded in at least five different fields.

10. Change the microscope field and repeat this step. Remember to check the focus and that there is no flow before recording each new field.

11. Record a final, blank screen after the last field of the sample for 10–15 s, preferably with a text saying "End of sample XXX" where "XXX" stands for the sample ID.

12. Record a message "End of recording" directly after the last field of the last sample on the recording medium.

Sperm concentration

Principle

Diluted and immobilized spermatozoa are easy to count under the microscope. The difficult part is to ascertain that the aliquot examined is adequate and representative for the entire semen sample. Spermatozoa should not be lost by sedimentation, aggregation or by adhesion to the walls of the sample container, pipette tips or test tubes, and there must be no dilution errors. Therefore, thorough mixing both before semen dilution and before the counting chamber is loaded is essential.

It is also important that the dilution is exact. Positive-displacement pipettes are necessary to measure exact volumes of semen samples since they are more viscous than watery solutions.

The next critical step is ensuring an accurate sub-sample volume (in practice, this is achieved by the depth of the counting chamber). To achieve a correct depth the coverslip must be mounted tight, and in order to examine the expected volume of the diluted specimen, the chamber must be filled correctly.

With a "wet" preparation depth of about 20 μm and a diameter of the field of vision of about 500 μm in the microscope, the observed number of spermatozoa per microscope field gives the appropriate dilution in Table 3.2. The correct area of the microscopic field can be determined using a stage micrometer. Measure the diameter of the microscope field and calculate the field area using the formula: Area $= \pi \cdot r^2$.

Table 3.2 Diluting the ejaculate for determining sperm concentration by hemocytometry. The most common dilutions are shown in bold.

Spermatozoa per microscopy field 40× objective	Dilution	Semen μl	Diluent μl
Swim up	1 + 1 (1 : 2)	100	100
<15	1 + 4 (1 : 5)	100	400
15–40	**1 + 9 (1 : 10)**	50	450
40–200	**1 + 19 (1 : 20)**	50	950
>200	1 + 49 (1 : 50)	50	2450

Thus, "standard" dilutions for semen are 1 + 19 and 1 + 9; for "swim-up" preparations with <10 million/ml, a dilution of 1 + 1 can be used.

Dilutions can be stored for a maximum of four weeks in tested vials at 4°C, but should preferably be assessed the same day. The problems that can occur upon prolonged storage are sperm clumping and sperm adhesion to the test tube walls.

Specimen

- Well-mixed, liquefied semen

Equipment and materials (see also Appendix 2)

- Vortex mixer
- Microscope with 10×, 20×, and 40× phase contrast objectives

- Humid chamber for hemocytometers
- Counting chamber: hemocytometer with Improved Neubauer ruling with proper coverslips
- Positive-displacement pipetter: 0–50 µl; with tips (ideally sterile)
- Calibrated, adjustable air-displacement pipetter: 200–1000 µl with tips (ideally sterile)
- Centrifuge
- Tally counter
- Calculator

Disposable materials
- Working/calculation sheet
- Test tubes with air-tight caps, e.g. Technicon autoanalyzer vials

Reagents
Diluent for sperm concentration

50.0 g	$NaHCO_3$
10.0 ml	36–40% formaldehyde solution (a saturated formaldehyde solution)

1. Dissolve the constituents in distilled water (>10 MΩ/cm) and dilute to 1000 ml.
2. Filter the solution to eliminate crystals into a clean bottle (filter paper for retention of coarse and gelatinous precipitates).
3. Store the diluent at 4°C (maximum 12 months).
4. The diluent should not contain any solid particles.

Quality control
- Calibration of pipettes should be carried out regularly. Pipettes showing erroneous results should be recalibrated according to the manufacturer's instructions, or sent for repair and recalibration. Results of calibration controls, as well as repairs and adjustments should be recorded in a separate log for each pipette
- Counting chambers should be checked for accuracy when new, and regularly after use (risk for wear causing changed chamber depth)
- Comparison of duplicate assessments for each sample analyzed
- For novices: Repeated training with experienced staff, and using archive material with known results
- For all staff members: IQC monitoring of the variation between staff members and over time (imprecision)
- For the laboratory as one unit: EQA monitoring of the laboratory's performance in relation to other laboratories (accuracy)

Procedure
1. The dilution is prepared according to Table 3.2 (if there are quality issues with the dilution step, it is advisable to make duplicate dilutions from each sample). Using

a positive-displacement pipette, the exact volume of well-mixed semen is taken and added to the diluent. To avoid transfer of additional semen on the outside of the pipette tip it is essential to carefully wipe off all fluid from the outside of the tip (*without* extracting any volume from the inside of the tip) before the tip is emptied in the diluent.

2. A special hemocytometer coverslip is mounted on the hemocytometer with Improved Neubauer ruling so that interference patterns are seen between the surfaces where the coverslip is attached. Several Newton's rings/fringes or iridescent lines should be visible when the coverslip is properly attached.

3. Immediately before withdrawing the aliquot of diluted spermatozoa, the tube of diluted specimen must be mixed for at least 10 s on a vortex mixer. First, take one aliquot of about 10 μl (the volume should be sufficient to fill one side of the hemocytometer) and load it into one side of a hemocytometer with Improved Neubauer ruling. Then take a second aliquot of the diluted specimen and load it into the other side of the hemocytometer. Each chamber must be completely filled, but not over-filled.

4. Place the chamber horizontally in a humid box for 10–15 min to allow sedimentation of the spermatozoa onto the grid of the counting chamber.

5. Spermatozoa are usually counted under a 20× phase contrast objective (for 40× it is often necessary to obtain a long working distance objective). One "large square" in the Improved Neubauer ruling hemocytometer chamber is limited on all sides by triple lines (Figure 3.5, see below). The *middle* of the three lines defines the large square. When spermatozoa are lying on or in contact with the borders of the square only spermatozoa on or in contact with the upper or the left border should be counted; those on or in contact with the lower or the right border must not be counted.

   a. Decide the number of squares that should be counted. First, count the number of spermatozoa in the large square in the upper, left corner of the central grid area. Based on this number, determine how many squares will be counted in each side of the chamber:

<10 spermatozoa	count all the grid (25 squares in each chamber)
10–40 spermatozoa	count 10 squares in each chamber
>40 spermatozoa	count 5 squares in each chamber (e.g. 4 corners and center)

   The goal is that typically more than 200 spermatozoa should be counted in each chamber and that this number is sufficient for a comparison between the two counts. If the total number of cells counted is less than 200 when all 25 large squares have been assessed, another of the 8 peripheral areas surrounding the central grid can be counted (Figure 3.5A).

   b. Only if a free sperm head can be recognized with certainty, should it be included in the count. If more than 20% of sperm heads lack tails the free heads should be counted separately and noted in the laboratory report. "Pinheads" should be counted separately and commented upon in the report form. Immature germ cells should not be counted (these will be assessed in the differential morphology count), but round cells and inflammatory cells can be counted separately to determine their respective concentrations.

c. Only spermatozoa where the head is located on the upper, or left limiting lines of a square (marked "OK" in Figure 3.5B) should be included for that square; do *not* count spermatozoa located on the lower, or right limiting lines (marked "out" in Figure 3.5B).

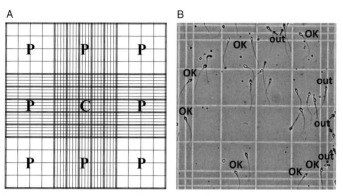

Figure 3.5 (A) Overview of the entire Improved Neubauer ruling hemocytometer with the central field (marked "C") surrounded by 8 peripheral fields (marked "P"), each of which has the same size as the central field. (B) Appearance of one of the 25 large squares of the central grid of a counting chamber in an Improved Neubauer ruling hemocytometer under phase contrast optics. Each central chamber consists of the 25 "large squares" (in a 5 × 5 pattern). Each "large square" is surrounded by triple lines and contains 16 small squares. The middle of the three lines limits each large square. Spermatozoa where the head is in contact with the upper or left line are counted ("OK" in figure), while those whose head is in contact with the left and lower line are not included ("out" in the figure). The small squares facilitate counting when there are many spermatozoa on the grid. Each central field (25 large squares) measures 1 mm × 1 mm, and has a depth of 0.1 mm (100 µm), giving a volume of 0.1 mm^3 = 0.1 µl = 100 nl. (Note that the Makler chamber has the same area as the central field of the improved Neubauer ruling hemocytometer, but a depth of only 0.01 mm (10 µm). Hence the volume is 0.01 µl = 10 nl, or one-tenth of that of the hemocytometer.)

Calculations and results

The duplicate counts are compared as described in Appendix 7. The total number of assessed spermatozoa (sum) and the difference between the two counts are calculated. An assessment is only accepted if the difference is equal to, or less than the value obtained in Table A7.3. Otherwise, the counts are discarded, and a new hemocytometer preparation made and assessed.

To get the concentration of spermatozoa in the original semen sample, the *sum* of the accepted duplicate counts (total number of spermatozoa in both chambers) is divided by the appropriate factor from Table 3.3, and the result expressed as millions of spermatozoa per ml ($\times 10^6$/ml). The total sperm number ($\times 10^6$/ejaculate) is obtained by multiplying the ejaculate volume (ml) and sperm concentration.

Sperm concentration should be expressed as "millions per milliliter" or $\times 10^6$/ml, and sperm count (total number of spermatozoa in the ejaculate) as "millions per ejaculate" with only 1 decimal place. However, for concentration or total count values <1 $\times 10^6$ two significant figures should be used, e.g. 0.094785 $\times 10^6$ could be expressed as 95 000 (per ml or ejaculate).

If reporting a result of "no spermatozoa" it is preferred that the result is not presented as 0.0 $\times 10^6$/ml, but that an asterisk (*) is written in the place for concentration and total sperm number. As a free comment, it should be stated if no, or perhaps just occasional motile or immotile, spermatozoa have been observed in the ejaculate, or in the centrifuged pellet.

Table 3.3 Conversion factors for use in calculating the results for sperm concentration determined using hemocytometry. Divide the total number of spermatozoa counted in the two hemocytometer chambers by the appropriate factor to give the concentration of spermatozoa in the original semen sample in millions of spermatozoa per milliliter (i.e. $\times 10^6$/ml).
A: Factors for use when only the central grid (5 × 5 large squares) has been assessed.

Dilution	Number of counted squares per chamber		
	25	10	5
1 + 1	100	40	20
1 + 4	40	16	8
1 + 9	20	8	4
1 + 19	10	4	2
1 + 49	4	1.6	0.8

B: Factors for use when at least one more field of 25 large squares than the central grid has been assessed.

Dilution	Number of 25-square fields counted							
	2	3	4	5	6	7	8	9
1 + 1	200	300	400	500	600	700	800	900
1 + 4	80	120	160	200	240	280	320	360
1 + 9	40	60	80	100	120	140	160	180

Interpretation guidelines

Besides incomplete sample collection and varying abstinence time there are many other external factors that can influence the total number of spermatozoa in the ejaculate, e.g. fever, some drugs and occupational exposure. Interpretation of sperm concentration and total number of spermatozoa in the ejaculate is the responsibility of the requesting clinician.

Notes

If counting chambers not made of glass are used, it is essential to ascertain that the optical properties of the material do not make the spermatozoa difficult to observe [15].

Sperm vitality

Principle

An intact cell membrane hinders the uptake of the stain eosin Y, while a dead cell (i.e. with damaged cell membrane) takes up the red stain. Nigrosin is a background stain that provides contrast for the unstained (white) live cells.

Specimen

- An aliquot of liquefied, well-mixed semen, ideally at 30 (maximum 60) min after ejaculation

Equipment and disposable materials

- Microscope with 100× oil immersion objective, bright-field not phase contrast (see Appendix 2)
- Microscope slides
- Coverslips, 22 × 50 mm or 24 × 50 mm, #1 thickness

Reagents

Stain: An equivalent stain is available commercially (Sperm VitalStain, Nidacon International).

0.67 g   eosin Y (C.I. 45380, Europe M 15935)
10.0 g   nigrosin (C.I. 50420, Europe M 15924)
0.90 g   sodium chloride
100 ml   distilled water

1. Dissolve the eosin Y and sodium chloride in 100 ml distilled water with gentle heating.
2. Add the nigrosin.
3. Bring the solution to boil and allow it to cool to room temperature.
4. Filter the solution through filter paper (e.g. Munktell Class II).
5. Store in a sealed glass bottle.
6. The staining solution should be at room temperature when used.

- Mounting: Use Merck Entellan mountant, or other equivalent medium for quick and permanent mounting.

Quality control

- For novices: Repeated training with experienced staff and using archive material with known results
- For all staff members: IQC monitoring of the variation between staff members and over time (imprecision)
- For the laboratory as one unit: EQA monitoring of the laboratory's performance in relation to other laboratories (accuracy)

Procedure

1. Mix 50 µl of well-mixed, undiluted, liquefied semen with 50 µl of eosin-nigrosin stain and incubate for 30 s.
2. Place 12–15 µl of the mixture on a clean microscope slide and make a smear.
3. Let the smear air dry and examine it directly or, preferably, mount it permanently the same day and examine after the mountant has dried (e.g. overnight). Mounted smears can be stored at room temperature.
4. Assess at least 200 spermatozoa at 1000× (or 1250×) magnification under oil immersion with a high-resolution 100× bright-field objective. Use properly adjusted bright-field optics (Köhler illumination), *not* phase contrast optics. White (unstained) sperm heads are classified as "live" and those with any pink or red stain are classified as "dead" with the exception of spermatozoa that show only a slight pink staining in the neck region ("leaky necks"); this is not considered a sign of cell death (Figure 3.6; see color plate section).

Figure 3.6 See color plate section. A sperm vitality preparation using the one-step eosin-nigrosin stain seen under bright-field optics (Köhler illumination) showing three dead (red) spermatozoa and one live (white) spermatozoon with a "leaky neck."

5. The WHO does not recommend duplicate counting for vitality assessment. However, if it is done, then duplicates should be compared in the same way as for motility and morphology (Table A7.1).

Calculations and results

The proportion of live spermatozoa is calculated by dividing the number of live spermatozoa counted by the total number of spermatozoa assessed.

The proportion of live spermatozoa is given as an integer percentage (i.e. without decimal points).

Interpretation guidelines

Sperm vitality measured with a staining method is clinically important when very few or no spermatozoa are motile. Ciliary dyskinesia (immotile cilia syndrome or Kartagener's syndrome) is a rare genetic disorder due to defects in the ciliary structure, affecting all cilia in the body of the affected individual, including the sperm tail. In addition to having live but totally immotile spermatozoa, chronic respiratory infections and *situs inversus* are not uncommon findings in these men.

If the immotile spermatozoa are dead then cytotoxic antisperm antibodies, or other negative effects of active inflammatory reactions can be suspected.

Notes

The proportion of live spermatozoa is usually slightly higher than the proportion of motile spermatozoa in the sample.

WHO recommendations for vitality staining [11] can cause spermatozoa to die due to too low an osmolarity [16]. The present method has been established not to do that [17].

Sperm morphology

Introduction

It was only since the early 1900s that the importance of sperm morphology in male fertility potential and its role in the fertilization process was recognized and researchers started to include this variable in the semen analysis. However, even at that early stage, contradictory reports were published on the importance and role of sperm morphology. In 1921 Hühner [18] made the statement that "If there are many active moving spermatozoa per microscopic field present, sperm morphology is of no importance and the presence of many abnormal spermatozoa will have no influence on the outcome of the post coital test." This was contradicted by Cary in 1930 [19], who stated that "morphology of human spermatozoa bears a definite relation to their success of migration through cervical mucus." This statement was repeated by Cary and Hotchkiss [20] when they wrote "Abnormal forms may process motility but are rarely if ever found in the upper levels of cervical mucus and we must consider them ineffectual for fertilization." This was also supported by a statement by

Moench and Holt [21] in 1932 that "Morphology of the sperm head seems to be the most reliable indicator of fertilizing power of these cells."

With the introduction of strict criteria for assessing human sperm morphology [22,23] these last three statements became more evident as supported by a literature analysis performed by Coetzee *et al.* [24]. It is therefore clear that the assessment of sperm morphology characteristics is very important for the complete evaluation of the semen sample. Sperm morphology evaluation can be divided into two categories: (a) the morphological evaluation of spermatozoa, and (b) the evaluation of semen cytology. Both must be regarded as important aspects.

Accurate evaluations of sperm morphology cannot be done if the following, although very basic, principles and steps are not followed as described below.

Sperm morphology – preparation of smears

Equipment (see also Appendix 2)
- Air-displacement pipette, 0–20 μl

Disposable materials
- Microscope slides with frosted ends
- Coverslips, 24 × 50 mm, #1 thickness

Procedure
The slides for the morphology smears must be clear from any debris or grease; if not, they must be thoroughly cleaned before use, first by washing in a detergent, rinsing in clean water, and then rinsing in alcohol and drying. This is to ensure that the semen smear will stick to the glass slide.

Coverslips must also be washed with alcohol, if indicated [25]. A small drop of well-mixed, liquefied semen (see Notes) is placed on the slide using either a positive-displacement or an air-displacement pipette. A small drop of semen must be used so that a very thin smear is prepared with no more than 5–10 spermatozoa being present per visual oil immersion field, at 1000–1250× magnification.

Smears are prepared by either the feathering or apposed slides techniques (Figure 3.7). Smears are left to air dry before fixing (see below).

Feathering technique

Figure 3.7 Diagram of two alternative techniques for making smears for sperm morphology assessment.

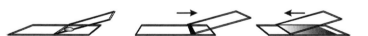

Apposed slides technique

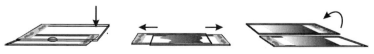

Notes

Thin smears are essential so that each spermatozoon can be visualized separately, and so that all spermatozoa will be in the same focal plane so their true form can be observed.

The thickness of the smear and thus the number of sperm per visual field can be controlled by altering the size of the semen drop and by adjusting the angle and speed of the slide used to make the smear.

With a high sperm concentration a small drop of semen (but not <6 μl) should be used. With a lower sperm concentration the size of the drop is increased, but to not more than 15 μl. Changing the angle between the two slides and of the speed at which the feathering is performed will change the thickness of the smear.

When feathering, it is important that the semen drop should be pulled over the semen smear slide. Pushing the drop may cause artifacts such as loose heads and broken or bent tails.

If the sperm concentration is very low ($<2 \times 10^6$/ml), an aliquot of the semen sample can be centrifuged (maximum 1000 g) and the pellet resuspended in a small amount of clean seminal plasma (i.e. the supernatant) to make the morphology smear.

With viscous samples it may be difficult to prepare good, thin smears unless alternative methods are used, such as the treatment of the sample with alpha-amylase or chymotrypsin [25], or alternatively a part of the semen specimen can be diluted with 170 mM NaCl solution and used to make smears [1].

Semen smears should always be prepared in duplicate. This is so that one smear can be stored for later reference purposes, or other studies, or in case the first staining was not successful.

Sperm morphology – fixation of smears

Specimen

- Semen smears that have been left to air dry (see above)

Equipment (see also Appendix 2)

- Staining dishes or Coplin jars

Materials

The fixation procedure will depend on the staining method used; for the modified Papanicolaou staining method use analytical grade absolute ethanol or methanol.

Procedure

Note: The fixation procedure will depend on the staining method used.

For the modified Papanicolaou staining procedure the best technique is to leave the smears until they appear to be just air-dried, i.e. only a few minutes, and then fix them immediately by immersion in analytical grade ethanol or methanol for at least 10–15 min.

The smears can be kept in the fixative for longer periods of time if needed, up to several days.

Fixed smears can be directly stained or taken out of the fixative and stored for later staining or use.

Notes

If smears are specially prepared for cytological evaluation they can be fixed immediately using a 50 : 50 mixture of ethanol and diethyl ether (caution: highly flammable).

Sperm morphology – staining of smears

Background

For routine work, a staining method such as the modified Papanicolaou procedure [11,26] is recommended. This method gives good staining of both spermatozoa and the so-called round cells, such as the precursors or germinal epithelium cells, and the various types of leukocytes. The Papanicolaou stain is a basophilic/acidophilic composition stain. Therefore, the nucleus of the spermatozoa and other cells stain an intense blue, while the sperm acrosome appears light blue, due to the effect of the hematoxylin under acid conditions. The sperm tails stain blue or, if staining conditions are very good, even red, while the midpiece can also stain red but mostly stains blue-green. Cytoplasmic residues at the head/neck junction will usually stain blue-green. Papanicolaou staining also gives a very good staining and definition of non-spermatozoal cells present in semen, due to the fact that in 1942 Papanicolaou [26] modified the Shorr stain method, which was specially developed for the staining of vaginal epithelium cells.

For special procedures, rapid staining methods such as the Diff-Quik® or Hemacolor® can be used [11,25]. Over-staining of the spermatozoa with the rapid staining methods and intense background staining of the seminal plasma are negative aspects of this method, as well as the fact that the spermatozoa undergo swelling, altering their morphological appearance. The background effect can be overcome by making very thin smears or by washing the semen samples before making the smears, but this can lead to additional morphological changes, or the presence of severely altered or decondensed spermatozoa. Spermac® [27] has the advantage of a short staining procedure, and also provides detailed differential staining of the acrosome, post-acrosomal region and tail. Spermac® stains the tails and intact acrosomes green and the visual part of the sperm head nucleus red. Due to its intense staining it is also very suitable for photography.

Equipment (see also Appendix 2)

- Staining dishes (glass)
- Stainless steel slide staining racks

Disposable materials

- Analytical grade ethanol
- Ethanol 95%, 80%, 70%, 50%
- Harris' hematoxylin (Papanicolaou solution 1a, Merck 9253)
- Orange G solution (OG6, Papanicolaou solution 2a, Merck 6888)
- Polychrome solution (EA50, Papanicolaou solution 3b, Merck 9272)
- Absolute 1-propanol
- Xylol (xylene) solution

The modified Papanicolaou staining procedure

1. Allow smears to air dry.

2. Fix for at least 10–15 min in analytic grade absolute ethanol.

3. Transfer one slide to the staining rack and the other to the slide filing box or cabinet. Slides should be stored in the dark at room temperature.

4. If all slides are collected, or if staining rack is full, proceed to staining by taking the rack through the sequential solutions and dyes as below.

5. Staining dishes should be adequately filled so that the whole slide will be immersed. For this reason it is recommended that staining racks where slides can be placed horizontally i.e. on their sides, should be used. Up to 20 slides can be placed back-to-back in each staining rack.

6. Proceed with staining according to the procedure in Table 3.4 (a "dip" corresponds to an immersion of about one second).

Table 3.4 Sequential steps for sperm morphology staining; with comments.

Step	Reagent	Exposure	Comment
a.	80% ethyl alcohol	10 dips	Slides transferred directly from the ethanol fixation without drying must pass through at least one container with 50% ethanol.
b.	70% ethyl alcohol	10 dips	Air-dried smears require longer rehydration time (2–3 min in 50% ethanol) if slides have been kept dry for several days.
c.	50% ethyl alcohol	10 dips	
d.	Distilled water	10 dips	
e.	Harris' hematoxylin[a]	5 min	If the nuclear staining is weak, a new stain solution should be prepared or exposure time increased.
f.	Rinse in running water	3 min	To remove unbound hematoxylin.
g.	0.5% HCl[b]	2 dips	This step can be checked in the microscope – unspecific staining should be removed.
h.	Rinse in running water	5 min	To readjust pH after acid treatment – sperm nuclei becoming blue (instead of reddish).
i.	Scott's water[c]	1 min	This step is essential when the pH of the water is too acidic (pH 4–5).
j.	Rinse in running water	1–5 min	
k.	50% ethyl alcohol	10 dips	To prepare for cytoplasmic staining with the ethanol soluble stains Orange G6 and EA 50 (or 65), water is removed by baths with increasing ethanol concentration. Ethanol after each staining bath is to remove surplus stain.
l.	70% ethyl alcohol	10 dips	
m.	80% ethyl alcohol	10 dips	
n.	95% ethyl alcohol	10 dips	

Table 3.4 (cont.)

Step	Reagent	Exposure	Comment
o.	Orange G6	5 min	
p.	95% ethyl alcohol	5 dips	
q.	95% ethyl alcohol	5 dips	
r.	EA 50 or 65	5 min	
s.	95% ethyl alcohol	5 dips	
t.	95% ethyl alcohol	5 dips	
u.	95% ethyl alcohol	5 dips	
v.	Absolute 1-propanol[e]	5 dips	To remove ethanol in order to be able to use a mountant not soluble in ethanol. For alternatives to xylol (xylene) see footnote "e."
w.	1-propanol and xylol (1 : 1)[d,e,]	5 dips	
x.	Xylol[e]	10 dips	
y.	Xylol[e]	10 dips	
z.	Xylol[e]	10–20 min	

(Modified from Eliasson, 1974; personal communication.)
[a] Harris' hematoxylin can be replaced with Mayer's hematoxylin.
[b] 1 ml concentrated HCl in 200 ml H_2O.
[c] 20 g $MgSO_4 \cdot 7H_2O$ and 2 g $NaHCO_3$ in 1000 ml H_2O, a small crystal of thymol can be added to avoid microbial growth.
[d] The function of the xylol (or xylene) series is to withdraw (dehydrate) all the water from the semen smears. If the xylol becomes milky, due to the presence of the water, replace immediately with fresh xylol.
[e] Important note: since xylene is toxic, especially for lungs due to the fixation of cilia, a fumehood or extraction cabinet must be used when performing the staining procedure. Health and Safety regulations can require that xylene is not used. Xylene can be exchanged for e.g. propanol or Neo-Clear® (Merck KGaA, Germany). Steps v–z are necessary to exchange the ethanol for another solvent for mountants that are insoluble in ethanol (e.g. DPX). These steps can be omitted if ethanol-soluble mountants are used. Ethanol-soluble mountants can be applied before the smears have air-dried after the last ethanol dip.

7. Mount the slides immediately with DPX (BDH) or other equivalent mountant. Leave mounted smears overnight for the mountant to set, or place in a low-temperature dry oven to enhance the drying process.

Sperm morphology – mounting of stained smears

Procedure

Place a thin line of mountant on the middle line over the length of the *coverslip* (24 × 50 mm is the most convenient size), starting and ending about 5 mm from the ends of the coverslip.

Take the semen-smear slide directly from the last xylol staining dish and place it smear-side down, directly onto the mountant.

Leave for some period of time so that the weight of the slide spreads the mountant to the sides of the coverslip.

Carefully press out any air bubbles with the aid of a pair of forceps, and center the coverslip so that its edge is about 5 mm away from the end of the slide. This will allow for the back-to-back storage of two slides in one slot of a storage box.

Notes

If a smear is technically difficult to read, then it might be that the smear was made too thick, or that the staining solutions were old or over-used. In such situations the reserve smear should be stained with fresh solutions and assessed.

If the smear was dislodged during the staining process, the smear was either too thick, or the slide was not clean enough.

Small, black-blue, fern-like crystals on the stained smears indicate that the hematoxylin solution is old or needs to be filtered.

Sperm morphology – evaluation

Background

For the evaluation of sperm morphology the whole spermatozoon must be considered. A spermatozoon without any morphological "defects" has been considered as morphologically "normal," although it is now recommended that the term "normal" should *not* be used to describe such spermatozoa, but rather to describe them as "typical." The definition for a morphologically typical spermatozoon is based on the modal form seen after spermatozoa have migrated through good, peri-ovulatory cervical mucus either *in vivo*, or *in vitro*. The spermatozoa seen in such a population are very homogeneous, and were used by Menkveld [22] and Menkveld *et al.* [23] to describe the "ideal" form. This principle was first adopted in the 1992 WHO manual [28], and confirmed as the standard method in the 1999 WHO manual [11].

Definition of the "typical" sperm morphology

According to the Tygerberg strict criteria [11,22,23] a typical spermatozoon is therefore defined as one having an oval form with a smooth contour and a clearly visible and well-defined acrosome with homogeneous, light-blue staining. The tail should be apically inserted without any abnormalities of the neck/midpiece and tail region and no cytoplasmic residues at the neck/midpiece or tail regions. The typical-sized acrosome should cover 30–60% of the anterior part of the sperm head. The typical-sized sperm head will measure between 3.0 and 5.0 μm in length and 2.0–3.0 μm in width. The midpiece should not be longer than 1.5× the length of a typical head and about 1 μm thick. The tail should be about 45–50 μm long and without any sharp bends. No cytoplasmic material can be present at the head/neck junction or along any part of the tail. For a spermatozoon to be classified as morphologically typical, the whole spermatozoon must be typical; borderline or slightly atypical spermatozoa are considered to be atypical.

Identification of morphologically atypical spermatozoa

Atypical spermatozoa are those that deviate from the defined criteria for morphologically ideal spermatozoa, due to differences in size, structure, or form. This assessment relates only to the main regions of the spermatozoon. For routine evaluations, differentiation between different abnormalities within the head or between different tail defects is not performed. If a specific abnormality/atypical form is dominant, or even common (e.g. affecting at least 20% of the spermatozoa in the specimen), this should be mentioned in the report form.

Main classes of sperm defects

1. Head defects: These include abnormalities due to size and/or form, and/or structure:
   a. "Size," where the sperm head is too small or too large. This is considered as the primary criterion for abnormality as long as the spermatozoa approximate the oval form.
   b. "Form" includes spermatozoa with an elongated or tapering form. The term tapering, i.e. spermatozoa having a narrowed head form due to flattening of the sides, might lead to confusion because it could be visualized by many investigators as a spear-point-like sperm. This is only one of the forms that can be included under the category of tapered. A more appropriate term would be elongated spermatozoa, since the so-called pear-shaped or pyriform spermatozoa should also be included in this category.
   c. "Structure" includes acrosome defects due to size, i.e. too large, >60% of normal head size, or too small, <30% of normal head size. Acrosome defects can also include staining defects of the acrosomes; including acrosomes showing vacuoles or cysts. In some patients, a very special defect has been observed where a cyst protrudes from the anterior acrosome area outside of the acrosome, forming a nipple-like structure (hence called a "nipple defect"), which was originally described in the bull. In humans it is regarded as a severe sperm morphology defect.
   d. "Duplications," where two or more spermatozoa are joined together at any location of the neck, midpiece or tail by cytoplasmic material, but not covering the sperm head itself. The classification of sperm-head duplications takes precedence over any other classification of sperm-head abnormalities.
   e. "Amorphous" includes all spermatozoa with head abnormalities that do not fall in any of the previously mentioned groups; this includes those spermatozoa with slight abnormalities.

2. Neck/midpiece defects: This category includes bent necks (i.e. the neck/midpiece forms a definitive angle with the sperm head). Thickened necks and midpieces are also included, as well as irregular or bent midpieces, asymmetrical tail insertions, or abnormally thin midpieces (i.e. where the mitochondria have shifted either to the neck region, not to be confused with the presence of cytoplasmic material or residues, or towards the principal piece of the tail). Different combinations of these aberrations can also be present.

3. Tail defects: This category includes tails bent at >90° at any part of the tail. A bend at the midpiece/tail junction is considered as a tail defect and not a neck/midpiece defect. Other abnormalities are short tails, coiled tails or irregular tails, or combinations of these. A frequency of >20% of coiled tails should be reported on the report from. In most cases, coiled tails will not be due to artifacts, such as hypo-osmotic stress or aging, but due to a definite abnormality where the coils of the tail are actually covered by one membrane. In the bull this abnormality is known as the DAG defect, named after the bull in which it was first described [29].

4. Cytoplasmic residues: Cytoplasmic droplets are better referred to as cytoplasmic residues, which can persist either protruding behind the sperm head at or around the neck/midpiece connection or on the tail itself. There is currently controversy as to whether the presence of cytoplasmic material or cytoplasmic droplets can be regarded as a normal phenomenon [30], but because they are seldom seen in stained semen smears they are regarded as abnormalities for sperm morphology evaluation. Although no cytoplasmic material should be present, a smooth droplet/residue of <30% of the normal-sized sperm head is still regarded as normal. The presence of cytoplasmic residues on spermatozoa is associated with sperm immaturity and the production of excessive reactive oxygen species (ROS) [25].

Other categories

1. Loose heads: Loose heads are not counted as an abnormality. The presence of >20 loose heads per 100 spermatozoa should be recorded on the report form.

2. Unknown cells: All cells that cannot be positively identified as either sperm precursors or inflammatory cells are placed in this group, and can also be mentioned on the report form.

3. Pinheads: So-called pinheads are also not included in the sperm morphology evaluation, since they typically do not contain any DNA or head structures (some can contain a small amount of chromatin). Again, a high prevalence, >20% relative to the sperm population, should be noted separately.

Teratozoospermia Index (TZI)

Each morphologically abnormal spermatozoon will have any one of the four types of abnormalities described above – or any combination of two to all four abnormalities. To reflect this, the Teratozoospermia Index (TZI) was introduced as an indication of the mean number of abnormalities (actually, defective regions) per abnormal spermatozoon [11,25,28].

Sterilizing defects

In some men persistent sperm morphology abnormalities are present as a consequence of genetic factors, such as the failure of the acrosome to develop, causing the "small round-head defect" or "globozoospermia" defect. These men are considered as sterile as far as normal in-vivo conception is concerned. The condition can be overcome by using ICSI, but success rates are very low. Another example is men with the so-called short tail syndrome. These conditions must be clearly recorded on the record form.

Equipment and disposable materials (see also Appendix 2)

- Microscope with bright-field illumination and at least three magnification options: a low power magnification (LPM) with an objective of 10×, 15×, or 20×; a high power magnification (HPM) option with a 40× objective, and a 100× oil immersion objective. The oil immersion 100× objective should be the highest quality plane-corrected objective available. Eyepieces should be 10×, 12.5×, or 15× with wide-field magnification

- Eyepiece with a built-in micrometer (or eyepiece reticle)
- Tally counter, minimum of 5 channels
- Immersion oil
- Lens cleaning paper

Quality control

- In order to be able to use reference limits obtained from published studies, it is essential that each analyst is properly trained, that the laboratory perform regular IQC, and that the laboratory participates in an EQA program (EQAP) employing the same criteria, methods, and standards as the centers that published the original data

Sperm morphology evaluation procedure

1. Scan the smear with the LPM objective to observe the spreading of the spermatozoa in the smear, the staining quality and the presence of round cells. If round cells are observed move to the 40× objective to identify the type of round cells present.

2. Identify suitable areas for the performance of the sperm morphology evaluation.

3. When a suitable area is identified under LPM, a small drop of immersion oil is placed on the slide, without removing the slide from the microscope stage.

4. Bring the oil immersion objective into place.

5. Sperm morphology evaluation should ideally be performed in more than one area to increase the accuracy of the evaluation. Experience has shown that in some cases a non-random distribution of sperm abnormalities can be present, and an unrepresentative evaluation might be obtained if this is not done.

6. Assess at least 200 spermatozoa. The WHO manual [11] suggests that counting one series of 200 spermatozoa is better than two counts of 100. Although it is preferable to count 200 spermatozoa twice to reduce counting error and variability, this may not always be practicable due to the quality of the smear or time constraints. However, according to the WHO manual when the diagnosis and treatment of the patient crucially depends on the percentage of morphological normal spermatozoa present, 200 spermatozoa should be assessed twice to increase the precision [11].

7. Record the morphological appearance of each spermatozoon as normal or abnormal. Assign four buttons on the counter for each of the four types of abnormalities. When a spermatozoon is scored as abnormal, the button for the specific abnormality is depressed; if more than one defect is present the buttons for each defect are depressed simultaneously. In this way all the defects of the spermatozoon will be scored, but the abnormal spermatozoon will only be counted once.

8. If there is any uncertainty about the size of a spermatozoon (especially if it is too large) it should be measured with the aid of the micrometer eyepiece.

Sperm morphology plates are shown in Figure 3.8 (see color plate section).

Figure 3.8 See color plate section. Sperm morphology color plates. (1) Sperm staining methods and sperm morphology patterns. (1A) Papanicolaou staining – elongated spermatozoa. (1B) Hemacolor® (Merck) rapid staining. Same patient as in 1A. Note slight swelling of spermatozoa, leading to rounder and larger forms, as well as background staining. (1C) Spermac staining®. Acrosomes and tail stain green and nucleus stains red. (1D) Normal morphology pattern of spermatozoa bound to the zona pellucida of a hemizona assay. (1E) Globozoospermia.

Spermac staining®. Note small round heads only with red staining, indicating the absence of the acrosomes. (1F) Stress pattern. All the spermatozoa are elongated. This condition can return to normal if cause of stress can be removed. Spermac staining®. (2) Specific sperm abnormalities. (2A–F) N = morphological ideal or normal spermatozoon; NM = neck/midpiece defect; T = tail defect; CR = cytoplasmic residue defect; V = vacuole(s). (2A) AL = large acrosome; HP = pyriform head. (2C) HL = head large (2E) MS = mitochondria shift to wards head; TC = coiled tail (DAG defect after a bull called DAG, where this abnormality was first diagnosed). (2F) HEL = head medium elongated; WBC = polymorphonuclear white blood cell; NMAS = asymmetrical implantation of the neck. (3) Specific sperm abnormities – continued. (3A–F) N = morphological ideal or normal spermatozoon; NM = neck/midpiece defect; T = tail defect; CR = cytoplasmic residue defect. (3A) HR = round head. (3C) CT = coiled tail. (3D) HSEL = slightly elongated head; NMAS = asymmetric implantation of the neck. (3E) Heterogeneous picture with small- and large-headed spermatozoa. HS = small head; HL = large head. (3F) HL = large head. (4) Semen cytology – non-spermatozoal cells possible in semen. (4A) Secondary spermatocyte. (4B) Polymorphonuclear white blood cells. (4C) Macrophage with phagocytosed spermatozoa. (4D) Monocyte with phagocytosed sperm head (SH). (4E) Prostate cell. (4F) Epithelium cell.

Calculations and results

The proportion of typical spermatozoa is calculated by dividing the number of spermatozoa assessed as "typical" by the total number of spermatozoa assessed. The result is given as an integer percentage (no decimal places).

Concerning the abnormalities seen, while the total of typical and abnormal cells will add up to the total number assessed, the sum of all abnormalities will be greater than the total number of spermatozoa that have been assessed.

To calculate the TZI, the sum of all recorded abnormalities is divided by the total number of *abnormal* spermatozoa (i.e. the total number of spermatozoa assessed – number of normal spermatozoa).

Since any given spermatozoon can have between one and four abnormalities, the TZI result will always be between 1.00 and 4.00.

Interpretation of results

The obtained results of the percentage of morphologically normal spermatozoa, expressed as % typical, can be used to classify the semen sample into the following three prognostic groups [31]:

≥15% = normal group
5–14% = G-group (good prognosis)
≤4% = P-group (poor prognosis group)

Notes

Since the TZI is considered an important measure of human sperm morphology, it is recommended that standard sperm morphology assessments include recording of the four basic types of abnormalities. In the 1999 WHO manual [11] only three of the four abnormal categories was used to calculate the TZI, for some reason cytoplasmic residues were not included in the calculation. The European Society of Human Reproduction and Embryology (ESHRE) manual [1] states that this is a wrong interpretation of the TZI, and therefore recommends that the original TZI score should be calculated according to the standard protocol as described in the 1992 WHO manual, with a clear indication that this earlier, correct definition has been used [28].

The microscope objectives should be arranged on the nosepiece in such a way that the LPM objective is in between the HPM objective and the oil immersion 100× objective.

This allows for alternating between the different magnifications when scanning the smear, and reduces the possibility of accidentally turning the 40× objective into a drop of immersion oil.

For evaluating sperm morphology a microscope with very good quality optics should be used, equipped with bright-field illumination and a 100× oil immersion, non-phase contrast objective, giving a total magnification of at least 1000×, but preferably 1250×. The use of the highest possible magnification is important; if this is not used only the grossest abnormalities will be observed.

If, for screening purposes, spermatozoa are only scored as typical or abnormal, only two channels of the laboratory counter are used.

Semen cytology in stained smears

Background
The evaluation of semen cytology is an important part of a semen analysis, and is performed using the fixed and stained smear used for sperm morphology evaluation.

Principle
The Papanicolaou stain adapted for spermatozoa is also useful to identify leukocytes and immature germ cells.

Specimen
- The same stained and mounted slides as for sperm morphology assessment

Equipment (see also Appendix 2)
- Microscope with 10×, 40×, and 100× objectives
- Coplin jars for fixation and/or staining of slides
- Staining dishes and racks, if required for the chosen staining method

Disposable materials
- Microscope slides with frosted ends
- Coverslips, 24 × 50 mm, #1 thickness
- Fixative (as per intended method), e.g. freshly-mixed 1 : 1 ethanol:diethyl ether (e.g. in a stoppered measuring cylinder)
- Stain(s) as per intended method

Procedure
1. For the evaluation of semen cytology, i.e. the investigation for the presence of round cells, such as leukocytes, germinal epithelium cells (precursors), as well as micro-organisms, a thicker smear can be prepared.
2. A small drop of egg albumin can be added to the semen drop to assure a better adherence of the cellular matter to the slides. Instead of the addition of albumin, poly-L-lysine coated slides can be used.

3. The slides are fixed immediately in a 1 : 1 mixture of ethanol:diethyl ether, and stained together with the slides for the sperm morphology evaluations.

4. The slides are screened at a low magnification (10× or 20× objective).

5. If any cells or organisms are observed, turn to the 40× objective to make a better identification.

6. Polymorphonuclear leukocytes and precursor cells are especially important. The presence of these cells is recorded separately as the estimated number of cells per high power (40× objective) field. To be able to calculate the concentration in semen of these cell types, the number of spermatozoa in the same fields must be counted.

Calculations and results

The presence of leukocytes (polymorphonuclear neutrophils) is expressed as number of cells/100 spermatozoa, and with the help of the sperm concentration as concentration ($\times 10^6$/ml).

The presence of precursors (germinal epithelium cells) is expressed in the same way.

Interpretation of results

The presence of $\geq 1 \times 10^6$/ml white blood cells is regarded by the WHO manual as leukocytospermia [11], but there is no known cut-off indicating that medical treatment of an infection is necessary. See also the section below on interpretation guidelines for "Identification of peroxidase-positive cells."

Identification of peroxidase-positive cells

Principle

Inflammatory cells in semen, i.e. neutrophil, basophil and eosinophil granulocytes, can be identified cytochemically due to their containing peroxidase. Using barbital-carbazol, cells with peroxidase activity stain brown while other cells are unstained (Figure 3.9; see color plate section) [32]. By determining the number of stained cells in a counting chamber, the concentration of inflammatory cells in the semen sample can be determined.

Figure 3.9 See color plate section. Appearance of brown-stained peroxidase-positive cell (inflammatory cell) in semen under phase contrast optics (40× objective).

Specimen

- Fresh, liquefied and well-mixed semen, ideally within 30–60 min after ejaculation

Equipment (see also Appendix 2)

- Microscope with 40× objective (bright-field or phase contrast optics)
- Hemocytometer (Improved Neubauer ruling) with special coverslips
- Positive-displacement pipetter, 0–50 μl or 0–100 μl
- Air-displacement pipette, 0–50 μl or 0–100 μl
- Humid chamber

Disposable materials

- Pipette tips to match the air-displacement pipette
- Tips for the positive-displacement pipette
- Eppendorf tubes, 1.5 ml

Reagents (see also Note 2, below)

- Distilled water (dH$_2$O)
- Stock solution 1 M HCl

Barbital acetate buffer, stock solution

5.90 g barbital sodium
3.89 g sodium acetate trihydrate
6.90 g sodium chloride

- Dissolve in 100 ml dH$_2$O while mixing at 37°C
- Adjust pH to 7.35 with 1 M HCl
- Add dH$_2$O to final volume 1000 ml
- Store at room temperature for up to 6 months

Carbazol solution

50 mg carbazol
30 ml dimethyl sulfoxide (DMSO) in a screw-top tube (e.g. a 50-ml centrifuge tube)

- Add the carbazol to the DMSO, mix until completely dissolved
- Pipette 1200-µl aliquots into separate small test tubes and seal with lids
- Store at −20°C for up to 5 weeks

Hydrogen peroxide solution, 0.25% (w/v)

7.1 ml hydrogen peroxide stock solution (35%, w/v)

- Add dH$_2$O to 1000 ml, store at 4°C for up to 12 months

Calibration

- No specific calibration required

Quality control

- If there is any doubt about the results, prepare a fresh working solution. Stock solution left out of the refrigerator or in bright light should be discarded

Procedure

1. Immediately before testing: Thaw a tube of carbazol solution.
2. Prepare the staining solution by mixing 10 ml of dH$_2$O and 10 ml of barbital acetate stock solution in a large (50 ml) centrifuge tube.
3. Add 120 µl hydrogen peroxide solution to the staining solution.
4. Add the thawed carbazol solution (1200 µl) to the staining solution.

5. Put lid on the staining solution and mix carefully by turning the sealed tube upside down several times. Use within 15 min.

6. Transfer 100 µl of semen into a 1.5-ml Eppendorf tube using the positive-displacement pipetter, and add 900 µl of the staining solution using the air-displacement pipetter. Cap the tube and mix the cell suspension for at least 20 min on a bench-top orbital shaker.

7. Load ~10 µl into each side of the hemocytometer with its coverslip attached, and allow the cells to sediment for 10–15 min by resting horizontally in a humid chamber.

8. Count as for sperm concentration (using a dilution factor of 1 : 10 [1 + 9]) under bright-field microscope optics (phase contrast can be used to facilitate observation of the hemocytometer grid); assess the entire central grid area (25 × 25 large squares) in the two counting chambers.

Calculations and results

The total number of observed cells with brown staining over the two chambers is divided by the factor of 20 to give the concentration of peroxidase-positive cells in million/ml in the original semen sample. Report the result with no more than one decimal place.

Interpretation guidelines

According to WHO recommendations, more than 1×10^6/ml peroxidase-positive cells is considered abnormal [11]. Recent studies indicate that even lower concentrations of leukocytes might be important markers for inflammatory disorders that can be significant in regard to a man's fertility potential [25,33,34], although other studies have found no relationship between leukocytes in semen and either other semen parameters, or clinical signs of inflammatory disorders [35].

Notes

1. An alternative "screening" procedure could include a first step mixing 10 µl semen and 10 µl working solution on a microscope slide and covering it with a coverslip. If examination under bright-field microscopy (40× objective) shows more than 1 peroxidase-positive cell per 5 fields, then a fresh mixture of 10 µl semen and 10 µl working solution is made on a porcelain spotting plate. From that mixture, a 4.5-µl aliquot is transferred to a Makler chamber and its coverglass applied until inference fringes are seen at the four support pillars. The chamber is examined under bright-field optics using a 20× objective (40× if possible), and the peroxidase-positive cells are counted in the whole grid. Divide the number of cells per grid area by 5 to obtain the concentration in the original semen in millions per milliliter (this automatically allows for the 1 + 1 dilution).

2. A benzidine-cyanosine stain is commercially available: the LeucoScreen™ kit from FertiPro (Beernem, Belgium).

Examination of semen after vasectomy

Introduction

After vasectomy it is important to establish whether the surgical procedure has been successful, i.e. that the communication between the testis and the urethra has been completely severed. This is done by examining the ejaculate for the presence of spermatozoa. Since it takes some time to empty the male reproductive tract of spermatozoa, it is essential to wait and not start the semen investigation until 3–4 months after the surgery [36,37]. It is believed that it is important that the man has regular ejaculations during the period before the investigation [38].

Specimen

- Fresh ejaculate (examination starting 30 min after ejaculation)

Equipment (see also Appendix 2)

- As for general sperm concentration assessment
- Centrifuge
- Air-displacement pipette, 0–100 μl

Disposable materials

- Centrifuge tubes, 15 ml, conical bottom, non-toxic to spermatozoa
- Tips for air-displacement pipette
- Microscope slides
- Coverslips, 22 × 22 mm, #1½ or #2 thickness

Calibration

No specific calibration is required except for the same microscope adjustments as for examining a wet preparation.

Quality control

- The method is semi-quantitative only, aimed at establishing whether any spermatozoa are present in the ejaculate; no quality control is needed beyond the training required for working with wet preparations and the assessment of sperm concentration

Procedure

1. Make a wet preparation and scan through the entire area of the coverslip.
2. If no spermatozoa are detected in the wet preparation the entire semen sample should be centrifuged at approximately 1000 g for 20 min.
3. After centrifugation most of the supernatant seminal plasma is removed and the sperm pellet is resuspended in the remaining minimum volume of seminal plasma supernatant.
4. A new wet preparation is made from the resuspended pellet and covered with a 22 × 22 mm coverslip.
5. Scan through the entire area of the coverslip (at least 400 fields) using phase contrast optics at a magnification of 400×.

Calculations and results

If motile or immotile spermatozoa are identified when the whole area of a coverslip (at least 400 fields under a 22 × 22 mm coverslip) is scanned, the numbers of motile and immotile spermatozoa are recorded on the semen sample report form [1].

Interpretation guidelines

In general, it is required that a man produces two to three consecutive complete semen samples without any detectable spermatozoa for him to be pronounced as "clear." The persistent presence of spermatozoa months after vasectomy combined with regular ejaculations can, in some cases, be due to partial surgical failure or possible re-canalization. Reappearance of spermatozoa after repeated absence might be due to re-canalization of the vas deferens [39].

Notes

Morphology staining of the smeared pellet is not suitable due to the small, but in these cases significant risk for contamination with spermatozoa from the staining solutions.

References

1. Kvist U, Björndahl L, eds. *Manual on Basic Semen Analysis*. Oxford: Oxford University Press 2002.
2. Mortimer D. *Practical Laboratory Andrology*. Oxford: Oxford University Press 1994.
3. Pound N, Javed MH, Ruberto C, *et al.* Duration of sexual arousal predicts semen parameters for masturbatory ejaculates. *Physiol Behav* 2002; **76**: 685–9.
4. Zavos PM, Goodpasture JC. Clinical improvements of specific seminal deficiencies via intercourse with a seminal collection device versus masturbation. *Fertil Steril* 1989; **51**: 190–3.
5. Kamischke A, Nieschlag E. Treatment of retrograde ejaculation and anejaculation. *Hum Reprod Update* 1999; **5**: 448–74.
6. MacLeod J, Gold RZ. The male factor in fertility and infertility. V. Effect of continence on semen quality. *Fertil Steril* 1952; **3**: 297–315.
7. Carlsen E, Andersson AM, Petersen JH, Skakkebaek NE. History of febrile illness and variation in semen quality. *Hum Reprod* 2003; **18**: 2089–92.
8. Cooper TG, Brazil C, Swan SH, Overstreet JW. Ejaculate volume is seriously underestimated when semen is pipetted or decanted into cylinders from the collection vessel. *J Androl* 2007; **28**: 1–4.
9. Björndahl L, Kvist U. Sequence of ejaculation affects the spermatozoon as a carrier and its message. *Reprod Biomed Online* 2003; **7**: 440–8.
10. MacLeod J, Gold RZ. The male factor in fertility and infertility. III. An analysis of motile activity in the spermatozoa of 1000 fertile men and 1000 men in infertile marriage. *Fertil Steril* 1951; **2**: 187–204.
11. World Health Organization. *WHO Laboratory Manual for the Examination of Human Semen and Sperm-Cervical Mucus Interaction.* 4th edn. Cambridge, UK: Cambridge University Press 1999.
12. Mortimer D. Laboratory standards in routine clinical andrology. *Reproductive Medicine Review* 1994; **3**: 97–111.
13. Sifer C, Sasportes T, Barraud V, *et al.* World Health Organization grade 'a' motility and zona-binding test accurately predict IVF outcome for mild male factor and unexplained infertilities. *Hum Reprod* 2005; **20**: 2769–75.
14. Verheyen G, Tournaye H, Staessen C, *et al.* Controlled comparison of conventional in-vitro fertilization and intracytoplasmic sperm injection in patients with asthenozoospermia. *Hum Reprod* 1999; **14**: 2313–19.

15. Kirkman Brown J, Björndahl L. Evaluation of a disposable plastic Neubauer counting chamber for semen analysis. *Fertil Steril* 2009; **91**: 627–31.

16. Björndahl L, Söderlund I, Johansson S, *et al.* Why the WHO recommendations for eosin-nigrosin staining techniques for human sperm vitality assessment must change. *J Androl* 2004; **25**: 671–8.

17. Björndahl L, Söderlund I, Kvist U. Evaluation of the one-step eosin-nigrosin staining technique for human sperm vitality assessment. *Hum Reprod* 2003; **18**: 813–16.

18. Hühner M. Methods of examining for spermatozoa in the diagnosis and treatment of sterility. *Int J Surg* 1921; **34**: 91–100.

19. Cary WH. Sterility diagnosis: The study of sperm cell migration in female secretion and interpretation of findings. *NY State J Med* 1930; **30**: 131–6.

20. Cary WH, Hotchkiss RS. Semen appraisal. A differential stain that advances the study of cell morphology. *JAMA* 1934; **102**: 587–90.

21. Moench GL, Holt H. Biometrical studies of head lengths of human spermatozoa. *J Lab Clin Med* 1932; **17**: 297–316.

22. Menkveld R. An investigation of environmental influences on spermatogenesis and semen parameters. Ph.D. dissertation, Faculty of Medicine, University of Stellenbosch, South Africa, 1987.

23. Menkveld R, Stander FSH, Kotze TJ vW, *et al.* The evaluation of morphological characteristics of human spermatozoa according to stricter criteria. *Hum Reprod* 1990; **5**: 586–92.

24. Coetzee K, Kruger TF, Lombard CJ. Predictive value of normal sperm morphology: a structured literature review. *Hum Reprod Update* 1998; **4**: 73–82.

25. Menkveld R. Chapter 9. The basic semen analysis. In: Oehninger S, Kruger TF, eds. *Male Infertility*. Oxon: Informa Healthcare 2007: 141–70.

26. Papanicolaou GN. A new procedure for staining vaginal smears. *Science* 1942; **95**: 438–9.

27. Oettlé EE. Using a new acrosome stain to evaluate sperm morphology. *Vet Med* 1986; **81**: 263–6.

28. World Health Organization. WHO *Laboratory Manual for the Examination of Human Semen and Sperm-Cervical Mucus Interaction*. 3rd edn. Cambridge, UK: Cambridge University Press 1992.

29. Oettlé EE, Menkveld R, Swanson RJ. Photographs with interpretations. In: Menkveld R, Oettlé EE, Kruger TF, *et al.*, eds. *Atlas of Human Sperm Morphology*. Baltimore, MD: Williams & Wilkins 1991: 15–65.

30. Cooper TG, Yeung CH, Fetic S, *et al.* Cytoplasmic droplets are normal structures of human sperm but are not well preserved by routine procedures for assessing sperm morphology. *Hum Reprod* 2004; **19**: 2283–8.

31. Kruger TF, Acosta AA, Simmons KF, *et al.* Predictive value of abnormal sperm morphology in in vitro fertilization. *Fertil Steril* 1988; **49**: 112–17.

32. Schaefer HE, Fischer R. {Specific staining of eosinophilic granulocytes with Biebrich scarlet}. *Klin Wochenschr* 1968; **46**: 396–7.

33. Lackner J, Schatzl G, Horvath S, *et al.* Value of counting white blood cells (WBC) in semen samples to predict the presence of bacteria. *Eur Urol* 2006; **49**: 148–52; discussion 52–3.

34. Punab M, Loivukene K, Kermes K, Mandar R. The limit of leucocytospermia from the microbiological viewpoint. *Andrologia* 2003; **35**: 271–8.

35. Rodin DM, Larone D, Goldstein M. Relationship between semen cultures, leukospermia, and semen analysis in men undergoing fertility evaluation. *Fertil Steril* 2003; **79** Suppl 3: 1555–8.

36. Bedford JM, Zelikovsky G. Viability of spermatozoa in the human ejaculate after vasectomy. *Fertil Steril* 1979; **32**: 460–3.

37. Lewis EL, Brazil CK, Overstreet JW. Human sperm function in the ejaculate following vasectomy. *Fertil Steril* 1984; **42**: 895–8.

38. Jouannet P, David G. Evolution of the properties of semen immediately following vasectomy. *Fertil Steril* 1978; **29**: 435–41.

39. Hancock P, McLaughlin E. British Andrology Society guidelines for the assessment of post vasectomy semen samples (2002). *J Clin Pathol* 2002; **55**: 812–16.

Extended semen analysis

Antisperm antibodies

Men (and women) with "antisperm antibodies" (ASABs) have reduced fertility [1] and hence testing should be mandatory for all subfertile men [2]. ASABs on spermatozoa will interfere with normal cell function, e.g. penetration into cervical mucus, capacitation, acrosome reaction and in-vitro fertilization [3,4]. However, the presence of ASABs is not an absolute indicator of subfertility since even men with high levels of ASABs can be fertile. Although clinical data are limited, at least 50% of the motile spermatozoa need to be coated with antibodies (assessed using mixed antiglobulin reaction [MAR] or immunobead test [IBT] methodology) before a test is considered to be clinically significant. In order to determine if the ASABs are interfering with sperm function, the consensus of opinion is that when these tests are positive (>50% sperm binding) additional tests (sperm–cervical mucus contact [SCMC] test, sperm–cervical mucus capillary tube test) should be done (see Chapter 5).

Although there are correlations between the presence and level of ASABs and specific characteristics of semen, e.g. men with antibodies have reduced sperm motility and higher levels of agglutination, these correlations are relatively weak and as such cannot be used to pre-screen which men should/should not be tested for ASABs [5].

There remains considerable controversy surrounding the testing of ASABs and their role in fertility [6,7,8]. Primarily, this is because there is still no clear information, despite considerable effort, as to the nature and identity of the antigens on the sperm surface that interfere with the reproductive process. Consequently, the testing that is performed detects antibodies on or to spermatozoa, but these antibodies may have no real functional significance. In addition, as a result of the lack of clarity of the nature of the antigens the testing for ASABs remains in its infancy and hence results need to be interpreted with caution. Historically, testing used agglutination and cytotoxicity assays, but now direct testing of the spermatozoa themselves, using either MAR or IBT, is the primary method employed.

ASABs in semen belong almost exclusively to two immunoglobulin (Ig) classes: IgA and IgG. There is evidence that IgA antibodies, particularly in the cases of men with vasovasostomy, have greater clinical importance than do IgG antibodies [9], although for subfertile men who have not had a vasectomy there is no clear data to suggest IgA is more significant than IgG. IgM antibodies, because of their large molecular size, are rarely found in semen – but if they are then they should be treated seriously as possible evidence of trauma within the male tract. The clinical significance of the location of where the antibodies bind to the spermatozoa (i.e. to the head, midpiece or tail) is also unclear, although binding restricted to the tail-tip is not associated with impaired fertility and can be present in fertile men [3].

The primary screening test for ASABs is performed on the fresh semen sample and makes use of either the IBT [10] or the MAR test. For these tests to be valid, at least 200 motile spermatozoa must be available for counting. The results from the IBT and the MAR test do not always agree. Additionally, data from proficiency testing (PT) shows some difficulties in classifying a positive versus a negative ASAB test [11], even when using the same method, e.g. indirect MAR [12].

Methods for traditional tests for sperm agglutinating antibodies (e.g. the Friberg "tray agglutination test" or TAT) and sperm immobilizing antibodies (e.g. the Isojima "sperm immobilization test" or SIT) have not been provided here. Detailed protocols for these techniques can be found elsewhere, e.g. Mortimer [13].

Outline of testing methods

Two different types of testing are used: *direct testing*, whereby the sperm sample itself is tested, and *indirect testing*, where reproductive tract fluids (seminal plasma, follicular fluid, cervical mucus) or serum are tested. In indirect testing the antibodies in these fluids are adsorbed onto prepared (i.e. seminal plasma free) donor spermatozoa, and these spermatozoa are then tested for antibody binding in a direct test format.

In both cases the beads/particles adhere to the motile and immotile spermatozoa that have surface-bound antibodies (or have adsorbed them), and the percentage of motile spermatozoa with beads bound is recorded.

Direct MAR test

This test is quicker and easier to perform than the IBT and is often recommended as a first-line screening test.

Principle

In the MAR test a "bridging" antibody (anti-IgG or -IgA) is used to attach the antibody-coated beads to unwashed, seminal spermatozoa bearing surface IgG or IgA. The direct IgG and IgA MAR tests are performed by mixing fresh, untreated semen separately with latex particles (or prepared erythrocytes) coated with human IgG or IgA. To this suspension is added a mono-specific anti-human-IgG or anti-human-IgA, and the formation of mixed agglutinates between particles and motile spermatozoa indicates the presence of IgG and IgA antibodies on the spermatozoa. As an internal control agglutination between beads serves as a positive control for antibody–antigen recognition. A variant of the MAR test (MarScreen®; www.sepalreproductivedevices.com) uses colored latex beads but its effectiveness in routine testing remains to be established.

Specimen

- Freshly ejaculated human semen which has liquefied

Equipment

- Microscope (phase contrast illumination, maximum total magnification 400×) with heated stage
- A 37°C temperature-controlled incubator
- Humidity chamber for incubating specimens
- Pipettes for 1–20 μl volumes

Disposable materials

- Clean glass slides and coverslips

Reagents

- SperMAR commercial test (FertiPro, Beernem, Belgium)

Calibration

- None required

Quality control

Tests should be run with controls. These can include ASAB-positive semen and ASAB-negative semen. This semen can be provided by men with and without ASABs, as detected by previous direct MAR testing. Positive spermatozoa can be produced by incubating washed spermatozoa with seminal plasma known to contain antibodies (see indirect MAR test, below). Alternatively positive and negative controls can be obtained from commercial companies.

Procedure

1. Place 3.5 μl of unwashed fresh semen on a clean microscope slide.

2. Add 3.5 μl IgG-coated latex particles and mix. Use IgA on a separate drop of semen when testing for IgA.

3. Add 3.5 μl antiserum against human IgG (antiserum to IgA when testing for IgA) to the semen-bead mixture and mix.

4. Cover the suspension with a 22 × 22 mm coverslip to provide a depth of approximately 20 μm.

5. Place the preparation in a humid chamber to settle at room temperature (2–3 min).

6. Examine the wet preparation under a phase contrast microscope at 200–400× magnification (bright-field optics can be used with colored beads). If spermatozoa have antibodies present on their surface, they will have latex beads adhering to them (Figure 4.1).

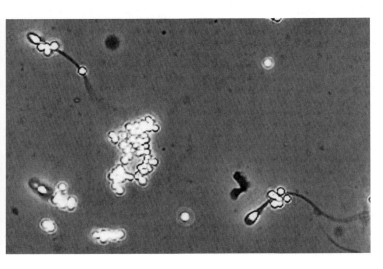

Figure 4.1 Example of beads binding to sperm in an antisperm antibody test.

Calculations and results

Motile spermatozoa with a few or even a group of particles attached are classed as positive. In the absence of coating antibodies the spermatozoa will be seen swimming freely between the particles. It is important to score moving spermatozoa as a spermatozoon may be immotile and have beads in close proximity (false negative). In some circumstances the motile spermatozoa will have beads attached but not show forward progressive movement; such cells should be regarded as positive-binding. At least 200 motile spermatozoa should be counted and the percentage of the motile spermatozoa that have particles attached is calculated. Record the class (IgG or IgA) and the site of binding of the latex particles to the spermatozoa (head, midpiece, tail).

Interpretation guidelines

ASABs are not an absolute indicator of subfertility. At least 50% of the motile spermatozoa need to be coated with antibodies before a test is considered to be clinically significant.

Notes

None required.

Indirect MAR test

Principle

The indirect MAR test is used to detect antisperm antibodies in heat-inactivated, sperm-free fluids (serum, seminal plasma or bromelain-solubilized cervical mucus [bromelain = EC 3.4.22.32]). Antibody-free spermatozoa bind ASABs from the test fluid and are then assessed as in the direct MAR test.

Specimen(s)

- *Cervical mucus:* Must be pre-treated (solubilized) using bromelain. Dilute mucus 1 + 1 with 10 IU bromelain/ml in sterile water, stir and incubate at 37°C for 10 min. When liquefaction is complete, centrifuge at 2000 g for 10 min and use the supernatant
- Inactivate any complement in the fluid (serum, seminal plasma or cervical mucus) by heating at 56°C for 30–45 min
- Dilute the heat-inactivated sample to be tested, e.g. 1 + 15 for the IgG-test and 1 + 3 for the IgA-test in swim-up medium, e.g. N-(2-hydroxyethyl)piperazine-N'-(2-ethanesulfonic) acid (HEPES) buffered cultured medium, ideally without albumin (unless verified as ASAB-free) or patient serum

Equipment

- Microscope (phase contrast illumination, maximum total magnification 400×) with heated stage
- A 37°C temperature-controlled incubator
- Water bath (for inactivating complement)
- Humidity chamber for incubating specimens
- Pipettes for 1–200 μl volumes

Disposable materials
- Clean glass slides
- Coverslips

Reagents
- SperMAR commercial test (FertiPro, Beernem, Belgium)
- Bromelain (EC 3.4.22.32) for cervical mucus solubilization
- HEPES-buffered medium for dilutions. (For example, Earl's buffered salt solution [EBSS]: NaCl [116.4 mM], KCl [5.4 mM], $CaCl_2$ [1.8 mM], $MgCl_2$ [1 mM], glucose [5.5 mM], Na lactate [19 mM], $MgSO_4$ [0.81 mM], HEPES [10 mM])
- ASAB-free donor spermatozoa: Prepare motile donor spermatozoa from a man lacking ASABs using DGC (see Chapter 7). Adjust the final motile sperm concentration to 20×10^6/ml in a HEPES-buffered medium with a maximum of 10 mg/ml of HSA that is known to be negative for ASABs (not serum)

Quality control
Tests should be run with controls. These can include ASAB-positive seminal plasma/serum and ASAB-negative seminal plasma/serum. This seminal plasma/serum can be provided by men with and without ASABs, as detected by previous direct MAR testing. Positive spermatozoa can be produced by incubating washed spermatozoa with seminal plasma known to contain antibodies (see indirect MAR test, below). Alternatively positive and negative controls can be obtained from commercial companies.

Procedure
Incubation of donor spermatozoa with fluid to be tested
1. Mix 100 μl sperm suspension with 100 μl diluted fluid to be tested.
2. Incubate at 37°C for 1 h.
3. Wash the spermatozoa by adding 2 ml HEPES-buffered media, mix well and centrifuge for 10 min at 400 **g**.
4. Remove the supernatant with a pipette.
5. Repeat the washing step on the pellet.
6. Remove the supernatant with a pipette and resuspend the sperm pellet in 50 μl medium by gentle pipetting or low-speed vortexing.

Procedure for the indirect MAR test
Perform the test as described for the direct MAR test using the pre-incubated donor spermatozoa instead of patient semen.

Calculations and results
Motile spermatozoa with a few or even a group of particles attached are classed as positive. In the absence of coating antibodies the spermatozoa will be seen swimming freely between

81

the particles. It is important to score moving spermatozoa as a spermatozoon may be immotile and have beads in close proximity (false negative). In some circumstances the motile spermatozoa will have beads attached but not show forward progressive movement; such cells should be regarded as positive-binding. At least 200 motile spermatozoa should be counted and the percentage of the motile spermatozoa that have particles attached is calculated. Record the class (IgG or IgA) and the site of binding of the latex particles to the spermatozoa (head, midpiece, tail).

Interpretation guidelines

ASABs are not an absolute indicator of subfertility since even men with high levels of ASABs can be fertile. At least 50% of the motile spermatozoa need to be coated with antibodies before a test is considered to be clinically significant. In order to determine if the ASABs are interfering with sperm function, the consensus of opinion is that when these tests are positive (>50% sperm binding), additional tests (sperm–cervical mucus contact [SCMC] test, sperm–cervical mucus capillary tube test) should be done (see Chapter 5).

Direct immunobead test

Principle

This assay is more complicated to perform than the MAR test but provides information about antibodies on spermatozoa which have been removed from potential masking components in seminal plasma.

In the IBT, beads coated with antibodies towards human IgG or IgA bind directly to washed spermatozoa displaying surface IgG or IgA. The direct IgG and IgA IBTs are performed by mixing washed spermatozoa with polyacrylamide spheres coated with covalently bound rabbit antihuman immunoglobulins. The formation of mixed agglutinates between particles and motile spermatozoa indicates the presence of IgG and IgA antibodies on the spermatozoa.

Specimen
- Freshly ejaculated human semen which has liquefied

Equipment
- Microscope (phase contrast illumination, maximum total magnification 400×) with heated stage
- A 37°C temperature-controlled incubator
- Humidity chamber for incubating specimens
- Pipettes for 1–20 μl volumes

Disposable materials
- Clean glass slides
- Coverslips

Reagents

- Immunobeads (Irvine Scientific). The buffers (see below) are also available commercially
- Dulbecco's phosphate buffered saline (PBS) with glucose and bovine serum albumin (BSA), or Tyrode's-BSA solutions
- Buffer I: Add 0.3 g Cohn fraction V BSA per 100 ml Dulbecco PBS or Tyrode's solution
- Buffer II: Add 5 g Cohn fraction V BSA per 100 ml Dulbecco PBS or Tyrode's solution
- Filter all solutions through 0.45 μm filters and warm to 37°C before use

Preparation of IgG and IgA immunobeads

1. Add 0.2 ml of stock bead suspension to 10 ml Buffer I in separate conical-base centrifuge tubes for each immunobead type (IgG, IgA).
2. Centrifuge at 500 *g* for 5–10 min.
3. Decant and discard the supernatant from the washed immunobeads.
4. Gently resuspend the beads in 0.2 ml Buffer II by gentle pipetting or low-speed vortexing.

Preparation of patient spermatozoa

1. Transfer an aliquot of well-mixed, liquefied semen to a conical centrifuge tube and add Buffer I to bring the final volume to 10 ml.
2. Centrifuge at 500 *g* for 5–10 min.
3. Decant and discard the supernatant from the washed spermatozoa.
4. Gently resuspend the sperm pellet in 10 ml of fresh Buffer I by gentle pipetting or low-speed vortexing.
5. Centrifuge again at 500 *g* for 5–10 min.
6. Decant and discard the supernatant.
7. Gently resuspend the sperm pellet in 0.2 ml Buffer II by gentle pipetting or low-speed vortexing.

Calibration

None required.

Quality control

Tests should be run with controls. These can include ASAB-positive semen and ASAB-negative semen. This semen can be provided by men with and without ASABs, as detected by previous direct immunobead testing. Positive spermatozoa can be produced by incubating washed spermatozoa with seminal plasma known to contain antibodies (see indirect MAR test, above). Alternatively positive and negative controls can be obtained from commercial companies.

Procedure

1. Place 5 μl washed test sperm suspension on a clean, dry microscope slide.
2. Add 5 μl IgG immunobeads to droplets of each test and mix.

3. Repeat steps 1 and 2 on different aliquots of sperm suspension with 5 µl of IgA immunobeads.
4. Cover the suspensions with a 22 × 22 mm coverslip to provide a depth of approximately 20 µm.
5. Place the preparation in a humid chamber to settle at room temperature (2–3 min).
6. Examine the wet preparation under a phase contrast microscope at 200–400× magnification. If spermatozoa have antibodies on their surface they will have immunobeads binding to them.

Calculations and results

Motile spermatozoa with a few or even a group of beads attached are classed as positive. In the absence of coating antibodies the spermatozoa will be seen swimming freely between the particles. It is important to score moving spermatozoa as a spermatozoon may be immotile and have beads in close proximity (false negative). In some circumstances the motile spermatozoa will have beads attached but not show forward progressive movement; such cells should be regarded as positive-binding. At least 200 motile spermatozoa should be counted and the percentage of the motile spermatozoa that have beads attached is calculated. Record the class (IgG or IgA) and the site of binding of the beads' particles to the spermatozoa (head, midpiece, tail).

Interpretation guidelines

ASABs are not an absolute indicator of subfertility since even men with high levels of ASABs can be fertile. At least 50% of the motile spermatozoa need to be coated with antibodies before a test is considered to be clinically significant. In order to determine if the ASABs are interfering with sperm function, the consensus of opinion is that when these tests are positive (>50% sperm binding) additional tests (sperm–cervical mucus contact test, sperm–cervical mucus capillary tube test) should be done (see Chapter 5).

Indirect immunobead test

Principle

The indirect IBT is used to detect antisperm antibodies in heat-inactivated, sperm-free fluids (serum, seminal plasma or bromelain-solubilized cervical mucus [EC 3.4.22.32]). Antibody-free spermatozoa take up antisperm antibodies present in the tested fluid and are then assessed as in the direct IBT.

Specimen(s)

- *Cervical mucus:* Must be pre-treated (solubilized) using bromelain. Dilute mucus 1 + 1 with 10 IU bromelain/ml in sterile water, stir with a pipette tip and incubate at 37°C for 10 min. When liquefaction is complete, centrifuge at 2000 *g* for 10 min and use the supernatant
- Inactivate any complement in the fluid (serum, seminal plasma or cervical mucus) by heating at 56°C for 30–45 min
- Dilute the heat-inactivated sample to be tested, e.g. 10 µl of the body fluid to be tested with 40 µl Buffer II

Equipment
- Microscope (phase contrast illumination, maximum total magnification 400×) with heated stage
- A 37°C temperature-controlled incubator
- Water bath (for inactivating complement)
- Humidity chamber for incubating specimens
- Pipettes for 1–200 µl volumes

Disposable materials
- Clean microscope slides and coverslips

Reagents
- Immunobeads and buffers as for the direct IBT
- Bromelain (EC 3.4.22.32) for cervical mucus solubilization
- HEPES-buffered media for dilutions
- ASAB-free donor spermatozoa: Prepare motile donor spermatozoa from a man lacking ASABs using DGC (see Chapter 7). Adjust the final motile sperm concentration to 20×10^6/ml in a HEPES-buffered medium without albumin or serum

Quality control
Tests should be run with controls. These can include ASAB-positive seminal plasma/serum and ASAB-negative seminal plasma/serum. This seminal plasma/serum can be provided by men with and without ASABs, as detected by previous direct MAR testing. Positive spermatozoa can be produced by incubating washed spermatozoa with seminal plasma known to contain antibodies (see indirect MAR test, previously). Alternatively positive and negative controls can be obtained from commercial companies.

Procedure
Incubation of donor spermatozoa with fluid to be tested
1. Mix 50 µl of the washed donor sperm suspension with 50 µl fluid to be tested.
2. Incubate at 37°C for 1 h.
3. Centrifuge the pre-incubated spermatozoa at 500 *g* for 5–10 min.
4. Decant and discard the supernatant.
5. Gently resuspend the sperm pellet in 10 ml fresh Buffer I by gentle pipetting or low-speed vortexing.
6. Centrifuge again at 500 *g* for 5–10 min.
7. Decant and discard the supernatant.
8. Repeat the washing steps 5 and 6 above.
9. Gently resuspend the sperm pellet in 0.2 ml Buffer II by gentle pipetting or low-speed vortexing.

Procedure for the indirect IgG and IgA immunobead test

Perform the test as described in the direct IBT with the pre-incubated donor spermatozoa instead of patient semen.

Calculations and results

Motile spermatozoa with a few or even a group of beads attached are classed as positive. In the absence of coating antibodies the spermatozoa will be seen swimming freely between the particles. It is important to score moving spermatozoa as a spermatozoon may be immotile and have beads in close proximity (false negative). In some circumstances the motile spermatozoa will have beads attached but not show forward progressive movement; such cells should be regarded as positive-binding. At least 200 motile spermatozoa should be counted and the percentage of the motile spermatozoa that have beads attached is calculated. Record the class (IgG or IgA) and the site of binding of the beads' particles to the spermatozoa (head, midpiece, tail).

Interpretation guidelines

ASABs are not an absolute indicator of subfertility since even men with high levels of ASABs can be fertile. At least 50% of the motile spermatozoa need to be coated with antibodies before a test is considered to be clinically significant. In order to determine if the ASABs are interfering with sperm function, the consensus of opinion is that when these tests are positive (>50% sperm binding) additional tests (sperm–cervical mucus contact test, sperm–cervical mucus capillary tube test) should be done (see Chapter 5).

Microbiological examination of the semen sample

Bacterial infections

Bacterial infection of the male reproductive tract can affect spermatogenesis and the secretory function of the accessory glands and may contribute to subfertility [14,15,16,17]. The main infectious agents are *Neisseria gonorrhoeae*, dominating in Africa and the Far East, and *Chlamydia trachomatis*, which dominates in Europe and the USA. *Ureaplasma urealyticum* and *Escherichia coli* are also often found in semen.

Examination of the ejaculate

Infections can be asymptomatic and signs of infection are not always observed by microscopic examination of the ejaculate. However, both macroscopic and microscopic assessment of the semen sample can reveal infection. Such observations are:

1. Brown or reddish color of semen due to the presence of erythrocytes.

2. A large number of microorganisms.

3. Excessive numbers of leukocytes ($>1 \times 10^6$/ml).

4. A high proportion of dead spermatozoa.

5. Most of the spermatozoa are covered by antisperm antibodies.

6. Biochemical analyses of the ejaculate can also reflect infection. Examples are:

A decrease in the secretion of markers of accessory gland function.

Excessive generation of reactive oxygen species (ROS) due to a high amount of leukocytes.

Increased levels of various immunoglobulins, cytokines and growth factors [18,19].

Upon suspicion of inflammation, microbiological evaluation of the semen sample should be performed by a laboratory specialized in the field. The patient must be instructed to wash his hands and penis before masturbation, and the sample should be collected in a sterile container. Sterile pipettes and pipette tips must be used upon withdrawal of samples or when preparing dilutions. The time before microbiological culturing of the semen sample should be as short as possible, and not exceed 3 hours.

Viral infections

Sexually transmitted viruses such as human immunodeficiency virus (HIV), cytomegalovirus (CMV), human papillomavirus (HPV), herpes simplex virus (HSV), human herpes virus (HHV), Epstein–Barr virus (EBV) and hepatitis B virus (HBV) can all be detected in human semen by polymerase chain reaction (PCR) or ligase chain reaction (LCR) technologies. The clinical implications for fertility status are not clear, but an association between virus DNA and reduced sperm concentration, and proportion of spermatozoa with normal morphology has been found [20].

Details of the microbiology, diagnosis, and treatment of infections, as well as handling and preparation of infectious specimens are described in detail in the excellent monograph by Elder, Baker, and Ribes [16].

Notes

1. Lysozymes and zinc in the seminal plasma have antibacterial properties, and a negative bacterial culture does not rule out an infection.

2. Microorganisms in semen can be due to contaminants from the patient's skin or from the air, thus having no clinical relevance.

Leukocytes in semen

Semen contains a number of different types of non-sperm cells. These can be classed either as leukocytes or non-leukocytes, the latter consisting primarily of germ cells, e.g. spermatids. Leukocytes, predominantly neutrophils, are present in almost all human ejaculates [21,22,23].

There is a considerable controversy about the role of leukocytes in semen. The initial concept was that leukocytes were a negative factor for fertility and a clear sign of infection. However, several large studies have revealed there to be no significant relationship between either the types or concentration of leukocytes (determined using monoclonal antibody staining) and semen parameters or, more importantly, in-vivo conception [21,22,23]. In fact, a positive relationship has been observed in non-pathological samples between the presence of leukocytes and sperm morphology [24]. However, leukocytes do produce significant amounts of reactive oxygen species which, particularly when limited antioxidant protective mechanisms are available, can be highly detrimental to sperm function [23], e.g. in washed sperm preparations.

Surprisingly, there is no consensus on what is a "normal" number of leukocytes in semen. There are data on mean levels in infertility clinic patients (390 000/ml ejaculate) [23] (but limited information is available from fertile control subjects). The WHO reference range is set at 1×10^6 leukocytes/ml as the threshold for leukocytospermia, but the evidence to support this value is relatively weak, with some authors believing it to be too low while others say it is too high. Historically, men with $>1 \times 10^6$ leukocytes/ml of semen were thought to have a significant likelihood of a genital infection compared to men with $<1 \times 10^6$ leukocytes/ml of semen [25]. However, with more sophisticated modern methods to detect subclinical genital infections, this cut-off point is of little value [26].

Leukocytes can be detected and quantified in stained preparations otherwise made for morphological examination (Papanicolaou staining procedure). In such preparations leukocytes can be differentiated from spermatids and spermatocytes by differences in staining coloration, as well as by the distinctive nuclear size and shape (Figure 4.2). However, the more accurate way to detect leukocytes is to use specific assays, such as the detection of peroxidase-positive cells (see Chapter 3) and the use of monoclonal antibodies against leukocyte-specific antigens [21,27].

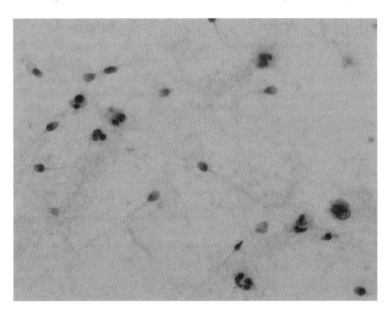

Figure 4.2 Example of leukocytes stained with Papanicolaou.

Immunocytochemical staining for the pan-leukocyte antigen CD45

Principle
The principle is that the pan-leukocyte monoclonal antibody recognizes the leukocytes. Visualization is via a secondary antibody. Leukocytes are stained reddish-brown.

Specimen
- Prepared semen samples

Equipment
- Bright-field microscope (at least 200× total magnification) with built-in grid reticule
- Air-displacement pipettes

- Tally counter
- Centrifuge

Disposable materials
- Slides
- Coverslips

Reagents
1. Dulbecco's phosphate buffered saline (PBS).
2. TRIS-buffered saline (TBS): Dissolve 60.55 g TRIS-base and 85.20 g NaCl in ~800 ml reagent water; adjust to pH 8.6 using 1 N HCl, and then make up to 1 liter with reagent water.
3. Hematoxylin.
4. Tetramisole (levamisole) 1.0 M: Dissolve 2.4 g (–)-tetramisole HCl in 10 ml purified water.
5. Substrate: To 9.7 ml of pH 8.2 TRIS buffer add 2 mg naphthol AS-MX phosphate, 0.2 ml dimethylformamide, and 0.1 ml of 1.0 M tetramisole. Then add 10 mg Fast Red TR salt and filter just before use.
6. Fixative: acetone alone, or to 95 ml acetone add 95 ml absolute methanol, and 10 ml 37% (v/v) formaldehyde.
7. Primary antibody: A mouse monoclonal antibody against the common leukocyte antigen (CD45), widely available commercially (e.g. Santa Cruz Biotechnology Inc.).
8. Secondary antibody: Anti-mouse rabbit immunoglobulins; the dilution used will depend on antibody titre and source (e.g. 1 : 25 dilution of the Z259 antibody manufactured by DAKO Corp.).
9. Alkaline phosphatase:anti-alkaline phosphatase complex (APAAP): Widely available commercially (e.g. Sigma Aldrich).

Calibration
The primary calibration is in calculating the final concentration of leukocytes (see below).

Quality control
For QC purposes peripheral blood leukocytes can be used. These cells will stain with the pan-leukocyte marker. As a negative control the primary antibody can be omitted.

Procedure
Preparing the spermatozoa
1. Mix an aliquot of liquefied semen (approximately 0.5 ml) with 5× the volume of phosphate buffered saline (PBS) in a centrifuge tube.
2. Centrifuge at 500 *g* for 5 min at room temperature, remove the supernatant, and suspend the sperm pellet in 5× its volume of PBS.
3. Centrifuge at 500 *g* for 5 min at room temperature.

4. Repeat this procedure, and suspend the pellet in PBS to the original volume of the semen sample.

5. Dilute the suspension 2–5× further in PBS depending on the concentration of spermatozoa.

Preparing the sperm smears

6. Prepare smears of two 5 µl aliquots of the suspension and allow to air dry onto clean glass slides. These can be fixed and stained immediately or wrapped in foil after fixing and stored at −70°C until subsequent analysis (up to several weeks).

7. Fix the air-dried cells in absolute acetone for 10 min (or the acetone above fixative for 90 s).

8. Wash twice with TBS and allow to drain.

Antibody labeling

9. Cover each aliquot of fixed cells with 1 µl primary monoclonal antibody and incubate for 30 min in a humidified chamber at room temperature.

10. Wash the slides twice with TBS and allow to drain.

11. Cover the cells on the smear with 10 µl secondary antibody and incubate for 30 min in a humidified chamber at room temperature.

12. Wash twice with TBS and allow to drain.

13. Add 10 µl APAAP to each smear.

14. Incubate for 1 h in a humidified chamber at room temperature.

15. Wash twice in TBS and allow to drain.

16. Incubate with 10 µl alkaline phosphatase substrate for 20 min at room temperature.

17. Counterstain and mount: Wash the slides with TBS and counterstain for a few seconds with hematoxylin; wash in tap water and mount in an aqueous mounting system.

18. Assessment: The entire cell suspension is examined and both CD45-positive cells and spermatozoa are counted until 200 CD45-positive cells have been counted.

Calculations and results

The concentration of CD45-positive cells is calculated relative to that of spermatozoa: If N is the number of CD45-positive cells counted in the same fields as 100 spermatozoa, and S is the concentration of sperm in millions/ml, then the concentration (C) of the given cell type in millions/ml can be calculated from the formula $C = S \times (N/100)$.

Interpretation guidelines

There is no consensus of what is a "normal" number of leukocytes in semen. There are data on mean levels in infertility clinic patients (390 000/ml ejaculate) [23] (but limited information is available from fertile control subjects).

Assessment of immature germ cells in semen

These include round spermatids and spermatocytes but rarely spermatogonia. They are often degenerating and, on a wet semen smear, difficult to distinguish from some leukocytes. However, they can be identified in stained semen smears based on differences in staining coloration, as well as by the distinctive nuclear size and shape. Alternatively the number of immature germ cells in semen can be calculated from the difference between the number of round cells in the semen sample and the number of leukocytes (examined using monoclonal antibodies). Using the latter method Aitken and colleagues showed that the median number of germ cells per ml of semen was 435 000 [23]. Interestingly, although there is limited data, the concentration of immature cells may be negatively associated with fertility [28].

Biochemical test – prostate: assessment of zinc in seminal fluid

Background
Zinc ions are secreted by the human prostate into the prostatic fluid. The secretion is androgen dependent. Zinc in semen is used as a marker for the prostatic fluid contribution to the ejaculate. Zinc contributes to the stabilization of the sperm nucleus.

Principle
A colorimetric assay for determination of zinc was developed by Wako Chemicals GmbH, and validated for seminal fluid by Johnsen and Eliasson [29,30].

The reagent, 2-(5-bromo-2-pyridylazo)-5-(N-propyl-N-sulfopropylamino)-phenol (5-Br-PAPS), binds a zinc ion and turns into a blue-violet color absorbing light at the wavelength of 560 nm.

Specimen
- Sperm-free, seminal plasma obtained from liquefied whole semen by centrifugation (3000 g for 20 min); supernatant decanted and stored at –20°C up to 12 months

Equipment
- Microtiterplate reader (spectrophotometry)
- Vortex mixer
- Balance, 0.1-mg accuracy
- Pipettes for 5–50 µl, 50–200 µl, 30–300 µl, and 200–1000 µl
- Multi-stepper pipette for 100 µl and 1000 µl
- Test tube racks
- Measurement flasks 100 ml
- Magnetic stirrer
- Large flask (500–1000 ml)

Disposable materials
- Polystyrene "Ellermann" test tubes (10 × 75 mm; 3 ml) with stoppers
- Microtiterplate flat bottom, 96 wells
- Tips for pipettes 0.5–300 µl
- Tips for pipettes 200–1000 µl
- Gloves

Reagents

1. 50 µmol/l zinc calibrator:
   a. Dissolve 288 mg of $ZnSO_4 \cdot 7H_2O$ in 100 ml water.
   b. Dilute further ($\times$ 200) by taking 500 µl of the above solution to 99.5 ml water to get a standard concentration of 50 µmol/l; store at –20°C or at +4 to +8°C up to 6 months.
2. Zinc kit: Wako Chemicals. Stable at room temperature for one year.
3. Color reagent A (2 $\times$ 60-ml bottles); color reagent B (1 $\times$ 30-ml bottle).
4. 5-Br-PAPS: 2-(5-bromo-2-pyridylazo)-5-(N-propyl-N-sulfopropylamino)-phenol.

Calibration

Mix 4 parts of color reagent A with 1 part of color reagent B (see table below).

Total number of semen samples, QC samples, and calibrator	Volume reagent A	Volume reagent B
10	4.8	1.2
15	5.6	1.4
20	6.4	1.6
25	7.2	1.8
30	8.0	2.0
35	8.8	2.2
40	9.6	2.4
45	10.4	2.6
50	11.2	2.8

Make a fresh solution for every new series.

Quality control

Internal quality control (IQC) samples

1. Make a pool of sperm-free seminal plasma from 100–300 patient samples (see "Specimen" above); thaw individual stored aliquots and mix together in a 500- to 1000-ml flask with a magnetic stirrer. Label sealable test tubes with IQC batch ID and date; pipette 50–100 µl of the well-mixed aliquot into each tube, cap and store at –20°C until use.
2. Determine zinc concentration in 10 replicates at 5 different occasions. Calculate the 95% confidence interval for zinc concentration. The mean results of the QC samples should be within the 95% interval in order to approve a series of analyses.

Procedure

Precautions: All materials (calibrators, samples, QC samples, and reagents) must be handled according to safety rules. Personal protection (clothes, latex gloves) shall be used during all work. All disposables shall be handled according to rules.

All procedures are carried out at "ambient" temperature, i.e. 15–35°C.

1. Thaw seminal fluid samples and one internal QC sample, mix well with vortex.

2. Dilute samples and QC samples in total 1 : 200 in duplicates. Use positive-displacement pipette for seminal plasma. Make two serial dilutions to minimize deviations, for instance: add 900 µl water and 100 µl seminal plasma or 100 µl QC sample to test tubes in duplicates and mix thoroughly with vortex. In the second step, take 50 µl of this dilution to a new Ellermann tube and add 950 µl water.

   If you also perform a series of fructose determinations, you can save the first serial dilution for fructose determination. If low semen volume does not allow this dilution scheme it is essential to note that in the report form. In cases of low semen volume, you could use 5 µl semen and add 995 µl water in a test tube. Note that the uncertainty in the final result increases when starting with small volumes.

3. Preparation of calibrators.

Calibrator No.	Molarity µM	µl Zinc 50 µM	µl water
S1	0	0	1000
S2	5	100	900
S3	10	200	800
S4	20	400	600
S5	40	800	200

4. Add in duplicate, 40 µl of each calibrator, diluted seminal plasma and diluted QC samples, into wells of a 96-well plate. Note that every sample should be well mixed by vortex before pipetting.

5. Add 200 µl of the fresh chromogen reagent to each well. Avoid the formation of bubbles. Use reverse technique for pipetting (before filling the pipette, press the pipette knob into bottom level and then fill. When pushing out into the well – stop at *first* "stop").

6. Mix for 5 min on a 96-well plate shaker.

7. Read the plate at 560 nm wavelength.

Calculations and results

1. Read the zinc concentration in mmol/l for each sample from the standard curve.

2. Samples with values higher than the highest standard should be reanalyzed at higher dilution.

3. Check that the mean of the QC samples is within the decided interval to approve this series of results.

4. Multiply all values by the dilution factor (200) to get the zinc concentration in undiluted seminal plasma. Use one decimal place: 1.461 is given as 1.5 mmol/l.

5. Multiply by the ejaculate volume in ml with one decimal, which will give the total amount of secreted zinc in the ejaculate in µmoles. Use one decimal, e.g. semen volume 3.2 ml × 1.461 = 4.675 is given as 4.7 µmol/ejaculate.

Interpretation guidelines

A total content of 2.4 μmol zinc or more in the ejaculate indicates a normal prostatic contribution to the ejaculate.

Values below 2.4 μmol indicate low contribution of the androgen-dependent prostatic fluid to the ejaculate. This can be seen after a short time of abstinence, particularly in hypogonadal men, men treated with for instance finasteride, and men with prostatic inflammation. The latter may also cause an increased concentration of inflammatory cells. Furthermore, incomplete collection of the ejaculate, for instance missing the first ejaculate portion, often results in a combination of few spermatozoa and low zinc.

The zinc concentration is also used in split-ejaculate fractions together with fructose concentration to determine the relative contribution from the prostatic and the seminal vesicles, respectively, to the different fractions.

Notes

1. Make sure that no air bubbles are present in the wells. To empty a bubble: insert a pipette tip (20–200 μl) into the bubble.

Biochemical test – seminal vesicles: quantitative assessment of fructose in seminal plasma

Background

Fructose in semen emanates mainly from the seminal vesicles, with a minor contribution from the corresponding secretory epithelium in the ampullary part of the vas deferens. The secretion is androgen dependent. Fructose in semen is used as a marker for the secretory contribution of the seminal vesicles to the ejaculate or to characterize the origin of split-ejaculate fractions. A normal secretory contribution of fructose means that these parts of the Wolffian ducts (seminal vesicles and ampulla) are intact and display an androgen-dependent secretion that is emptied at emission/ejaculation [30,31,32].

Principle

Fructose reacts, in the presence of hydrochloric acid under heat, with indol and produces a colored complex that can be measured at the wavelength of 470 nm.

Specimen

- Sperm-free seminal plasma obtained from liquefied, whole semen by centrifugation (3000 g for 20 min); supernatant decanted and stored at –20°C up to 12 months

Equipment

- Microtiterplate reader
- Printer to reader
- Micropipettes for 5–50 μl, 50–200 μl, 30–300 μl and 200–1000 μl
- Multi-stepper pipette for 50–1000 μl
- Vortex

- Balance, 0.1 mg accuracy
- Water bath
- Thermometer, precision ±1°C
- 1 stop-watch, precision ±1 min/hour
- Measurement flask or cylinder 100 ml
- Test tube racks

Disposable materials

- Ice
- Eppendorf tubes 1.5 ml
- Polystyrene "Ellermann" test tubes (10 × 75 mm; 3 ml) with stoppers
- Parafilm
- Microtiterplate, flat bottom, 96 wells
- Pipetter tips 0.5–300 µl 5–200 µl and 200–1000 µl

Reagents
Three groups of reagents

1. Two deproteinizing solutions:
   63 mM $ZnSO_4 \cdot 7H_2O$: Add 1.8 g into 100 ml water.
   0.1 M NaOH: Add 0.4 g in 100 ml water.

2. Color reaction solution:
   2 µM indole reagent + 16 µM benzoic acid: Dissolve 200 mg benzoic acid in 90 ml water, shaking in a water bath with temperature 60°C, then dissolve 25 mg indole in this solution and fill up to 100 ml. Store at +4°C.

3. Fructose stock solution – for calibrators:
   22.4 mM fructose – stock solution: Add 403 mg fructose to 100 ml pure water (stable for 6 months at +4 to +8°C).

Calibration

Dilute the stock solution 1/10 to get the highest calibrator (2.24 mmol/l). Dilute in series 1 : 2 (1 + 1) with water to achieve the additional calibrators of 1.12, 0.56, 0.28 and 0.14 mmol/l, respectively, and use pure water as standard 0 mmol/l.

Calibrator No.	mM	Fructose solution	Pure water
S1	0.00	0	0.5 ml
S2	0.14	0.5 ml of 0.28 mM (S_3)	0.5 ml
S3	0.28	0.5 ml of 0.56 mM (S_4)	0.5 ml
S4	0.56	0.5 ml of 1.12 mM (S_5)	0.5 ml
S5	1.12	0.5 ml of 2.24 mM (S_6)	0.5 ml
S6	2.24	100 µl/ml of fructose-stock solution 22.4 mM	900 µl

Quality control

Internal quality control (ICQ) samples:

1. Make a pool of sperm-free seminal plasma from 100–300 patient samples (see "Specimen" above); thaw individual stored aliquots and mix together in a 500- to 1000-ml flask with a magnetic stirrer. Label sealable test tubes with IQC batch ID and date; pipette 50–100 μl of the well-mixed aliquot into each tube, cap and store at –20°C until use.

2. Determine fructose concentration in 10 replicates at 5 different occasions. Calculate the 95% confidence interval for fructose concentration. The mean results of the QC samples should be within the 95% interval in order to approve an analysis series.

Procedure

Precautions: All materials (calibrators, samples, QC samples, and reagents) must be handled according to safety rules. Personal protection (clothes, latex gloves) shall be used during all work. All disposables shall be handled according to rules.

Check water-bath temperature, 50°C.

1. Thaw seminal fluid and one internal QC sample; mix well with vortex.

2. Dilute each sample ×40. Add 25 μl of well-mixed seminal fluid and QC samples with a positive-displacement pipette to 975 μl water in Ellermann tubes and mix on vortex.

   a. Note: If dilutions have been prepared for zinc assessment, use the first (1 : 10 dilution of seminal plasma) and dilute this 1 : 4. To 300 μl pure water add 100 μl of the 1 : 10 diluted seminal plasma.

   b. When low semen volume: Make a 1 : 40 dilution with 7 μl seminal fluid and add 273 μl of pure water in an Ellermann tube. Note that the uncertainty increases when starting with small volumes. If other dilutions are used: always make careful notes in your protocol of dilutions other than standard ones.

3. Add 50 μl $ZnSO_4$ and 50 μl NaOH to Eppendorf tubes. The number of tubes is calculated as duplicates of the seminal plasma samples and QC samples.

4. Transfer 200 μl of diluted seminal fluid samples in duplicate, diluted QC samples in duplicate and duplicates of each calibrator (0–2.24 mM) to Eppendorf tubes, close lids, vortex each sample and incubate for 15 min at room temperature.

5. Centrifuge all Eppendorf tubes at 7000 g for 5 min.

6. Take off 100 μl of each supernatant and transfer to acid-proof test tubes.

7. Add 100 μl indole reagent to each tube and mix. Then add 1 ml of 37% (= concentrated) hydrochloric acid to each tube. Seal all tubes with acid-proof stopper.

8. Incubate for 20 min in water bath heated to +50°C, and cool in ice water for 15 min.

9. Within the ventilated hood: Transfer 250 μl of all semen fluid samples, QC samples and calibrators to a 96-well plate.

10. Cover the top of the plate with acid-proof transparent plastic film (to avoid corrosion of the spectrophotometer).

11. Read the plate in the 96-well plate reader at 470 nm.

12. Remove the plate *immediately* after reading and leave spectrophotometer open for 10 min to allow the acid fumes to evaporate.

Calculations and results

1. Read the fructose concentration in mmol/l for each sample from the calibration curve.
2. Note that samples with values higher than the highest standard should be reanalyzed at higher dilution.
3. Check that the mean of the QC samples is within the decided interval to approve this series of results.
4. Multiply by the dilution factor (40) to get the fructose concentration in undiluted seminal fluid. Use one decimal (e.g. 11.5 mmol/l).
5. Multiply by the ejaculate volume in ml with one decimal, which will give the total amount of secreted fructose in the ejaculate in μmol. Use one decimal, e.g. volume 3.2 ml × 11.5 mmol/l = 36.8 μmol/ejaculate.

Interpretation guidelines

A content of 13.0 μmol fructose or more per ejaculate indicates normal secretory contribution from the seminal vesicles to the ejaculate [30].

A content under 13.0 μmol indicates a low androgen-specific contribution of vesicular fluid to the ejaculate. This can be seen after a short time of abstinence, in partially hypogonadal men, and in men where emission or ejaculation of fluid is impaired. Emission can be hindered by neuromuscular diseases, post-surgery and by drugs and also by obstructions due to obstruction in the ejaculatory ducts or temporarily by an inflammation in the vesicles or in the prostate.

Very low content of fructose, in combination with low semen volume and azoospermia, could be due to a total obstruction of the Wolffian ducts as can be seen in agenesis of the Wolffian ducts.

The fructose concentration is also used in split-ejaculate fractions together with zinc concentration to determine the relative origin of the fractions.

Qualitative assessment of fructose in semen

Background
See previous section on quantitative assessment of fructose in seminal plasma.

Principle
The assay is a simple, semi-quantitative, colorimetric test for any keto-hexose [33].

Specimen
- Well-mixed, liquefied semen

Equipment
- Hotplate to be used at 55°C
- Porcelain spotting plate
- Air-displacement pipetter 10–100 μl

Disposable materials

- Pipetter tips, 10–100 µl

Reagents

1. Test reagent: Dissolve 0.4 g of p-methyl-aminophenol sulfate ("metol") and 8.0 g of urea in 20 ml of 40% sulfuric acid. Store in a brown glass bottle covered with aluminum foil to minimize photo-oxidation. Keep at +4°C when not in use. Stable for 2–3 months. Discard if there are any signs of contamination or sedimentation.

2. Fructose standard: Stock solution = 2.7 mg of fructose dissolved in 100 ml of reagent water (i.e. 27 µg/ml, equivalent to 15 mmol fructose/l, an average seminal plasma value). This stock is kept at +4°C when not in use and discarded if there are any signs of contamination or sedimentation.

3. Working solution is a 100 times dilution of the stock solution, made using reagent water. It is prepared daily and any unused portion is discarded at the end of the day.

Calibration and quality control

None required as this is a qualitative test only. If the working fructose standard fails to show a blue color in the test then both it and the reagent should be discarded and fresh solutions prepared.

Procedure

1. Pre-heat a white porcelain spotting plate to 55°C on an electric hotplate.
2. Dilute the test sample 1 : 100 with reagent water.
3. a. Place 20-µl and 50-µl aliquots of the test sample in separate wells on the spotting plate.
   b. In another well place 50 µl of reagent water as a blank and 50 µl of the working fructose standard in another.
4. Allow all wells to evaporate to dryness.
5. Add one drop (about 50 µl) of the reagent solution to each well.
6. Heat for 10 min.
7. Examine each well for the development of a distinct blue coloration or a blue ring, indicative of the presence of fructose (or any other keto-hexose).

Calculations and results

The intensity of the blue coloration is proportional to the keto-hexose (fructose) concentration; aldohexoses such as glucose do not react. Positive reactions in the 20- and 50-µl test sample wells correspond to a semen-fructose concentration of ≥1080 and ≥2700 µg/ml, respectively (i.e. ≥6 and ≥15 mmol/l, respectively).

Interpretation guidelines

See previous section on quantitative assessment of fructose in seminal plasma.

Biochemical test – epididymis: assessment of neutral α-glucosidase in seminal fluid

Background

Neutral iso-enzyme α-glucosidase is an androgen-dependent enzyme secreted from the epididymis. The total activity of *neutral* α-glucosidase in semen is an indicator of the amount of excretion from the cauda epididymis emitted at ejaculation. However, in seminal plasma there are also significant amounts of an acidic iso-enzyme, originating from the prostate [34].

Principle

The prostatic iso-enzyme is inhibited with the detergent sodium dodecyl sulfate (SDS) whereafter selective measurement of the epididymal form is possible. The enzymatic action of α-glucosidase is assessed by measuring the cleavage of the *p*-nitrophenol part of α-D-glucopyranoside. The chromogene *p*-nitrophenol is yellow and its yellow color is augmented by the addition of sodium carbonate. Castanospermine inhibits all α-glucosidase activity and is used as a control for non-specific degradation of the substrate [30,35].

Specimen

- Sperm-free seminal plasma obtained from liquefied whole semen (preferably within 60 min after ejaculation) by centrifugation (3000 g for 20 min); supernatant decanted and stored at –20°C for up to 12 months

Equipment

- Microtiterplate reader, 405 nm (spectrophotometry)
- Eppendorf tube vortex
- Balance, precision d = 0.001 g
- Pipettes for 5–50 μl, 50–200 μl, 30–300 μl and 200–1000 μl
- Multi-stepper pipette for 100 μl and 1000 μl
- Test tube racks
- Measurement flasks 100 ml
- Magnetic mixer on heated stage
- Water bath
- Thermometer, precision ±1°C
- 1 stop-watch, precision ±1 min/hour
- Measuring cylinders 100 ml

Disposable materials

- Eppendorf tubes 1.5 ml
- Polystyrene Ellermann test tubes (10 × 75; 3 ml) with stoppers
- Microtiter plate flat bottom, 96 wells

- Pipetter tips 0.5–300 μl, 200–1000 μl and 1–10 ml
- Gloves

Reagents

1. 0.1 M phosphate buffer, pH 6.8: Prepare 0.1 M K_2HPO_4 (8.7 g in 500 ml pure water) and 0.1 M KH_2PO_4 (dissolve 6.8 g in 500 ml pure water) and mix equal volumes of each until pH is 6.8. To increase pH, add K_2HPO_4; to decrease pH, add KH_2PO_4.

2. 0.1 M phosphate buffer pH 6.8 with 1% sodium dodecyl sulfate (SDS): Add 1 g SDS to 100 ml of the 0.1 M phosphate buffer pH 6.8. Note that the solution precipitates at low temperature but dissolves upon mild warming.

3. 5 mM p-nitrophenol (stock solution): Dissolve 0.139 g PNP (Sigma 104–8) in 100 ml pure water. Warm up to +60°C to dissolve. Store in light protected vessel at 4°C. Make a fresh solution every 3 months.

4. 0.1 M Na_2CO_3 solution – color reagent 1: Dissolve 5.3 g Na_2CO_3 in 500 ml pure water.

5. 0.1 M Na_2CO_3 solution with 0.1% SDS: Add 0.5 g SDS to 500 ml of 0.1 M Na_2CO_3 solution.

6. 16.6 mM p-nitrophenyl α-D-glucopyranoside (PNPG) in 1% SDS:
   Dissolve 0.100 g PNPG (Sigma N1377) in 20 ml 0.1 M phosphate buffer pH 6.8 with 1% SDS, cover the vessel with a lid and warm up and stir the solution on a hot magnetic stirring plate at, but not above, 50°C for 10 min. Some crystals may remain undissolved. Keep at 50°C before use within 30 min and at +37°C (not below) when using.

7. Castanospermine 1 mM: Add 5.3 ml pure water to flask of 1 mg Sigma C3784 to get the working solution of 1 mM. Freeze in aliquots at –20°C.

Calibration

The calibration solutions are made ready just before the incubation is stopped.
1. Make solutions A and B:
   a. Solution A: Add 200 μl of 5 mM p-nitrophenol (PNP) to 9.8 ml Na_2CO_3 solution with 0.1% SDS.
   b. Solution B: 0.1 M Na_2CO_3 solution with 0.1% SDS.
2. Make a dilution to obtain calibrators C0 to C5 according to the table below:

Calibrator No.	Activity U/l (μmol product formed)	Solution A μl	Solution B μl
C0	0 (0)	0	1000
C1	12.4 (20)	200	800
C2	24.8 (40)	400	600
C3	37.2 (60)	600	400
C4	49.6 (80)	800	200
C5	61.9 (100)	1000	0

Quality control

Internal quality control (ICQ) samples: Make a pool of seminal plasma and freeze in 50- to 100-μl aliquots. Determine the α-glucosidase activity in 10 replicates at 5 different occasions.

Calculate the 95% confidence interval for the assessed α-glucosidase activity. The mean results of the QC samples in each batch should be within the 95% interval in order to approve an analysis series.

Procedure

Precautions: All materials (calibrators, samples, QC samples, and reagents) should be handled according to laboratory safety rules. Personal protection (clothes, latex gloves) should be used during the work. All used material (disposable) should be handled according to local safety regulations.

1. Make sure that the PNPG solution is kept at +50°C.
2. Thaw the seminal plasma samples, one internal QC sample and an aliquot of the inhibitor castanospermine using a water bath at +37°C.
3. Vortex each tube with seminal plasma and withdraw in duplicate 15 µl with a positive-displacement pipette and place in new 1.5-ml Eppendorf tubes. Also shake tubes with internal control and inhibitor. Add 15 µl of well-mixed QC sample into duplicate tubes labeled (a) QC and (b) castanospermine blank.
4. Add 8 µl of 1 mM castanospermine solution to the "castanospermine blank" tubes and vortex.
5. Add 100 µl of the PNPG solution to all tubes and apply the tube stoppers. Note that the PNPG should be warm otherwise it will precipitate and needs to be rewarmed up to +50°C in order not to allow the temperature to fall below +37°C. Vortex all tubes.
6. Incubate at +37°C for 120 min in water bath. Control temperature and time.
7. Prepare the calibrators and make ready just before the incubation is stopped.
8. Add 1000 µl of 0.1 M Na_2CO_3 solution to stop the reaction and augment the yellow color.
9. Pipette 250 µl of calibrators and samples to a 96-well plate and read the plate at the wavelength of 405 nm.

Notes

Make sure that no air bubbles are present in the wells. To empty a bubble: insert a pipette tip (20–200 µl) into the bubble.

Calculations and results

1. Plot the results for the calibrators. On the X-axis plot µmoles and the corresponding activity (see calibration above) and plot the absorbance on the Y-axis. Note: The activity corresponding to a given amount of product formed is only valid when the method is performed as described here. Since 1 unit (U) of glucosidase activity equals the formation of 1 µM of product (p-nitrophenol) per min at +37°C, the correction factor for 15 µl seminal plasma in a total volume of 1115 µl incubated for 120 min equals: 1115/15/120 = 0.6194. Thus, 100 µmol formed multiplied by the factor 0.6194 corresponds to 61.9 U/l.
2. Samples with values higher than the highest calibrator should be reanalyzed at higher dilution.
3. Subtract the mean value for the castonospermine tubes from each mean activity value from seminal fluid and QC samples. This eliminates product not caused by the α-glucosidase activity.

101

4. Check that the means of the QC samples are within the decided interval to approve this series of results.

5. Report the neutral α-glucosidase activity with one decimal place, e.g. 12.47 is given as 12.5 U/l, or use 12.5 mU/ml since seminal plasma is measured in milliliters.

6. Multiply by the ejaculate volume in ml with one decimal, which will give the total amount of secreted α-glucosidase activity in the ejaculate in milli Units (mU). Use one decimal, e.g. volume 3.2 ml times 12.47 = 39.904 is given as 39.9 mU/ejaculate.

Interpretation guidelines

Values above 20 mU/ejaculate mean a 95% probability for normal passage through the epididymis (meaning no obstruction). A combination of normal levels of zinc, fructose and neutral α-glucosidase indicates a representative ejaculate with secretory contributions from all major sources to the ejaculate.

Values below 20 mU/ejaculate indicate disturbed emission of fluid through the Wolffian ducts (vas deferens – ejaculatory ducts) which can be caused by neuromuscular impairment or obstructions.

Azoospermia with low values for neutral α-glucosidase and low values for fructose indicates a high obstruction in the ejaculatory ducts or agenesis of the Wolffian ducts.

A low value for neutral α-glucosidase combined with normal values for zinc and fructose indicates a representative ejaculate delivered after successful vasectomy.

Contrastingly, absence of spermatozoa combined with low neutral α-glucosidase activity and low fructose level does not primarily indicate successful vasectomy but for an obstruction between the seminal vesicles and the urethra. Thus such an ejaculate is not indicative of vasectomy success.

Sequence of ejaculation

Introduction

Ejaculation is a sequential emptying of epididymal and vas deferens contents (sperm) and secretions from the prostate and seminal vesicles. Normally, sperm are expelled first together with prostatic fluid, while the later 2/3 of the ejaculate volume is dominated by seminal vesicular fluid [36,37,38,39].

Pathological changes in the sequence of ejaculation can occur. Sperm exposed to abnormal amounts of seminal vesicular fluid have poorer motility, die faster and the chromatin is less stable.

Principle

The man is instructed to collect the individual fractions of the ejaculate in the order they are expelled and in separate containers (Figure 4.3). If the man empties more fractions than vials provided in the collection device, all the last fractions are collected in the last vial.

In the separately collected fractions, semen volume, sperm concentration and biochemical markers for prostatic secretion (zinc), seminal vesicular fluid (fructose) and epididymis (α-glucosidase) can be assessed.

A

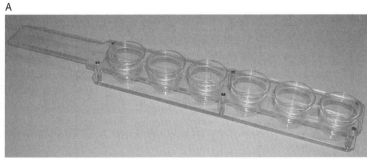

B

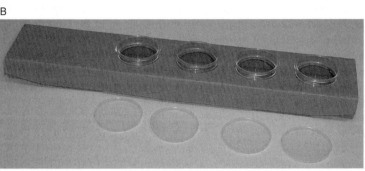

Figure 4.3 Examples of (A) a 6-vial plastic reusable device, and (B) a 4-vial corrugated cardboard disposable device, for the collection of split-ejaculates.

Specimen

Ejaculate fractions collected at the laboratory after, ideally, a 3-day period of prior sexual abstinence.

Equipment

Device with four to six collection vials linked together (e.g. mounted in a plastic ruler or in a disposable holder made of corrugated cardboard) [40].

Disposable materials

- Semen collection vials
- Disposable collection vial holder

Calibration

None required.

Quality control

No specific quality controls besides those required for sperm counting and biochemistry.

Procedures

The patient collects the sequential ejaculate fractions. The correct order of the vials must be confirmed with the patient. The vials should be numbered in sequential order in addition to the usual ID marking of the vials.

Coagulum formation will not occur in fractions dominated by prostatic fluid. For those fractions, investigations can start immediately (5–10 min warming in the incubator if motility is to be assessed). For coagulated fractions, 30 min at 37°C usually dissolves the coagulum, with exceptions for fractions with an extreme composition (lack of proteases of prostatic origin).

Calculations and results

1. For each fraction, calculate concentrations and total amount of sperm, zinc and fructose, as well as the zinc–fructose molar ratio.
2. Calculate the relative distribution of sperm, zinc and fructose: Add up the total numbers for each parameter and calculate the percentage found in each fraction. Example: Sperm number in each of the fractions was 75, 40, 14, 8 and 2 million sperm. Total number of sperm in the ejaculate was 139 million; the first fraction contained 75/139 = 54%, the second contained 29%, etc. If possible graphic presentations (3D bar diagrams) can be used to present data in addition to tabulated results (see also Appendix 6).

Interpretation guidelines

The first 1/3 of the ejaculate should contain the main bulk of sperm and also the dominant part of the prostatic secretion (Figure 4.4). High admixture of seminal vesicular fluid in the fractions with high proportion of sperm provides a reasonable explanation for poor motility in an earlier sample with isolated motility problems. It could either be a high concentration of fructose in the first sperm-rich fractions, or it could be that most sperm are expelled in the later ejaculate fractions.

Notes

The patient might benefit from training with the collection technique, which is easiest if disposable, cardboard collection vial holders are used.

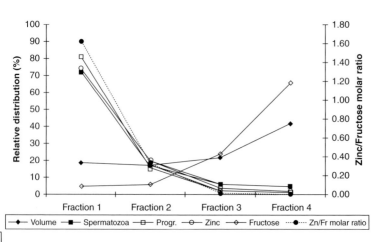

Figure 4.4 Example graph showing the distribution of spermatozoa, zinc, and fructose within a 6-portion split-ejaculate.

Computer-aided sperm analysis (CASA)

Despite greatly improved technology since its first introduction in 1985, computer-aided sperm analysis (CASA) is still not widely used in routine diagnostic andrology laboratories. This has been attributed to unrealistic expectations of the technology, and early attempts to sell CASA systems as automated semen analyzers [41]. A detailed discussion of CASA is beyond the scope of this chapter and interested readers are referred to relevant review articles [13,42,43,44,45], and especially to reports from expert consensus workshops [46,47,48]. Much of the responsibility for the persistent misuse of CASA technology must lie with its users who, rather than promoting the measurement of traditional semen characteristics known to have only limited clinical predictive value, should have applied the advanced capabilities of CASA technology to assess sperm characteristics with greater biological significance; notably, ones based on sperm movement characteristics ("kinematics," see below).

It is well-established that it is dynamic sub-populations of motile spermatozoa with appropriate movement characteristics that determine whether a man's spermatozoa can penetrate his partner's cervical mucus, or penetrate the cumulus–oocyte complex and fertilize the oocyte [13,47,48]. Standardized protocols that apply CASA technology to investigate such sperm functional potential must be promoted (see Chapter 5).

Because the technical limitations of CASA technology can dramatically affect the correct use of CASA instruments, even to the extent of rendering results completely meaningless, it is essential that users understand both the technology and its limitations, and adhere to the consensus recommendations for its correct application (see Appendix 4).

Kinematic measures of human sperm motility

Although it is the sperm tail which creates motility, the modern CASA system still cannot analyze flagellar beating, and hence we must continue to analyze motility by tracking the sperm head, which was the basis for all sperm kinematic measures in routine use (see Figure 4.5) [49]. Analyses of sperm movement derived from tracking the head can provide a great deal of useful information on sperm movement in semen [49], and it was from observations on flagellar beating that descriptions of hyperactivated motility were based [43].

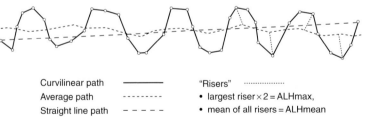

Curvilinear path ————	"Risers" ··········
Average path - - - - - - - -	• largest riser × 2 = ALHmax,
Straight line path – – – – –	• mean of all risers = ALHmean

Figure 4.5 Illustration showing how the currently-used kinematic measures are derived from the 2-dimensional projection of a spermatozoon's real 3-dimensional trajectory. (Modified from ref. 54.)

Curvilinear velocity (VCL)

VCL is calculated from the sum of the straight-lines joining the sequential positions of the sperm head along the spermatozoon's track. VCL is therefore the two-dimensional projection of the true three-dimensional helical path of the spermatozoon, as revealed by the time resolution of the imaging method used – making it highly sensitive to the frame rate (see Figure 4.6) [50]. VCL values (sometimes referred to as "track speed") are reported in µm/s to one decimal place.

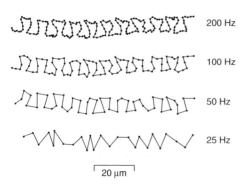

200 Hz

100 Hz

50 Hz

25 Hz

20 μm

Figure 4.6 Illustration of the effect of image sampling frequency (frame rate) on the perceived curvilinear velocity (VCL) of a spermatozoon. (Modified from ref. 11.)

Average path velocity (VAP)

VAP is the velocity along the "average" path of the spermatozoon. However, because the average path is derived by CASA machines using a variety of algorithms [40,42,48], the precise method used for its derivation must always be stated. For example, 5-point smoothing is *not* adequate for progressive human spermatozoa when tracked at 50 or 60 images/s; there, frame rates typically require more like 11-point smoothing or, better, adaptive smoothing algorithms. VAP values are reported in μm/s to one decimal place.

Straight-line velocity (VSL)

VSL is the linear or "progression" velocity of the spermatozoon, and is calculated from the straight-line distance between the start and end of the observed track. VSL values are reported in μm/s to one decimal place.

Three progression ratios, all expressed as integer percentages, can be calculated from the three velocity measurements described above:

Linearity $LIN = VSL/VCL \times 100$
Straightness $STR = VSL/VAP \times 100$
Wobble $WOB = VAP/VCL \times 100$

Amplitude of lateral head displacement (ALH)

ALH is calculated from the amplitudes of the lateral deviations of the sperm head about the cell's axis of progression (average path). Different CASA programs use either an average value (ALHmean) calculated from the individual measurements made over the length of the track, or the maximum value (ALHmax) of all the measurements. Traditionally ALH measurements were expressed as the width across the whole track [49], i.e. twice the average or maximum measurement, and this has been retained as the convention for ALH measurements, which are expressed in μm to one decimal place.

Beat cross frequency (BCF)

BCF is the number of times that the curvilinear track crosses the average path per unit time. It is expressed in Hz, to one decimal place. In reality, BCF is a derivation of the true flagellar beat frequency and the frequency of rotation (ROF) of the head. Although it cannot be analyzed by automated CASA systems, the ROF is the number of times the sperm head rotates through 360° per unit time (a human spermatozoon swimming in seminal plasma will usually rotate through 180° at the apex of each lateral deviation of the head about the axis of progression). BCF values are also subject to the image sampling rate, as well as to aliasing errors (see [43] for further explanation); hence, reported values greater than half the frame rate must be considered suspect.

CASA and semen analysis

Sperm concentration

As concluded by the ESHRE Special Interest Group in Andrology [47], this must not be a primary reason for acquiring a CASA instrument because the current technology does not provide accurate, reproducible values for sperm concentration unless the imaging method can differentiate spermatozoa from other cells and debris by a specific staining method (e.g. fluorescent staining of DNA with quantitative determination of nucleus size [51]). Consequently, anyone using a CASA instrument for this purpose must establish that their protocol provides accurate results compared to established, reliable techniques (e.g. hemocytometry method, see Chapter 3).

Sperm motility percentage(s)

Again, the ESHRE Special Interest Group in Andrology has concluded that this aspect of semen analysis should not be considered a primary reason for acquiring a CASA instrument [48]. Current CASA instruments cannot be relied upon to distinguish between debris and dead spermatozoa in semen while tracking live spermatozoa at the same time – and therefore should not be used to determine the *proportion* of motile spermatozoa. However, CASA could be used to determine the *concentration* of progressively motile spermatozoa in routine semen analysis, since this value can be determined accurately if care is taken with specimen preparation, instrument use and appropriate user-defined criteria.

Sperm morphology

The current generation of CASA instruments remains unable to analyze human sperm morphology, including assessment of the midpiece and tail regions as required by current WHO guidelines [30], and for the determination of the Teratozoospermia Index (TI) (see Chapter 5). While most modern CASA systems are able to provide reliable morphometric analysis of human sperm heads, it seems that few routine laboratories employ this technology [44], primarily because it provides little or no benefit in time compared to trained technicians. Consequently, the ESHRE Special Interest Group in Andrology does not currently support the use of CASA instruments for the clinical assessment of human sperm morphology [48]. Slide preparation and staining procedures are critical for obtaining reliable results.

CASA and the assessment of sperm functional potential

Although CASA analysis results have been correlated with in-vivo fertility [52,53], it is generally understood that using CASA to define specific sub-populations of potentially functional spermatozoa, rather than considering population-averaged kinematic measures, will provide more meaningful results for patient diagnosis and management [43,48].

Sperm–mucus penetration

We have long known that spermatozoa with the "right" motility (i.e. good kinematics) are better able to penetrate cervical mucus [43], and hence quantifying this sub-population should be a major benefit at semen analysis. The following Boolean criteria have been proposed for identifying spermatozoa with "good mucus penetrating ability," where straightness is abbreviated as "STR" [54]:

$$VAP \geq 25 \text{ μm/s AND } STR \geq 80\% \text{ AND } ALH \geq 2.5 \text{ μm AND } ALH < 7.0 \text{ μm.}$$

The fourth term serves to exclude spermatozoa whose motility has been compromised by ROS-induced damage, which can cause a quasi-hyperactivation pattern of movement.

Analysis of sperm hyperactivation

Hyperactivated motility is a high-energy pattern of movement characterized by the development of high-amplitude flagellar waves, but with little net space gain (Figure 4.7). It occurs in all Eutherian spermatozoa studied, is a concomitant of capacitation *in vitro*, and has been observed in free-swimming spermatozoa in the oviduct *in situ* [43]. The physiological importance of hyperactivation is generally accepted, but the clinical significance of its assessment is still under investigation (see Chapter 5).

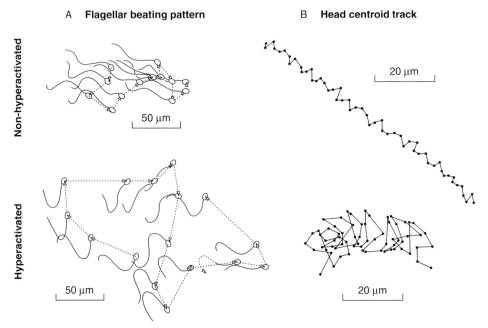

Figure 4.7 Sperm hyperactivation. Panel (A) shows the changes in flagellar beating that underlie hyperactivated motility (modified from ref. 4), while panel (B) shows the changes in head-derived tracks (modified from refs. 50 & 55).

The identification of hyperactivated motility using sperm head-derived tracks is suboptimal [43], but routine flagellar analysis remains impractical. Validated criteria for identifying hyperactivated human spermatozoa using the IVOS instrument (Hamilton Thorne Biosciences, Beverly, MA, USA) operating at 60 Hz frame rates have been established and validated, where "LIN" is the linearity [53,55]:

$$VCL \geq 150 \text{ μm/s AND } LIN \leq 50\% \text{ AND } ALH \geq 7.0 \text{ μm.}$$

Use of these – or other – criteria in other CASA systems must be independently validated using flagellar analysis studies.

Quality control for CASA

Quality control (QC) is extremely important in all measurement systems employed in medical laboratories, and each laboratory using CASA must have appropriate QC procedures in place.

It has been suggested that QC for sperm motility analysis should use appropriate video recordings in conjunction with the "playback" feature of the CASA instrument to ensure that all the motile spermatozoa are being identified using each set of system parameters. However, this approach is not logical as it fails to control for the most important aspects of instrument operation that can affect reliable tracking and analysis of spermatozoa (since the correct derivation of kinematic values from a track by the software should not be in doubt). Moreover, it is likely that different setup parameters will need to be used for video recordings compared to "live" specimens – and that system setup parameters have not been changed can easily be verified by inspecting the setup screen (although, in fact, most systems allow supervisors to prevent technical operators from changing these parameters). It is, therefore, more important to follow a daily QC procedure similar to the following:

1. Basic system operation and magnification calibration can be verified by analyzing known-concentration preparations of microscopic beads as surrogates for sperm heads, e.g. Accu-Beads® from Hamilton Thorne Biosciences (Beverly, MA, USA). The concentration of beads obtained from the CASA instrument must be within the stated reference range.

2. Verify that the CASA instrument's imaging system (illumination intensity and focus) and setup parameters are properly matched. This will ensure that:

   a. spermatozoa will be correctly identified;

   b. debris particles will not contribute undue numbers of spurious spermatozoa; and

   c. moving spermatozoa will be tracked reliably.

To do this, analyze a field from a *live* specimen and then use the "playback" function to make sure that:

1. the great majority of the spermatozoa in the field have been identified correctly (e.g. at least 90% of visually identifiable sperm tracks or immotile heads have been tagged by the system);

2. debris has not been excessively identified as spurious sperm heads (e.g. <10% of the number of sperm identified should be suspect); and

3. all the moving cells have been tracked, and that the tracks appear intact (i.e. not fragmented into shorter lengths). A track that was truncated due to colliding with another cell or piece of debris is not considered a tracking problem.

Then check 10–20 individual tracks (e.g. using the "Edit Tracks – Zoom" function for a Hamilton Thorne IVOS) and verify that only occasional track points have been lost (e.g. no more than 2 missed points, either individually or in sequence), and that adjacent short tracks are not fragments of the same, longer track. The latter can be identified from the image numbers for the track points that make up each track; a complete intact track will contain points from the first image through to the end of the sequence, e.g. 30 points.

Note: This procedure must be repeated for each variation of illumination and optics used.

References

1. Chamley LW, Clarke GN. Antisperm antibodies and conception. *Semin Immunopathol.* 2007; **29**: 169–84.
2. World Health Organization. *WHO Laboratory Manual for the Examination of Human Semen and Sperm-Cervical Mucus Interaction.* 2009; in press.
3. Chiu WW, Chamley LW. Clinical associations and mechanisms of action of antisperm antibodies. *Fertil Steril* 2004; **82**: 529–35.
4. Lombardo F, Gandini L, Lenzi A, Dondero F. Antisperm immunity in assisted reproduction. *J Reprod Immunol* 2004; **62**: 101–9.
5. Barratt CL, Dunphy BC, McLeod I, Cooke ID. The poor prognostic value of low to moderate levels of sperm surface-bound antibodies. *Hum Reprod* 1992; **7**: 95–8.
6. Helmerhorst FM, Finken MJ, Erwich JJ. Antisperm antibodies: detection assays for antisperm antibodies: what do they test? *Hum Reprod* 1999; **14**: 1669–71.
7. Hjort T. Antisperm antibodies. Antisperm antibodies and infertility: an unsolvable question? *Hum Reprod* 1999; **14**: 2423–6.
8. Mahmoud A, Comhaire F. Antisperm antibodies: use of the mixed agglutination reaction (MAR) test using latex beads. *Hum Reprod* 2000; **15**: 231–3.
9. Meinertz H, Linnet L, Fogh-Andersen P, Hjort T. Antisperm antibodies and fertility after vasovasostomy: a follow-up study of 216 men. *Fertil Steril* 1990; **54**: 315–21.
10. Bronson RA, Cooper GW, Rosenfeld DL. Sperm-specific isoantibodies and autoantibodies inhibit the binding of human sperm to the human zona pellucida. *Fertil Steril* 1982; **38**: 724–9.
11. Matson PL. External quality assessment for semen analysis and sperm antibody detection: results of a pilot scheme. *Hum Reprod* 1995; **10**: 620–5.
12. Bohring C, Krause W. Interlaboratory variability of the indirect mixed antiglobulin reaction in the assessment of antisperm antibodies. *Fertil Steril* 2002; **78**: 1336–8.
13. Mortimer D. *Practical Laboratory Andrology.* New York: Oxford University Press 1994.
14. Keck C, Gerber-Schäfer C, Clad A, *et al.* Seminal tract infections: impact on male fertility and treatment options. *Hum Reprod Update* 1998; **4**: 891–903.
15. Weidner W, Krause W, Ludwig M. Relevance of male accessory gland infection for subsequent fertility with special focus on prostatitis. *Hum Reprod Update* 1999; **5**: 421–32.
16. Elder K, Baker D, Ribes J. *Infections, Infertility and Assisted Reproduction.* Cambridge, UK: Cambridge University Press 2005.
17. Ochsendorf FR. Sexually transmitted infections: impact on male fertility. *Andrologia* 2008; **40**: 72–5.
18. Eggert-Kruse W, Kiefer I, Beck C, *et al.* Role for tumor necrosis factor alpha (TNF-alpha) and interleukin 1-beta (IL-1beta) determination in seminal plasma during infertility investigation. *Fertil Steril* 2007; **87**: 810–23.
19. Politch JA, Tucker L, Bowman FP, *et al.* Concentrations and significance of cytokines and other immunologic factors in semen of healthy fertile men. *Hum Reprod* 2007; **22**: 2928–35.
20. Bezold G, Politch JA, Kiviat NB, *et al.* Prevalence of sexually transmissible pathogens in semen from asymptomatic male infertility patients with and without leukocytospermia. *Fertil Steril* 2007; **87**: 1087–97.
21. Tomlinson MJ, Barratt CL, Cooke ID. Prospective study of leukocytes and leukocyte subpopulations in semen suggests they are not a cause of male infertility. *Fertil Steril* 1993; **60**: 1069–75.
22. Aitken RJ, Buckingham D, West K, Wu FC, Zikopoulos K, Richardson DW. Differential contribution of leukocytes and spermatozoa to the generation of reactive oxygen species in the ejaculates of oligozoospermic patients and fertile donors. *J Reprod Fertil* 1992; **94**: 451–62.
23. Aitken RJ, West K, Buckingham D. Leukocytic infiltration into the human ejaculate and its association with semen

quality, oxidative stress, and sperm function. *J Androl* 1994; **15**: 343–52.

24. Tomlinson MJ, White A, Barratt CL, Bolton AE, Cooke ID. The removal of morphologically abnormal sperm forms by phagocytes: a positive role for seminal leukocytes? *Hum Reprod* 1992; **7**: 517–22.

25. Comhaire F, Verschraegen G, Vermeulen L. Diagnosis of accessory gland infection and its possible role in male infertility. *Int J Androl* 1980; **3**: 32–45.

26. Eggert-Kruse W, Zimmermann K, Geißler W, Ehrmann A, Boit R, Strowitzki T. Clinical relevance of polymorphonuclear (PMN-) elastase determination in semen and serum during infertility investigation. *Int J Androl* 2009; **32**: 317–29.

27. Nahoum CR, Cardozo D. Staining for volumetric count of leukocytes in semen and prostate-vesicular fluid. *Fertil Steril* 1980; **34**: 68–9.

28. Tomlinson MJ, Barratt CL, Bolton AE, Lenton EA, Roberts HB, Cooke ID. Round cells and sperm fertilizing capacity: the presence of immature germ cells but not seminal leukocytes are associated with reduced success of in vitro fertilization. *Fertil Steril* 1992; **58**: 1257–9.

29. Johnsen Ø, Eliasson R, Evaluation of a commercially available kit for the colorimetric determination of zinc in human seminal plasma. *Int J Androl* 1987; **10**: 435–40.

30. World Health Organization. *WHO Laboratory Manual for the Examination of Human Semen and Sperm-Cervical Mucus Interaction*. 4th edn. Cambridge, UK: Cambridge University Press 1999.

31. Cooper TG, Weidner W, Nieschlag E. The Influence of inflammation of the human male genital tract on secretion of the seminal markers α-glucosidase, glycerophosphocholine, carnitine, fructose and citric acid. *Int J Androl* 1990; **13**: 329–36.

32. Dreden P, Richard P, Gonzales J. Fructose and proteins in human semen. *Andrologia* 1989; **21**: 576–9.

33. Jungreis E, Nechama M, Paz G, Homonai T. A simple spot test for the detection of fructose deficiency in semen. *Int J Androl* 1989; **12**: 195–8.

34. Paquin R, Chapdelaine R, Dube JY, Tremblay RR. Similar biochemical

properties of human seminal plasma and epididymal α-1,4-glucosidase. *J Androl* 1984; **5**: 277–82.

35. Cooper TG, Yeung CH, Nashan D, *et al.* Improvement in the assessment of human epididymal function by the use of inhibitors in the assay of α-glucosidase in seminal plasma. *Int J Androl* 1990; **13**: 297–305.

36. MacLeod J, Gold RZ. The male factor in fertility and infertility. III. An analysis of motile activity in the spermatozoa of 1000 fertile men and 1000 men in infertile marriage. *Fertil Steril* 1951; **2**: 187–204.

37. Lindholmer C. Survival of human spermatozoa in different fractions of split ejaculate. *Fertil Steril* 1973; **24**: 521–6.

38. Björndahl L, Kjellberg S, Kvist U. Ejaculatory sequence in men with low sperm chromatin-zinc. *Int J Androl* 1991; **14**: 174–8.

39. Björndahl L, Kvist U. Influence of seminal vesicular fluid on the zinc content of human sperm chromatin. *Int J Androl* 1990; **13**: 232–7.

40. Björndahl L, Kvist U. Sequence of ejaculation affects the spermatozoon as a carrier and its message. *RBM Online* 2003; **7**: 440–8.

41. Davis RO, Katz DF. Computer-aided sperm analysis: technology at a crossroads. *Fertil Steril* 1993; **59**: 953–5.

42. Boyers SP, Davis RO, Katz DF. Automated semen analysis. *Curr Probl Obstet Gynecol Fertil* 1989; **XII**: 167–200.

43. Mortimer ST. A critical review of the physiological importance and analysis of sperm movement in mammals. *Hum Reprod Update* 1997; **3**: 403–39.

44. Mortimer D, Mortimer ST. Value and reliability of CASA systems. In: Ombelet W, Bosmans E, Vandeput H, *et al.*, eds. *Modern ART in the 2000s*. Carnforth: Parthenon Publishing 1998.

45. Mortimer ST. CASA–practical aspects. *J Androl* 2000; **21**: 515–24.

46. Mortimer D, Aitken RJ, Mortimer ST, Pacey AA. Workshop report: clinical CASA – the quest for consensus. *Reprod Fertil Dev* 1995; **7**: 951–9.

47. ESHRE Andrology Special Interest Group. Consensus workshop on advanced diagnostic andrology techniques. *Hum Reprod* 1996; **11**: 1463–79.

48. ESHRE Andrology Special Interest Group. Guidelines on the application of CASA

technology in the analysis of spermatozoa. *Hum Reprod* 1998; **13**: 142–5.

49. Serres C, Feneux D, Jouannet P, David G. Influence of the flagellar wave development and propagation on the human sperm movement in seminal plasma. *Gamete Res* 1984; **9**: 183–95.

50. Mortimer D, Serres C, Mortimer ST, Jouannet P. Influence of image sampling frequency on the perceived movement characteristics of progressively motile human spermatozoa. *Gamete Res* 1988; **20**: 313–27.

51. Zinaman MJ, Uhler ML, Vertuno E, *et al.* Evaluation of computer-assisted semen analysis (CASA) with IDENT stain to determine sperm concentration. *J Androl* 1996; **17**: 288–92.

52. Irvine DS, Macleod IC, Templeton AA, *et al.* A prospective clinical study of the relationship between the computer-assisted assessment of human semen quality and the achievement of pregnancy in vivo. *Hum Reprod* 1994; **9**: 2324–34.

53. Macleod IC, Irvine DS. The predictive value of computer-assisted semen analysis in the context of a donor insemination programme. *Hum Reprod* 1995; **10**: 580–6.

54. Mortimer D, Mortimer ST. Laboratory investigation of the infertile male. In: Brinsden PR, edn. *A Textbook of In-Vitro Fertilization and Assisted Reproduction.* 3rd edn. London: Taylor & Francis Medical Books 2005: 61–91.

55. Mortimer ST, Swan MA. Effect of image sampling frequency on established and smoothing-independent kinematic values of capacitating human spermatozoa. *J Androl* 1999; **14**: 997–1004.

Sperm function tests

Introduction

During the last three decades of the twentieth century, extensive research on a global basis was directed towards developing tests that might be able to identify particular aspects of sperm pathophysiology that resulted in dysfunction, and hence could help diagnose male factor infertility. In June 1995 the ESHRE Special Interest Group in Andrology held a Consensus Workshop on *Advanced Diagnostic Andrology Techniques* in Hamburg that seemed to mark a point of closure for much of the research in this field [1]. Certainly the widespread availability of ICSI from the mid-1990s has led to much less interest in trying to diagnose what might be the etiology of a man's infertility, and very few diagnostic andrology laboratories nowadays offer testing of sperm fertilizing ability.

This chapter will summarize the current status of what were the mainstream sperm function tests, and provide experimental protocols for anyone who might need to employ them, either for diagnostic or research purposes. Sections are also included on two areas where there is continued expanding interest: the involvement of reactive oxygen species (free radicals) in sperm function and competence and the use of tests of sperm chromatin.

Reactive oxygen species (ROS)

Background

Mammalian spermatozoa have been shown to produce oxygen radicals and to export them to the extracellular medium [2,3,4,5,6]. The main source of oxygen radicals in spermatozoa appears to be the mitochondria, as the result of the monovalent reduction of molecular oxygen during oxidative phosphorylation [3].

Spermatozoa have a relatively high content of polyunsaturated fatty acids in their membrane and in particular of docosahexaenoic acid (DHA), which makes them especially vulnerable to lipid peroxidation induced by oxygen radicals [7]. DHA is thought to play a major role in regulating membrane fluidity in spermatozoa, and is the main substrate of lipid peroxidation, accounting for 90% of the overall rate of lipid peroxidation in human spermatozoa [7]. Oxidation of phospholipid-bound DHA has been shown to be the major factor that determines the motile lifespan of spermatozoa *in vitro* [6], as well as membrane damage and DNA oxidation [8,9]. The rate of lipid peroxidation of spermatozoa in vitro is determined by: (a) oxygen concentration and temperature in the extracellular medium; (b) ROS production; (c) the activity of antioxidant enzymes in spermatozoa; and (d) the content of phospholipid-bound DHA [5,7]. The equilibrium between these factors determines the overall rate of lipid peroxidation and oxidative stress *in vitro*. During the process of sperm maturation, spermatozoa retain a critical level of DHA resulting in: (a) optimal membrane fluidity required to support sperm motility and the early steps of fertilization; and (b) minimal risk of oxidative damage to the sperm membranes and DNA [10].

Mammalian sperm metabolic strategy is geared towards maximal production of adenosine triphosphate (ATP) in the flagellum through anaerobic glycolysis rather than maximal efficiency through the Krebs cycle, thus minimizing the flux of reducing β-nicotinamide adenine dinucleotide (NADH) equivalents through the inner mitochondrial membrane and the production of oxygen radicals. Therefore, this metabolic strategy can be considered as an additional antioxidant mechanism of paramount importance in spermatozoa.

Oxygen radicals produced by spermatozoa include the superoxide anion (O_2^-); its conjugated acid, the hydroperoxyl radical ($HO_2^\bullet$); hydrogen peroxide (H_2O_2), produced mostly through the dismutation of the superoxide anion by superoxide dismutase; and the hydroxyl radical ($OH^\bullet$) produced by the reaction of the superoxide anion with hydrogen peroxide in the presence of heavy metals [5]. Oxygen radicals, as a group, are currently designated as reactive oxygen species (ROS).

Most ROS found in semen are produced by immature spermatozoa and by leukocytes. Although ROS levels produced by activated leukocytes could be several orders of magnitude higher than those produced by spermatozoa, immature spermatozoa may produce comparable levels of ROS in the presence of pro-inflammatory factors [11]. Since transient in-vitro exposure of immature spermatozoa to leukocytes has been shown to result in the production of very high levels of ROS after PMA stimulation and the removal of leukocytes from the sperm suspension [10], formyl-methionyl-leucyl-phenylalanine- (FMLP-) and phorbol 12-myristate 13-acetate- (PMA-) stimulated ROS production in semen is no longer recommended. In addition to the ROS produced by immature spermatozoa and leukocytes, semen may also contain ROS produced by the epithelial cells of the epididymis [12]. ROS levels in semen derived from all these different sources have been shown to be inversely correlated with normal sperm function and directly correlated with male infertility [13,14].

Principle

ROS are measured in semen by chemiluminescence using luminol as a substrate [15,16]. Luminol is a highly sensitive probe that reacts with a variety of ROS at neutral pH, and can be used to measure both extracellular and intracellular ROS. ROS have a very short lifespan and, therefore, must be measured quickly after semen collection. The free radical combines with luminol to produce photons that are then converted to an electrical signal which is then measured with a luminometer [8], with ROS generation being measured as counted photons per minute (cpm).

Specimen(s)

- Liquefied semen collected, ideally, at the laboratory after a 3-day period of prior sexual abstinence. A semen analysis should be performed on the specimen

Equipment (see also Appendix 2)

- Air-displacement pipettes, 0–10 µl and 100–1000 µl
- Positive-displacement pipette (400 µl) for taking semen aliquots
- Pipette controller

- Vortex mixer
- Luminometer, model LKB 953, Wallac Inc (Gaithersburg, MD, USA)

Disposable materials
- Disposable polystyrene tubes with caps, 17 × 20 mm (e.g. Fisher Scientific cat.no. 14–959–491)
- Polystyrene round-bottom tubes, 12 × 75 mm (e.g. Falcon #2003)
- Disposable serological pipettes, 1 ml, 2 ml and 10 ml

Reagents
1. Luminol stock solution: 100 mM solution of luminol (5-amino-2,3 dehydro-1,4 phthalazinedione; Sigma A8511) in DMSO (Sigma D8779). Dissolve 0.177 g of luminol in 10 ml of DMSO in a polystyrene tube; cover the tube in aluminum foil since luminol is light sensitive. This solution, which is a clear, straw color when prepared, can be stored at room temperature in the dark for up to 6 months. Discard if there is any change in color or turbidity.

2. Luminol working solution: 5 mM solution in DMSO. Mix 20 μl luminol stock solution with 380 μl DMSO in a foil-covered polystyrene tube. Prepare the solution fresh prior to use and store at room temperature in the dark until needed.

3. PBS solution: Dulbecco's phosphate buffered saline solution (e.g. PBS-1X, cat.no. 9235, Irvine Scientific).

Calibration
None required.

Quality control
1. Criterion for acceptance: Control reads $<0.02 \times 10^6$ cpm.
2. Criterion for rejection: Control reads $>0.02 \times 10^6$ cpm. The assay must be repeated and results shown to the Laboratory Director.
3. The control is run in 35 assays with a mean value of 0.32×10^6 cpm and a standard deviation of ±0.09.
4. The reagent lot numbers and expiration dates are recorded in the assay quality control book located in the laboratory.

Procedure
1. Turn on the LB953 luminometer and associated computer system; allow to warm-up for 10–15 min.
2. Label sufficient 6-ml polystyrene tubes as follows:

Blank	1 tube
Controls	2 tubes
Each patient	2 tubes per patient

3. Add reagents as follows:

   Blank   400 µl PBS
   Control   400 µl PBS + 10 µl luminol working solution
   Test   400 µl semen + 10 µl luminol working solution

   Note: To avoid contamination, change the pipette tip after each addition of luminol.

4. Gently vortex the tubes to uniformly mix the contents.
5. Place the appropriately labeled tubes in the luminometer in the following order: Blank, Control 1, Control 1, Patient 1 tube A, Patient 1 tube B, Patient 2 tube A, Patient 2 tube B, etc. Close the lid.
6. On the luminometer control screen:

   a. Highlight "Measure" and press "enter";

   b. On the next menu, highlight "Chemiluminescence" and press "enter";

   c. Highlight the number of tubes in the assay and press "enter"; this will allow the measurement to occur over a 15 min time frame for each tube;

   d. Record the filename and press "enter";

   e. Press the F10 key to start measurement.

7. When the assay run has finished, print a hard copy of the results by:

   a. Highlighting "Evaluation" and pressing "enter";

   b. Highlighting "Print Report" and pressing "enter."

Calculations and results

1. Calculate average values of the control tubes. Verify that the control value must be $<1 \times 10^6$ cpm before calculating the results.
2. Calculate the ROS generation for each patient:

   Patient average cpm – control average cpm = patient ROS result in cpm.

3. Because the results will be expressed as 10^6 cpm per 20 million spermatozoa, calculate the correction factor for each patient:

   Correction factor = 20/actual sperm concentration.

   e.g. if the sperm concentration is 8.5×10^6/ml, multiply the patient ROS cpm value by 2.35 (20/8.5).

4. Calculate the final result for each patient:

   Patient ROS result in cpm × correction factor.

   Express the final result as million counted photons per minute (cpm) per 20 million spermatozoa.

Interpretation guidelines

Normal range $<0.2 \times 10^6$ cpm per 20 million spermatozoa
Abnormal values $>0.2 \times 10^6$ cpm per 20 million spermatozoa

Notes

None.

Hyperactivation

Principle

Hyperactivated motility is a high-energy pattern of sperm movement seen in all Eutherian species. It is characterized by the development of high-amplitude flagellar waves, but their propagation along the sperm tail results in little net space gain (see Figure 4.7). It is a visible concomitant of sperm capacitation *in vitro*, and has been observed in free-swimming spermatozoa in the oviduct *in situ*, and is now generally accepted to have a physiological importance for fertilization both *in vivo* and *in vitro*, especially in the penetration of the zona pellucida [17,18].

The clinical value of human sperm hyperactivation assessment is still unclear, its investigation being confounded by several factors. There is both inter- and intra-individual variation in the proportion of human spermatozoa that exhibit hyperactivated motility, and spermatozoa do not remain in the hyperactivated state indefinitely [19].

Although hyperactivation is a flagellar phenomenon, the only practical means for assessing its prevalence in a capacitating sperm population requires the use of specialized CASA techniques (see the section on CASA in Chapter 4). Unless all appropriate assay conditions are met (including careful separation of the spermatozoa from seminal plasma, specific physiological requirements for the incubation medium, and an adequate analysis preparation depth so as not to constrain flagellar movement) hyperactivation studies will produce unreliable results [20,21].

Because the expression of spontaneous sperm hyperactivation is highly variable over time, even for sperm sub-populations within a single ejaculate (Figure 5.1), the need for multiple assessment time points has made the establishment of a robust clinical assay for hyperactivation difficult. However, two hyperactivation agonists, progesterone and pentoxifylline, have been employed to create a similar assay to the acrosome reaction following ionophore challenge (ARIC) test [22,23]. Exposure of prepared motile sperm populations to 1 µg/ml progesterone plus 3.6 mM pentoxifylline in a capacitating sperm medium for 60 min induces maximal levels of hyperactivation in the majority of men (Figure 5.2). This "HAmax" assay contributes significantly towards predicting cases with poor and good IVF fertilization rate (0–49% and 50–100%, respectively) even when

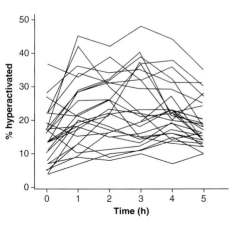

Figure 5.1 Illustration of the levels of spontaneous hyperactivation during the in-vitro capacitation of density-gradient-prepared spermatozoa from 25 different men.

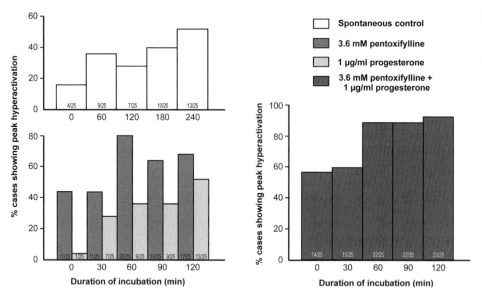

Figure 5.2 Proportions of the 25 cases showing sperm hyperactivation within 10% of the peak spontaneous hyperactivation seen for each man level at different time points after either no treatment (control), treatment with 3.6 mM pentoxifylline or 1 μg/ml progesterone, or treatment with both pentoxifylline and progesterone. Based on these results, the optimum test format for the "HAmax" assay was a 60-min incubation with the combined agonist treatment.

testing is performed weeks, or even months prior to the actual treatment cycle: discriminant function analysis $R^2 = 0.884$ with 100% sensitivity (22/22 cases) and 100% specificity (7/7 cases).

Specimen
- Liquefied semen collected, ideally, at the laboratory after a 3-day period of prior sexual abstinence. A semen analysis should be performed on the specimen

Equipment (see also Appendix 2)
- As for semen analysis
- As for sperm preparation using DGC
- Analytical balance
- CO_2 incubator, operating at 6.0% CO_2-in-air if close to sea level. If a CO_2 incubator is not available then gas the tubes with pre-mixed gas containing 6.0% CO_2, cap them tightly and mix by inversion to equilibrate with the gas, and place the tubes in a 37°C incubator with an air atmosphere
- Hamilton Thorne IVOS 60 Hz computer-aided sperm analyzer (CASA) system with the "Edit Tracks" and "Sort" function software options installed (see Chapter 4 for further details)

Disposable materials

- As for semen analysis
- As for sperm preparation using DGC
- Fixed-depth chambers for CASA analysis, ideally 50 μm MicroCell HAC chambers (Conception Technologies, San Diego, CA, USA), but 20 μm chambers such as the 2X-CEL (Hamilton Thorne Biosciences) can be used *for this particular assay* if deeper chambers are unavailable
- Falcon #2003 culture tubes

Reagents

1. As for sperm preparation using DGC.
2. A bicarbonate-based (not HEPES-buffered) "sperm medium" that supports human sperm capacitation (ideally Sydney IVF Fertilization Medium, Cook Medical; see www.cookmedical.com).
3. "HAmax" reagent: This is a 2 × concentrated solution of pentoxifylline and progesterone in sperm medium, which is mixed 1 + 1 with the prepared sperm suspension (also in the same medium). The HAmax reagent contains 7.2 mM pentoxifylline and 2 μg/ml progesterone dissolved in sperm medium with added human serum albumin to give 30 mg HSA/ml, and must be prepared for use each day.
4. Stock 1000 × progesterone solution: Dissolve 1.0 mg of progesterone (Sigma P6149) in 1.0 ml of absolute ethanol. Store tightly-capped at +4°C for up to 6 months from date of opening.
5. Daily use HAmax reagent:
   a. To 2.0 ml of sterile sperm medium, add 4.0 mg pentoxifylline (Sigma P1784), 4.0 μl of stock progesterone solution and 40 mg of human serum albumin (HSA) (Sigma A1653).
   b. Mix thoroughly by gentle inversion; do not shake, as this will cause frothing due to the protein content of the medium.
   c. Store loosely capped in a CO_2 incubator at 37°C until required. Discard any unused reagent at the end of the day.

Calibration

The IVOS must be properly calibrated in terms of its optics and stage temperature (37°C), and the "Sort" function must be configured to use the following validated criteria for identifying hyperactivated human spermatozoa using this instrument [21]:

$$VCL \geq 150 \text{ μm/s AND LIN} \leq 50\% \text{ AND ALH} \geq 7.0 \text{ μm.}$$

There are no other special calibrations required for the performance of this assay.

Quality control

1. Daily QC is required for the proper operation of the IVOS instrument.
2. A positive control sample (i.e. semen from a control donor who has known HAmax response) should be run for each batch of HAmax reagent.

Procedure

1. Prepare a selected motile population of spermatozoa using a standardized 2-layer discontinuous density gradient method (see Chapter 7) in sperm medium at 5×10^6 to 10×10^6 motile spermatozoa/ml.

2. Label two small Falcon #2003 culture tubes with the patient's name, the Andrology Lab Accession Number and the date, and either HA control or HAmax.

3. Transfer 0.5 ml of the washed sperm preparation into each tube.

4. a. To the HA control tube add 0.5 ml of sperm medium.

   b. To the HAmax tube add 0.5 ml of the HAmax reagent.

   c. Mix thoroughly but gently; do not vortex.

5. Incubate the tubes loosely capped at 37°C in the CO_2 incubator.

6. After the 60-min incubation, remove the tubes and perform a CASA analysis on each sperm population for the level of hyperactivated motility being expressed.
   Note: Remember to mix each tube thoroughly before taking the aliquots for making the CASA preparations. Do not mix too vigorously because this will cause frothing due to the high HSA content of the medium; do not vortex.

7. Once the CASA analyses have been completed discard the tubes.

Calculations and results

No calculations are required for this specific procedure. The "% hyperactivation" (%HA) reported by the IVOS is the proportion of the motile spermatozoa in the sample that demonstrated movement characteristics indicative of hyperactivated motility.

Report both the spontaneous (control) level of hyperactivation as well as the agonist-induced HAmax value. In those men who show rapid capacitation the spontaneous value might exceed the HAmax value (which can be reduced in cases of "burn-out" caused by the powerful agonists employed). The higher value is taken as the maximum likely level of hyperactivation typical of the sperm population assayed.

Interpretation guidelines and notes

1. Normal result: Control shows >20% spontaneous HA and HAmax >50%. Suitable for any form of treatment.

2. Good result: Spontaneous HA and HAmax >20%. Recommended treatment options would be natural intercourse or IUI (with or without ovarian stimulation) or IVF (unless otherwise contraindicated).

3. Low result: Spontaneous HA <20% and/or HAmax <20%. Recommended treatment options would be IUI (with or without ovarian stimulation), but if no pregnancy ensues after 3 cycles then proceed directly to ICSI.

4. Abnormal results: Spontaneous HA <20% and HAmax <10%; or if the results diverge by >20–30%. Recommended treatment option is ICSI.

   Note: Treatment option decisions must only be made by a medical infertility specialist with particular expertise in andrology.

Acrosome reaction testing

Principle

Because the fertilizing spermatozoon undergoes its acrosome reaction (AR) on the surface of the zona pellucida (ZP) in response to binding to the putative sperm receptor, the zona glycoprotein ZP3, studies of the spontaneous AR have little positive predictive value for clinical applications. Because human zonae are so scarce, the true physiological inducer of the AR cannot be used in diagnostic laboratory practice, and biologically active recombinant human ZP3 (rhuZP3) is still not yet available commercially. As a result, various assay protocols exist that employ biological agonists or inducers of the AR, with human follicular fluid (hFF), a calcium ionophore (most usually A23187), or progesterone being used most often [1]. Pentoxifylline does not itself induce the human sperm AR, but rather it sensitizes the response to calcium ionophore in cases where the sperm show poor responsiveness to A23187. Unfortunately, hFF is impossible to standardize for long-term or multi-center use as an agonist in this assay.

Good correlations have been found between the response of human spermatozoa to calcium ionophore and their fertilizing ability [24], and a modification of the original ARIC test (whose practical usefulness has been confirmed by numerous workers) is currently recommended [1].

Specimen

Liquefied semen collected, ideally, at the laboratory after a 3-day period of prior sexual abstinence. A semen analysis should be performed on the specimen.

Equipment (see also Appendix 2)

- As for semen analysis
- As for sperm preparation using DGC
- Air-displacement pipetter, 10 μl, 200 μl and 1000 μl capacities
- Analytical balance
- CO_2 incubator, operating at 6.0% CO_2-in-air if close to sea level. If a CO_2 incubator is not available then gas the tubes with pre-mixed gas containing 6.0% CO_2, cap them tightly and mix by inversion to equilibrate with the gas, and place the tubes in a 37°C incubator with an air atmosphere
- Fluorescence microscope equipped with the appropriate filter set for the particular acrosome probe used

Disposable materials

- As for semen analysis
- As for sperm preparation using DGC
- Falcon #2003 culture tubes
- 0.5-ml Eppendorf tubes

Reagents

1. A23187 stock: Dissolve 5 mg of A23187 (Sigma C5149) in 4.775 ml DMSO (Sigma D8779) to give a 2 mM stock solution. Store frozen at $-20°C$ in small aliquots in 0.5-ml Eppendorf tubes. Cover the tubes in aluminum foil to protect the A23187 from exposure to light.

2. ARIC reagent: Add stock A23187 to the "sperm medium" (see below) in a ratio of 1 : 200, i.e. to give a final concentration of 10 μM A23187 and 0.1% (v/v) DMSO.

3. Sperm medium: A bicarbonate-based (not HEPES-buffered) "sperm medium" that supports human sperm capacitation should include at least 10 mg/ml HSA (ideally Sydney IVF Fertilization Medium, Cook Medical, see www.cookmedical.com).

4. Fixative: Either 25% v/v glutaraldehyde (e.g. Sigma G6257) or absolute ethanol.

Calibration

None required.

Quality control

- A positive control sample (i.e. semen from a control donor who has known ARIC response) must be run each time the test is performed
- Each new batch of probe must be verified by using it in parallel with the previous batch on a positive control specimen

Procedure

1. Prepare a selected motile population of spermatozoa using a standardized 2-layer discontinuous density gradient method (see Chapter 7) in sperm medium at 1×10^6 motile spermatozoa/ml.

2. Label two small Falcon #2003 culture tubes with the patient's name, the Andrology Lab Accession Number and the date, and either ARIC control or ARIC.

3. Transfer 1.0 ml of the washed sperm preparation into each tube.

4. Incubate the tubes loosely capped at $37°C$ in the CO_2 incubator.

5. a. To the ARIC control tube add 5 μl of DMSO.

   b. To the ARIC test tube add 5 μl of the ARIC reagent.

   c. Mix thoroughly but gently; do not vortex.

6. Incubate both tubes for a further 15 min in the CO_2 incubator.

7. Remove a small aliquot from each tube and assess for sperm motility before stopping the effect of the ARIC reagent by adding 200 μl of fixative.

   Notes:

   a. Remember to mix each tube thoroughly – but not too vigorously – before taking the aliquots for motility assessment; do not vortex.

   b. Mix the tubes thoroughly again after adding the fixative; gentle vortex mixing is acceptable with fixed spermatozoa.

8. Prepare slides from the fixed sperm suspensions for staining using whichever probe has been selected.

9. Examine the preparations under epifluorescence and assess the proportion of acrosome-reacted spermatozoa according to the appropriate criteria for the probe being used (Figure 5.3; see color plate section). Count at least 100 spermatozoa per slide.

Figure 5.3 See color plate section. Photomicrographs of the same field of spermatozoa following agonist treatment to induce the acrosome reaction under either phase contrast optics (right panel) or epifluorescence for FITC-labeled PNA lectin (left panel). Note the fluorescent labeling over the equatorial segment of the acrosome denoting the acrosome-reacted status.

Calculations and results

1. a. Calculate the percentage of "acrosome-reacted spermatozoa" (AR+ve) in the Control and ARIC populations using the total numbers of spermatozoa counted in the replicate preparations.

   b. The ARIC value for each specimen is calculated as: ARIC AR+ve % – Control AR+ve %.

2. Two types of AR pathology can be defined from ARIC tests: "AR insufficiency" and "AR prematurity."

   a. AR prematurity: >20% of spermatozoa show spontaneous ARs after 3 h of incubation under capacitating conditions.

   b. AR insufficiency: <10% ARs inducible by ionophore treatment above the spontaneous background, indicating a likely impairment of fertilizing ability; 10–15% is a gray area, indicating a risk of sperm dysfunction.

   c. Normal result: >15% ARs inducible by ionophore treatment above the spontaneous background.

3. If the sperm motility is significantly lower in the ARIC sample compared to the Control, then this must be reported as a likely confounding factor for interpreting the results. Sperm death can be confirmed if the AR staining method includes assessment of sperm vitality.

Interpretation guidelines

1. Approximately 5% of infertility patients have an AR problem, about half have AR insufficiency and half have AR prematurity [1].

2. Both AR prematurity and AR insufficiency are good indicators of a likely clinical problem: a poor ARIC test result is a strong indicator of poor sperm fertilizing ability at IVF (although a good ARIC result does not necessarily indicate the absence of any problem with the physiological AR). The ARIC score has been reported to be a better predictor of pregnancy during IUI treatment than conventional semen characteristics [25].

3. Both problems can be treated by ICSI because there is no apparent relationship between AR function and ICSI outcome.

4. Given the overall prevalence of such problems, one cannot propose AR studies as an upfront diagnostic test such as semen analysis, although automation of test scoring, and simplified protocols using rhuZP3, might make such testing more amenable to routine clinical use in the future.

5. Extensive studies have demonstrated that the zona-induced acrosome reaction or "ZIAR" is an interesting assessment of sperm functional potential [26,27] which has been further correlated with sperm morphology [28,29]. However, the difficulty of running this assay in routine andrology laboratories continues to hinder its wider application and acceptance into routine pre-treatment evaluation.

Notes

The standardized ARIC test protocol provided above is based on the consensus protocol from the ESHRE Special Interest Group in Andrology [1], and has also been promoted by the WHO [30]. Their particular criteria were:

1. Spermatozoa must be separated from seminal plasma using a non-deleterious preparation method and suspended in a bicarbonate-based culture medium capable of supporting capacitation, supplemented with at least 10 mg/ml albumin (preferably HSA).

2. Pre-incubate the prepared sperm suspension under capacitating conditions for 3 h. While pre-incubation is not essential for responsiveness to A23187, it improves reproducibility and allows for the simultaneous assessment of spontaneous acrosome loss (i.e. AR prematurity).

3. Assess acrosomal status before and after a rather standard ionophore treatment of 10 μM A23187 for 15 min.

4. Given the extensive studies validating various techniques for visualizing the human sperm acrosome, either lectins (e.g. peanut, *Arachis hypogea*, or pea, *Pisum sativum* agglutinins, i.e. PNA or PSA), monoclonal antibodies, or the triple stain may be employed as probes for the acrosome reaction status of human spermatozoa [31,32,33,34]. Replicate (minimum two) slides must be scored for each determination, with at least 100 spermatozoa counted per slide.

5. A vitality assessment should be included to differentiate post-mortem acrosomal degeneration or loss from a true acrosome reaction unless the labeling technique gives an "equatorial segment only" pattern, which is typical of a true AR and rarely seen with degenerative acrosome loss. This information is very important if many spermatozoa die during the ARIC treatment step. Exclusion of the fluorescent dye Hoechst 33258 is preferred over a hypo-osmotic swelling (HOS)-type test [31,34].

6. As with any bioassay, a positive control sample is mandatory in each assay run, although a negative control is not essential. The positive control need not necessarily be from a proven fertile donor (although this is preferred), but it must be from a man proven to have a normal response in the test. Because cryopreservation alters sperm membranes, fresh semen must be used for the positive control.

Sperm–zona binding tests

Background

Sperm binding to the zona pellucida (ZP) is an essential recognition stage in the Eutherian fertilization process. After penetrating the cumulus oophorus, spermatozoa bind tightly to the zona pellucida through the ZP3 receptors present on the zona pellucida, which induces a signal transduction cascade within the spermatozoon, leading to the acrosome reaction. Acrosome-reacted spermatozoa are then considered to bind to another zona protein (ZP2) facilitating penetration of the zona matrix and progression into the perivitelline space. Much of the species-specificity of human fertilization occurs at the level of sperm–zona pellucida interaction, including induction of the physiological acrosome reaction in the fertilizing spermatozoon, which has led to great interest in the development of tests to assess sperm binding to the human zona pellucida [1].

Two types of sperm–zona pellucida binding test have been described in the literature. The original hemizona assay test made use of the two halves of a bisected oocyte, one as the test and the other half as the internal control [35,36]. In the second type of test, called the intact zona-binding assay [37], intact zonae are used, and these are exposed to sperm for the test subject and the control on the same oocytes. Zona binding tests assess tight sperm binding to the zona as the primary endpoint, and have a high predictive value for in-vitro fertilization in prospectively designed studies, as well as a high capacity for identifying male factor cases at risk for failed or poor fertilization, indicating the multiple sperm functions necessary for successful fertilization, of which many can be indicated by sperm morphology [1,38,39].

Materials – zonae pellucidae

Sources: Zonae pellucidae (ZPs) are from human oocytes and can be obtained from the following sources [40]:

1. Post-mortem derived ovaries: It is important that all applicable ethical and legal guidelines are followed. Ovarian oocytes can be obtained by macerating ovarian tissue in a Petri dish containing any culture medium used for human IVF. After the mincing of the tissue the fluid is examined under a stereozoom microscope and the oocytes, mostly immature, are collected by means of a small-bore pipette.

2. Inseminated but non-fertilized IVF oocytes: These are oocytes not showing any evidence of either two pronuclei or cleavage at 48–60 h post-insemination. After removal of any remaining cumulus cells by repeated pipetting using a fine glass pipette, they can be transferred into storage.

3. Recycled hemizonae: From the hemizona assay (see below).

Storage: ZPs can be stored in any of three ways:

1. Salt storage: A solution of 1.5 M $MgCl_2$, 0.01% polyvinylpyrrolidone (average MW = 40 000, e.g. Sigma PVP-40) and 40 mM HEPES buffer. Usually employed as 0.5 ml in an Eppendorf tube containing 10–30 oocytes.

2. Ammonium sulfate solution: Usually stored as 15–30 oocytes in 1 ml of a 1 M ammonium sulfate solution in a cryotube for 2–8 weeks.

3. DMSO: 2 M DMSO in PBS. 10–30 oocytes in this solution are loaded into a cryopreservation straw and the ends sealed, e.g. Critoseal haematocrit putty (Fisher Scientific) for polyethylene terephthalate glycol (PETG) straws. Straws are immediately frozen at –70°C and can be stored for 1–6 months before use.

The hemizona assay (HZA)

Principle
In this technique the zonae are bisected prior to use so that the halves can be used in parallel for patient spermatozoa and a matched control.

Specimens
- *Sperm preparations:* Two sperm samples are involved in the hemizona assay (HZA); one sample is obtained from a previously tested fertile male whose sperm–zona binding capacity is known (control) and a second semen sample is from the patient whose sperm–zona binding potential is to be evaluated (test). Motile sperm preparations are prepared as described in Chapter 7, and finally resuspended in a bicarbonate-buffered medium capable of supporting sperm capacitation (e.g. IVF medium) and adjusted to a concentration of 5×10^5 motile spermatozoa per ml
- *Zonae pellucidae:* ZPs stored using either technique are washed using 4×1-ml changes of the same culture medium as will be used for the assay over a period of 4 h at 37°C. Each oocyte is micro-bisected into two matching hemizonae using either a micromanipulation technique (preferred), manual cutting under high power stereozoom magnification, or by a laser procedure

Equipment (see also Appendix 2)
- As for standard semen analysis
- As for sperm preparation using density gradients
- Inverted microscope with 10× and 40× phase contrast objectives and micromanipulation arm
- CO_2 incubator, operating at 6.0% CO_2-in-air if close to sea level. If a CO_2 incubator is not available then gas the tubes with pre-mixed gas containing 6.0% CO_2, cap them tightly and mix by inversion to equilibrate with the gas, and place the tubes in a 37°C incubator with an air atmosphere
- Air-displacement pipette, 100 μl

Disposable materials
- As for standard semen analysis
- As for sperm preparation using density gradients
- Small and large Petri dishes (Falcon #3001 and #3003)
- Glass Pasteur pipettes
- Conical 15-ml tubes (e.g. Falcon #2095)
- Culture oil

Reagents
Sperm medium: A bicarbonate-based (not HEPES-buffered) "sperm medium" that supports human sperm capacitation; should include at least 10 mg/ml HSA.

Calibration

None required.

Quality control

The HZA incorporates an internal control by comparing the patient and positive control (sperm donor) results on matched hemizonae.

Procedure

1. For each assay, prepare:

   a. A 60-mm Petri dish with two 50-μl droplets of sperm suspensions, one from the test patient, and the other from the control donor, and cover with oil.

   b. Another Petri dish with two 50-μl droplets of medium only under oil.

2. Transfer the matching hemizonae, one into each of the sperm droplets.

3. Co-incubate the spermatozoa and hemizonae at 37°C under an appropriate CO_2-in-air atmosphere for 4 h.

   Note: Put the second dish into the CO_2 incubator to equilibrate alongside the assay dish.

4. Rinse each hemizona separately using clean medium by gently pipetting 4–6× through a finely-drawn micropipette (100 μm diameter) to dislodge all loosely attached spermatozoa and transfer it into the correct medium droplet in the second dish.

5. Hold the rinsed hemizonae in the culture medium droplets under oil until examination (within 1 h).

6. Using phase contrast microscopy at 400× magnification, count the number of spermatozoa that are tightly bound to each hemizona (Figure 5.4).

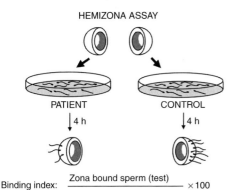

HEMIZONA ASSAY

PATIENT   CONTROL

4 h   4 h

Binding index: $\dfrac{\text{Zona bound sperm (test)}}{\text{Zona bound sperm (control)}} \times 100$

Figure 5.4 Diagrammatic illustration of the principle of the hemizona assay for studying human sperm-zona pellucida binding. (Courtesy of Dr. Franken, Department of Obstetrics & Gynaecology, University of Stellenbosch, Tygerberg Hospital, Tygerberg 7505, South Africa.)

Calculations and results

The HZA result, the "hemizona index" (HZI), is calculated from the absolute numbers of tightly bound sperm for each of test and control hemizonae as follows:

$$\text{HZI} = \frac{\text{Number of tightly-bound spermatozoa for the patient test}}{\text{Number of tightly-bound spermatozoa for the control}} \times 100\%$$

Interpretation guidelines

Clinical studies indicated a cut-off value of $\geq36\%$ as prognostic for IVF fertilization. With an HZI $\leq35\%$ the chances for poor IVF fertilization *in vitro* are 90–100%, whereas the chances for fertilization are 80–85% with an HZI $>35\%$. The observed false-positive rate is less than 15%. For further information see [40].

Notes

Indirect sperm–zona binding test at IVF

The ESHRE consensus workshop on advanced diagnostic andrology recommended that, in cases of total fertilization failure at IVF, the oocytes should be examined for the presence of spermatozoa bound to the zona pellucida [1]. Absence of zona-bound spermatozoa may indicate a sperm-binding defect. Although not as reliable as a sperm–zona binding test, this procedure will at least provide an indication as for the reason for the failure of fertilization and may be the only source of information as sperm–zona binding tests are not readily available in most laboratories, mainly due to lack of oocytes.

Standardization of sperm–zona binding tests

The hemizona assay and competitive sperm–zona binding tests both provide highly comparable results, confirming that sperm–zona binding tests are good predictors of both invitro fertilization and non-fertilization results. To better standardize both tests, and make the results even more comparable, the ESHRE consensus workshop proposed the following general guidelines [1]:

1. A protein-supplemented, bicarbonate-based, IVF culture medium should be used to resuspend selected (isolated) motile spermatozoa to a concentration of 100 000–250 000/ml. Patient and control donor preparations should be at the same motile sperm concentration.

2. Co-incubation of spermatozoa and zonae should take place in a drop of culture medium (e.g. 100 μl) under oil for 4 h at 37°C in an appropriate CO_2-enriched atmosphere.

3. After co-incubation with the spermatozoa, zonae should be washed thoroughly, after which the number of tightly bound spermatozoa is counted on the entire surface of the (hemi-)zona to avoid any skewing of results due to heterogeneous distribution of spermatozoa.

4. Results can be expressed as a percentage index of the test results relative to the control results.

5. Zona-intact oocytes intended for binding tests should preferably be stored in a hypertonic salt solution able to preserve the sperm-binding capacity of the zona pellucida for up to at least three months.

The competitive (intact) sperm–zona binding assay

Principle

In this method, the patient (test) and control (donor) sperm populations are labeled with different fluorochromes and then incubated together with the ZPs [37].

Specimens

- *Sperm preparations:* Two sperm samples are involved in the hemizona assay; one sample is obtained from a previously tested fertile male whose sperm–zona binding capacity is known (control), and a second semen sample is from the patient whose sperm–zona binding potential is to be evaluated (test). Motile sperm preparations are prepared as described in Chapter 7, in a bicarbonate-buffered medium capable of supporting sperm capacitation (e.g. IVF medium) and adjusted to a concentration of 5×10^5 motile spermatozoa per ml

- *Zonae pellucidae:* ZPs stored using either technique are washed using 4×1-ml changes of the same culture medium, as will be used for the assay over a period of 4 h at 37°C

Equipment (see also Appendix 2)

- As for standard semen analysis
- As for sperm preparation using density gradients
- Inverted microscope with 160× or 250× phase contrast magnification
- CO_2 incubator, operating at 6.0% CO_2-in-air if close to sea level. If a CO_2 incubator is not available then gas the tubes with pre-mixed gas containing 6.0% CO_2, cap them tightly and mix by inversion to equilibrate with the gas, and place the tubes in a 37°C incubator with an air atmosphere
- Air-displacement pipette, 100 µl

Disposable materials

- As for standard semen analysis
- As for sperm preparation using density gradients
- Small and large plastic Petri dishes (Falcon #3001 and #3003)
- Glass Pasteur pipettes
- Glass microcapillary pipettes, inner diameter 250 µm
- Conical 15-ml test tubes (e.g. Falcon #2095)
- Culture oil

Reagents

1. Sperm medium: A bicarbonate-based (not HEPES-buffered) "sperm medium" that supports human sperm capacitation should include at least 10 mg/ml HSA.

2. PBS+glucose: Dulbecco's phosphate buffered saline (PBS) containing 55 mM glucose. Filter sterilize through 0.22 µm membrane filter (e.g. Millipore Millex-GV) and store at +4°C for up to 1 month. Discard if there are any signs of precipitation or cloudiness.

3. Fluorescein isothiocyanate (FITC) label: Dissolve 1.0 mg of fluorescein isothiocyanate (FITC, Sigma F7250) in 0.1 ml of a 100 mM aqueous solution of KOH, and dilute within 15 s to 5 ml with sterile PBS+glucose. Store at 4°C in a Falcon #2003 tube wrapped in aluminum foil for up to 1 week.

4. Tetramethylrhodamine B isothiocyanate (TRITC) label: Dissolve 0.5 mg of tetramethylrhodamine B isothiocyanate (TRITC, Sigma T3163) in 0.1 ml of a 100 mM aqueous

solution of KOH, and dilute within 15 s to 5 ml with sterile PBS+glucose. Store at 4°C in a Falcon #2003 tube wrapped in aluminum foil for up to 1 week.

Calibration
None required.

Quality control
The assay incorporates an internal control by combining the fluorescently labeled patient and positive control (donor) spermatozoa, which are then tested on the same ZPs.

Procedure
1. Fluorochrome labeling of spermatozoa (based on [37]). For each sperm preparation:
   a. Centrifuge an aliquot of the washed sperm preparation at 600 g for 5 min. Carefully remove and discard the supernatant then resuspend the pellet in 0.3 ml of the appropriate fluorochrome labeling solutions (e.g. FITC for the patient test sample and TRITC for the control donor).
   b. Incubate at 37°C for 15 min.
   c. Centrifuge the sperm suspensions at 600 g for 5 min to recover the spermatozoa.
   d. Carefully remove and discard the supernatant, then resuspend the pellet in 10 ml of IVF medium.
   e. Centrifuge the sperm suspensions at 600 g for 5 min to recover the spermatozoa.
   f. Carefully remove and discard the supernatant, then resuspend the pellet in IVF medium to a final concentration of 1×10^5 motile spermatozoa per ml with fresh IVF medium.

2. Preparation of co-incubation drops:
   a. In a separate Petri dish for each patient being tested, dispense a number of 25-µl droplets of the labeled patient sperm preparation equal to the number of ZPs to be used in the test.
   b. To each patient sperm drop add 25 µl of the labeled control donor sperm preparation. Change the pipette tip between patients.
   c. Cover the drops with culture oil.
   d. Add a single ZP to each drop. Remember to change the pipette tip between patients.

3. Incubate in a CO_2 incubator at 37°C for 4 h. During this time prepare a small Petri dish with fresh IVF medium for each patient being tested, and put these dishes in the incubator adjacent to the test dishes to equilibrate.

4. Rinse each ZP in the appropriate wash dish by vigorous aspiration in and out of a finely drawn glass pipette to dislodge any loosely attached spermatozoa.

5. Transfer each ZP individually, when ready, onto a clean microscope slide and mount it under a square coverslip supported by four small pillars of high-vacuum silicone grease at its corners; compress the coverslip to flatten the ZP.

6. Examine the mounted ZP at magnification of 160× to 250× under an epifluorescence microscope using separate filter sets to visualize the FITC-labeled (green) and TRITC-labeled (red)

spermatozoa separately (see Appendix 2). Count the total number of each color of spermatozoa bound to the ZP.

7. Repeat steps 5 and 6 for each ZP.

Calculations and results

For each patient test, calculate the total numbers of patient and donor spermatozoa bound to all the ZPs used in that test. The result of each test, the "sperm-binding ratio," is calculated as:

$$\frac{\text{Total number of bound spermatozoa for the patient test ZPs}}{\text{Total number of bound spermatozoa for the donor ZPs}}$$

Interpretation guidelines

A sperm–zona binding ratio of ≥ 0.88 can be regarded as a normal value, in which case an IVF fertilization rate of $>50\%$ can be expected [37].

Notes

See notes for the hemizona assay (above).

Zona-free hamster egg penetration test

Although popular during the 1980s and early 1990s, the "hamster egg penetration test" (HEPT) – often referred to in the US literature as the "sperm penetration assay" (SPA) – is used in very few laboratories nowadays [1]. Since there is still widespread clinical and patient awareness of the test a brief overview has been included here. More extensive reviews and detailed laboratory protocols can be found elsewhere [30,34].

The HEPT is an integrated assessment of the ability of spermatozoa to capacitate *in vitro* and undergo the acrosome reaction, which leaves them in a fusogenic state able to bind to and fuse with the hamster oocyte oolemma. After the sperm head has been incorporated into the oocyte the nucleus decondenses, and visualization of this "swollen sperm head" is the test endpoint (Figure 5.5).

Because of substantial intra- and inter-sample heterogeneity in sperm populations, both in the time required for spermatozoa to undergo capacitation and in their susceptibility to undergoing spontaneous acrosome loss, results from protocols that rely on spontaneous ARs will perforce vary according to pre-incubation conditions. A wide range of protocols were developed employing strategies to induce ARs artificially in more-or-less capacitated sperm populations, including the use of the calcium ionophore A23187 – but with no one having been generally accepted as providing optimum, physiologically meaningful results [1,30,34].

Inconsistent terminology caused substantial confusion in understanding the HEPT's clinical relevance and very few papers reported prospective studies using clinically relevant endpoints such as the achievement of in-vivo conception or in-vitro fertilization. False negative results were common in many early studies based on spontaneous ARs, and false positive results were a persistent problem. General interpretation guidelines for HEPT results were not, therefore, possible; each laboratory had to interpret its results according to its own criteria.

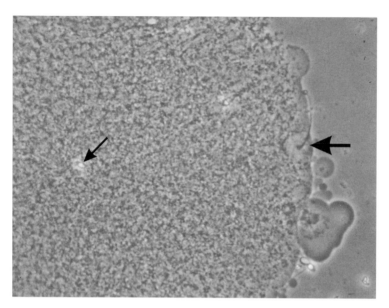

Figure 5.5 Photomicrograph (phase contrast optics) of a zona-free hamster oocyte showing a swollen sperm head (large arrow) denoting that the oocyte had been penetrated during the test. Note the still-attached sperm tail extending in the 12-o'clock direction from the center of the swollen sperm head. The head of a spermatozoon attached to the oolemma is indicated, for comparison of size, by the small arrow.

The ESHRE Special Interest Group in Andrology therefore concluded that, although its value as a research tool for assessing sperm function is unquestioned, the HEPT is not a frontline clinical diagnostic test [1] – a conclusion since echoed by other authorities [41].

Sperm chromatin testing

Principle

The integrity of the paternal genome is of paramount importance in the initiation and maintenance of a viable pregnancy. The presence in the embryonic genome of DNA strand breaks and/or nucleotide modifications coming from the paternal genome, that were not repaired by the oocyte or the embryo after fertilization, is incompatible with normal embryonic and fetal development.

DNA damage in spermatozoa can affect both nuclear and mitochondrial DNA, and can be induced by six main mechanisms: (a) apoptosis during the process of spermatogenesis; (b) DNA strand breaks produced during the remodeling of sperm chromatin during spermiogenesis; (c) post-testicular DNA fragmentation induced mainly by ROS within the male tract; (d) DNA fragmentation caused by endogenous endonucleases; (e) DNA damage caused by radio- and chemotherapy; and (f) damage induced by environmental toxicants [42]. Of these, post-testicular damage during epididymal sperm transport appears to play the major role in causing sperm DNA fragmentation, with ejaculated spermatozoa showing higher DNA fragmentation than epididymal and testicular spermatozoa [43,44,45,46,47].

DNA fragmentation induced by the hydroxyl radical results in the formation of 8-OH-guanine and 8-OH-2′-deoxyguanosine in the first stage and is followed by double-stranded DNA fragmentation thereafter [48]. While DNA damage of the first type could be repaired to some extent by the oocyte, double-stranded DNA damage is virtually irreversible. Since DNA fragmentation values in ejaculated human spermatozoa above 20%, as assessed by the terminal deoxynucleotidyl transferase (TUNEL) test [49], or above 30%, as assessed by the sperm chromatin structure assay (SCSA) test [50], are associated with low pregnancy rates, it might be expected that the remaining spermatozoa could fertilize oocytes and produce viable pregnancies. But, in addition to double-stranded DNA breaks, a significant proportion of all the spermatozoa could have DNA base modifications of the 8-OH-guanine and 8-OH-2'-deoxyguanosine type, resulting in a much lower chance of a spermatozoon with normal DNA achieving fertilization. This concept has been called the "iceberg effect" [50]. DNA damage related to acid- or alkali-labile sites or single-strand DNA breaks, such as those produced during chromatin remodeling, would not be normally expressed after fertilization, since it would require dissociation of both DNA strands during sperm decondensation.

Tests like the SCSA, DNA breakage detection – fluorescence *in situ* hybridization (DBD-FISH) [51], sperm chromatin dispersion (SCD) [52], Chromomycin A3 [53] or Comet assay [54,55] require an initial denaturation step in order to detect measurable DNA fragments or potential breaks in the DNA backbone. In contrast, TUNEL [56], *in situ*-nick translation (ISNT) [56] or Comet under neutral pH conditions [54], do not require a denaturation step, and measure actual single- (ISNT, TUNEL and Comet) and double-stranded (TUNEL and Comet) DNA breaks (see Figure 5.6, see color plate section).

Figure 5.6 See color plate section. Sperm chromatin assessment by TUNEL using fluorescence microscopy. All images are of the same field of spermatozoa: matching images of propidium iodide ("PI" as a general DNA stain; red), FITC (green), and PI+FITC fluorescence, with and without concurrent phase contrast optics, are shown in the left- and right-hand columns, respectively. See text for further explanation of the TUNEL assay. However, it is clear that some spermatozoa are not labeled by either fluorochrome, indicating the origin of possible artifact in this test. (Images courtesy of Madelaine From Björk, Andrology Laboratory, Karolinska University Hospital, Huddinge, Sweden.)

Since the intracellular pH of the oocyte is around 7.0, the susceptibility to DNA fragmentation measured by the first group of tests would be of little or no consequence for pronuclei formation or embryo development, since the sperm DNA strands will not dissociate at neutral pH. Moreover, this type of DNA damage is easily repaired by the oocyte. In contrast, a fertilizing spermatozoon with significant single- or double-stranded DNA damage could severely compromise the developmental potential of the resulting embryo, since this type of damage is virtually irreparable. Consequently, tests that measure real DNA damage will be better predictors of pregnancy than tests that measure potential DNA damage [45,57,58,59] – while tests that measure "potential" DNA damage generally have a very low predictive value [60]. Furthermore, since >90% of DNA consists of non-protein-coding regions or introns, the probability of DNA damage affecting protein-coding regions or exons, is very low – and hence spermatozoa carrying some DNA damage can produce viable pregnancies.

The TUNEL test has been found to have a high predictive value for pregnancy, especially for IUI treatment [57,59], in sharp contrast to the SCD/Halosperm kit, which did not correlate with pregnancy outcome [60]. It must be noted that, although the TUNEL test is frequently used to determine apoptosis in cells, TUNEL positivity is not always synonymous with apoptosis, since hydroxyl radical-induced DNA damage also results in double-stranded DNA fragmentation that is detected by the TUNEL test [61].

Despite the above-noted issues regarding predictive value, the SCSA remains the most robust test, and the one for which most clinical data are available and, indeed, many of the current indications for sperm DNA fragmentation testing were derived from SCSA testing. A low DNA fragmentation index (DFI) result (usually using a cut-off of 30%) is highly predictive for both natural fertility and pregnancy following IUI [62]. In addition, men over 45 have significantly higher levels of DNA fragmentation [63], and men who are homozygous null for glutathione-S-transferase M1 are less able to detoxify metabolites of carcinogenic, polycyclic aromatic hydrocarbons found in air pollution – making them more susceptible to adverse effects of air pollution [42]. This latter issue might explain, at least in part, why sperm DNA fragmentation can occur episodically in some men without an apparent cause [64]. A significant percentage of men with varicoceles have pathological levels of SCSA-measured sperm DNA fragmentation, which decrease significantly after varicocelectomy in as many as 65% of cases [65].

To summarize:

- While the presence of acid- or alkali-labile DNA breaks in the paternal genome above a critical threshold may not necessarily lead to failed pregnancy after ART, the presence of extensive double-stranded DNA breaks and high levels of 8-OH-guanine and 8-OH-2'-deoxyguanosine (as produced after hydroxyl radical-induced damage during sperm transit through the male tract) could severely compromise embryo development

- Even if there is significant sperm DNA damage, the probability for a viable pregnancy depends on: (a) the proportion of sperm with damaged DNA; (b) the extent of DNA fragmentation per cell; (c) the level of 8-OH-guanine and 8-OH-2'-deoxyguanosine in sperm DNA; (d) the type of DNA regions that are damaged (introns vs. exons); (e) the ability of the zygote and embryo to repair the damage; (f) the number of oocytes available; (g) the methodology used for processing the spermatozoa for IVF/ICSI, which should always follow the basic principle of *primum non nocere*; and (h) the type of test used to measure DNA fragmentation

- Some of these factors cannot be measured, e.g. whether the DNA damage affects exons or introns, or whether it was repaired by the oocyte and/or the embryo

- Although the combined assessment of sperm DNA fragmentation and nucleotide modifications might improve the predictive value of current tests for sperm DNA damage (especially those measuring double-stranded DNA breaks), tests to measure 8-OH-guanine and 8-OH-2'-deoxyguanosine are not yet available for application in a clinical setting

Consequently, the predictive value of sperm DNA fragmentation tests will always be subject to uncertainty, and cannot have a 100% negative predictive value, as was originally suggested by the "iceberg effect" model [50].

Given its high predictive value and the commercial availability of a test kit, the TUNEL test is therefore currently recommended for measuring sperm DNA fragmentation in routine laboratory use. Although the recommended mode of analysis is by flow cytometry, procedures for fluorescence, and light microscopy assessment are also provided.

The main *indications* for sperm DNA fragmentation testing are:

1. Idiopathic infertility.
2. Repeated pregnancy failure in IVF without an apparent cause.
3. Recurrent miscarriage.
4. Previous treatment with chemo- and/or radiotherapy.
5. Recent episode of high fever.
6. Clinical varicocele (grades 2 and 3).
7. Male age above 45 years.

TUNEL test for sperm DNA damage

Specimens

- An aliquot of liquefied, well-mixed semen from a specimen provided for semen analysis (see Chapter 3). At least 10 million spermatozoa are required for the assay

Equipment (see also Appendix 2)

- Air-displacement pipettes, 1–1000 μl
- Vortex mixer
- Microcentrifuge, for 1.5-ml Eppendorf tubes
- Either:
  a. Microscope with either epifluorescence and phase contrast optics or bright-field and phase contrast optics as per the intended assessment technique; or
  b. Flow cytometer.

Disposable materials

- 15-ml Falcon conical centrifuge tubes with caps
- Serological pipettes, 1 ml, 2 ml, 10 ml
- 1.5-ml Eppendorf tubes

Reagents

1. For each assay, prepare PBS solution: Dulbecco's phosphate buffered saline (e.g. PBS-1X; Irvine Scientific, cat.no. 9235).
2. Fixation solution: Paraformaldehyde (Sigma-Aldrich cat.no. P6148) at 4% (w/v) in PBS, pH 7.4, freshly prepared.
3. Permeabilization solution: 0.1% (v/v) Triton X-100 (Sigma-Aldrich ref. X100–100ML, cat.no. 066K0089) dissolved in 0.1% (w/v) sodium citrate in PBS, freshly prepared.
4. Labeling solution: TUNEL enzyme kit, Roche Diagnostics cat.no. 1168479910:
   a. Solution 1 = TUNEL enzyme solution
   b. Solution 2 = TUNEL label solution
5. Positive control reagent: DNAase I solution (Roche Diagnostics, cat.no. 09536282001).
6. Anti-fluorescein antibody: Fab fragment from sheep conjugated with horse-radish peroxidase (Roche Diagnostics, cat.no. 1684817).
7. Diaminobenzidine substrate: DAB substrate (Roche Diagnostics cat.no. 1718096).

Calibration

None required beyond ensuring that the flow cytometer is in proper working order.

Quality control

1. For IQC, run duplicates of each sample (test sample, positive, and negative control). Duplicates should be within 5% for flow cytometry, and within 10% for fluorescence and bright-field microscopy.

2. For EQC, send aliquots of fixed samples to a reference laboratory for analysis by TUNEL/ flow cytometry. Values at both laboratories should be within 10% for flow cytometry and within 15% for fluorescence and bright-field microscopy.

Procedure: TUNEL procedure

1. Specimen preparation:

   a. Take an aliquot of the liquefied semen sample that contains a total of 10×10^6 spermatozoa and place it in a 15-ml Falcon centrifuge tube.

   b. Add 2 volumes of PBS and centrifuge at 300 g for 10 min.

   c. Discard the supernatant and resuspend the pellet in 500 μl of PBS.

   d. Centrifuge at 300 g for 10 min.

   e. Discard the supernatant and resuspend the pellet in 100 μl of PBS.

2. Transfer the 100 μl of washed sperm suspension into a 1.5-ml Eppendorf tube.

3. Add 200 μl of PBS and mix thoroughly.

4. Centrifuge in Eppendorf microcentrifuge at 300 g for 2 min.

5. Discard the supernatant and resuspend the pellet in 200 μl of PBS.

6. Add 200 μl of fixation solution (final concentration of paraformaldehyde = 2%).

7. After incubation, add 200 μl of PBS to stop the fixation process. At this point, the sample can be stored at +4°C until further analysis.

8. Divide the fixed sample into 3 aliquots and transfer each into a different Eppendorf tube:

   a. test sample;

   b. positive control;

   c. negative control.

9. Centrifuge at 300 g for 2 min.

10. Discard the supernatant and resuspend the pellet in 200 μl of PBS.

11. Centrifuge at 300 g for 2 min.

12. Discard the supernatant and resuspend the pellet a second time in 200 μl of PBS.

13. Centrifuge at 300 g for 2 min.

14. Discard the supernatant and resuspend the pellet in 100 μl of permeabilization solution.

15. Incubate at +4°C for 2 min.

16. Add 300 μl of PBS and centrifuge at 300 g for 2 min.

17. Prepare the TUNEL reaction mixture by adding 10 μl of Solution 1 (TUNEL enzyme solution) to 90 μl of Solution 2 (TUNEL label solution).

18. Discard the supernatant from the positive control tube, and resuspend the pellet in 100 μl of DNAase I, and incubate at 15–25°C for 10 min.

19. Negative control and test sample:

   a. Discard the supernatants from the tubes.

   b. Test sample tube: Add 50 μl of the TUNEL reaction mixture.

   c. Negative control tube: Add 50 μl of TUNEL Solution 2 (TUNEL label solution) *only*.

20. Positive control tube: Add 50 μl of the TUNEL reaction mixture.

21. Incubate all the tubes at 37°C for 60 min in the dark (e.g. inside an incubator).

22. Add 300 μl of PBS to each tube and centrifuge at 300 g for 2 min.

23. Discard the supernatants and resuspend each pellet in 300 μl of PBS, then centrifuge again at 300 g for 2 min.

Proceed to the appropriate section below for the analysis method being employed.

Procedure: TUNEL analysis by flow cytometry

24. Discard the supernatants and resuspend the pellets in 500 μl of PBS.

25. Keep at +4°C in the dark until analysis by flow cytometry.

26. The following flow cytometry parameters are for a Becton Dickinson FACScan instrument (Becton Dickinson). Light scattering and fluorescence data are obtained at a fixed gain setting in logarithmic mode. Green fluorescence from FITC is detected in the FL1 sensor using a 550 nm dichroic long-pass filter and 525 nm band-pass filter. A minimum of 10 000 spermatozoa are analyzed per determination.

Procedure: TUNEL analysis by fluorescence microscopy

(See Figure 5.6 in color plate section)

24. Discard the supernatants and resuspend the pellets in 50 μl of PBS.

25. Keep at +4°C in the dark until analysis.

26. Smear on slide and place coverslip on top.

27. Set up the epifluorescence microscope for FITC: excitation wavelength in the range of 450 to 500 nm (e.g. 488 nm), and detection wavelength in the range of 515 to 565 nm.

28. Assess each slide according to the following procedure:

    a. Pick a field at random and, under epifluorescence, count the number of fluorescent spermatozoa in the field.

    b. Change to phase contrast optics and count the total number of spermatozoa in the field.

    c. Tally the results.

    d. Repeat steps 28a–c for different randomly selected fields until at least 200 (and preferably 500) spermatozoa have been counted by phase contrast microscopy.

Notes:

1. The numbers of spermatozoa counted in the negative control and test sample must be the same.

2. The proportion of fluorescent spermatozoa in the positive control should be in the range 95–100%.

Procedure: TUNEL analysis by bright-field microscopy

24. Discard the supernatants and resuspend the pellets in 50 μl of PBS.

25. Smear 50 μl of the sperm suspension on a clean microscope slide and air dry for 10 min.

26. Add 50 µl of the anti-fluorescein antibody solution.

27. Incubate in a humidified chamber at 37°C for 30 min.

28. Rinse each slide with 100 µl of PBS. Repeat this step twice more.

29. Add 50 µl of DAB substrate to each slide.

30. Wait 2 min at ambient temperature.

31. Place a 24 × 60 mm pre-cleaned coverslip on the slide.

32. Assess each slide according to the following procedure:

   a. Pick a field at random and, under bright-field (Köhler) illumination, count the number of DAB-stained spermatozoa in the field.

   b. Change to phase contrast optics and count the total number of spermatozoa in the field.

   c. Tally the results.

   d. Repeat steps 32a–c for different randomly selected fields until at least 200 (and preferably 500) spermatozoa have been counted by phase contrast microscopy.

Notes:

1. The numbers of spermatozoa counted in the negative control and test sample must be the same.

2. The proportion of DAB-stained spermatozoa in the positive control should be in the range 95–100%.

Calculations and results

1. Fluorescence microscopy: Subtract the number of fluorescent spermatozoa in the negative control (F_c) from the number of fluorescent spermatozoa in the test sample (F_s), divide by the total number of spermatozoa counted by phase contrast microscopy (N), and multiply by 100 to give the test result as a percentage:

$$\text{Test result}(\%) = [(F_s - F_c)/N] \times 100$$

2. Bright-field microscopy: Subtract the number of DAB-stained spermatozoa in the negative control (D_c) from the number of DAB-stained spermatozoa in the test sample (D_s), divide by the total number of spermatozoa counted by phase contrast microscopy (N), and multiply by 100 to give the test result as a percentage:

$$\text{Test result}(\%) = [(D_s - D_c)/N] \times 100$$

3. Flow cytometry: A minimum of 10 000 events are examined for each measurement at a flow rate of about 200 events/s on a Becton Dickinson FACScan instrument. Green fluorescence (TUNEL-positive cells) is measured using a 550 nm band-pass filter. Spermatozoa obtained in the plots are gated by using forward-angle light scatter (FSC) and side-angle light scatter (SSC) dot plot to gate out debris aggregates and other non-sperm cells. Data are processed using Becton Dickinson's CELLSOFT software and WinMDI (Windows Multiple Document Interface for Flow Cytometry) software. TUNEL-positive spermatozoa in the populations are measured in the corresponding histogram.

Interpretation guidelines

Normal values: <20% TUNEL-positive spermatozoa.
Abnormal values: >20% TUNEL-positive spermatozoa.

Notes

None.

Sperm survival assay

Principle

Assessments of human sperm survival *in vitro* are carried out for two purposes: (a) as a bioassay for determining the acceptability of culture media and contact materials in an assisted reproductive technology laboratory [66,67]; or (b) in an attempt to evaluate the longevity of a man's spermatozoa [68].

While well-validated protocols are available for the former application (see below), the latter application does raise some intriguing physiological questions. The prolonged incubation of human spermatozoa under capacitating conditions results in their capacitation, followed by a high level of spontaneous acrosome reactions due to the lability of the capacitated spermatozoon; and once having undergone the acrosome reaction the spermatozoa die [69]. Consequently, there is a dilemma as to whether a high sperm survival after a 24-h incubation is "good" or "bad," since in a medium optimized for sperm capacitation, a high proportion of dead spermatozoa after 24 h could be seen as revealing a high physiological response of the man's spermatozoa to the incubation conditions, whereas in a medium that is sub-optimal for sperm capacitation, and/or where the man's spermatozoa respond poorly to the capacitating conditions, a high level of sperm survival would *not* reflect a "good" result. However, notwithstanding this discussion, when a sperm survival test (SST) is carried out as part of an IVF treatment cycle under controlled conditions, it can yield useful information [68] – although that information might not necessarily be transferable to another laboratory using a different culture system.

The method provided below for the QC version of the SST is based on a protocol generously provided by Jieying Laboratory Inc. (Longueuil, Quebec, Canada). It is an optimized method where albumin is omitted from the culture medium so as to increase the sensitivity of the system to spermotoxic substances.

Specimen(s)

Either contact materials or culture media to be tested for sperm toxicity.

Note: The suspension of washed spermatozoa used in the assay is considered to be a reagent (see below), not a specimen.

Equipment

- As for sperm preparation using DGC
- Air-displacement pipetters, 1–20 µl and 1000 µl

- CO_2 incubator, operating at 6.0% CO_2-in-air if close to sea level. If a CO_2 incubator is not available then gas the tubes with pre-mixed gas containing 6.0% CO_2, cap them tightly and mix by inversion to equilibrate with the gas, and place the tubes in a 37°C incubator with an air atmosphere
- Either:
  - Phase contrast compound microscope configured for andrology (see Appendix 2); or
  - CASA instrument (see Chapter 4)
  - Laboratory counter (see Appendix 2)

Disposable materials
- As for semen analysis
- As for sperm preparation using DGC
- Sterile small Falcon culture tubes (#2003 or #2054)
- NUNC 4-well dishes

Reagents
- As for sperm preparation using DGC
- A suspension of washed spermatozoa, at a concentration of 5×10^6 motile spermatozoa/ml, prepared using DGC. (If cryopreserved semen is used, then swim-up can be used as an alternative sperm preparation procedure)
- "Sperm buffer": Any suitable HEPES-buffered sperm washing medium with ≥ 5 mg/ml HSA

Calibration
No calibration is required unless the motility assessments are being made using computer-aided sperm analysis (CASA), in which case the standard CASA calibration requirements must be met (see Chapter 4).

Quality control
Note: All media and contact materials used in the assay must have been tested and certified suitable for assisted conception use, i.e. non-spermotoxic or have passed the mouse embryo bioassay, and be free of endotoxin.

1. Positive control: An aliquot of the prepared sperm suspension in sperm buffer must be run in each assay. To be valid, this control must show >70% progressively motile spermatozoa at the end of the 18- to 24-h assay period. (If using cryopreserved spermatozoa, then the requirement is >40%.)
2. Negative control: An aliquot of the prepared sperm suspension in sperm buffer that has been adulterated with formaldehyde, or some other substance toxic to spermatozoa, must be run in each assay. To be valid, this control must have an SMI <0.50 at the end of the 18- to 24-h assay period.

Procedure: testing contact materials
1. Expose the test material (e.g. a dish or tube) to 0.5 ml of the sperm suspension at 37°C for 5 min.

2. Remove the sperm suspension using a sterile pipette tip, and transfer into a sterile small Falcon tube.

3. Incubate the tube at 37°C under an air atmosphere for 18–24 h.

Procedure: testing culture media

1. For each test medium, centrifuge a 500-μl aliquot of the sperm suspension at 500 $g \times$ 5 min.

2. Resuspend the spermatozoa in 500 μl of the test medium and incubate under the appropriate conditions:

   a. Bicarbonate-buffered media: Transfer the sperm suspension into a sterile NUNC 4-well dish and incubate in a CO_2 incubator (5.0–6.0% CO_2, as appropriate for the medium being tested; see the manufacturer's recommendations). An oil overlay is not necessary if using a Cook K-MINC-1000 mini-incubator.

   b. HEPES-buffered media: Transfer the sperm suspension into a sterile small Falcon tube and incubate in an air incubator.

3. Incubate at 37°C for 18–24 h.

Procedure: sperm motility assessment

1. For each of the positive and negative controls and each test sample preparation:

   a. Mix the sperm suspension thoroughly and take an aliquot to assess the sperm motility either visually (as per Chapter 3) or using CASA (see Chapter 4). Assess at least 200 spermatozoa, and determine the proportion of spermatozoa showing active forward progression.
   Note: For media that do not contain HSA, see Note 1, below.

   b. Repeat the motility assessment.

   c. Verify that the two replicate assessments are in agreement (see Chapter 3). If not, then repeat the assessment.

   d. Calculate the average % progressive motility for each control and test sample.

Calculations and results

The "sperm motility index" (SMI) is derived by dividing the % progressive motility in the test sample at the end of the incubation period by the % progressive motility in the positive control sample at the start of the incubation period.

1. Verify that the positive and negative controls meet the assay QC criteria. If not, then repeat the entire assay.

2. For each test sample, calculate the SMI as the ratio between the test sample's progressive motility and the positive control's progressive motility. For example:

   Test sample: Count A = 130/200; count B = 142/200; difference <10% so results are OK.

$$\text{Progressive motility} = 272/400 = 68\%$$

Positive control: Count A = 165/200; count B = 175/200; difference <10% so results are OK.

$$\text{Progressive motility} = 340/400 = 85\%$$

$$\text{SMI} = 68/85 = 0.80$$

Interpretation guidelines

SMI values <75% are taken to indicate sperm toxicity in the test material.

Therefore, the SMI result shown in the example above indicates that the test specimen passed the test, i.e. it did not show detectable toxicity to human spermatozoa.

Notes

1. Spermatozoa in a test medium that does not contain any HSA will likely show the "sticking-to-glass" phenomenon. In this case, the post-incubation sample must be diluted with an equal volume of Sperm Buffer (ideally containing at least 10 mg/ml of HSA) before analysis.

References

1. ESHRE Andrology Special Interest Group. Consensus workshop on advanced diagnostic andrology techniques. *Hum Reprod* 1996; **11**: 1463–79.
2. Alvarez JG, Storey BT. Spontaneous lipid peroxidation in rabbit epididymal spermatozoa. *Biol Reprod* 1982; **27**: 1102–8.
3. Holland MK, Alvarez JG, Storey BT. Production of superoxide and activity of superoxide dismutase in rabbit epididymal spermatozoa. *Biol Reprod* 1982; **27**: 1109–18.
4. Alvarez JG, Storey BT. Lipid peroxidation and the reactions of superoxide and hydrogen peroxide in mouse spermatozoa. *Biol Reprod* 1984; **30**: 833–41.
5. Alvarez JG, Touchstone JC, Blasco, L, Storey BT. Spontaneous lipid peroxidation and production of hydrogen peroxide and superoxide in human spermatozoa. Superoxide dismutase as major enzyme protectant against oxygen toxicity. *J Androl* 1987; **8**: 338–48.
6. Aitken RJ, Clarkson JS. Cellular basis of defective sperm function and its association with the genesis of reactive oxygen species by human spermatozoa. *J Reprod Fertil* 1987; **81**: 459–69.
7. Alvarez JG, Storey BT. Differential incorporation of fatty acids into and peroxidative loss of fatty acids from phospholipids of human spermatozoa. *Mol Reprod Dev* 1995; **42**: 334–46.
8. Fraga CG, Motchnik PA, Shigenaga MK, et al. Ascorbic acid protects against endogenous oxidative DNA damage in human sperm. *Proc Natl Acad Sci USA* 1991; **88**: 11003–6.
9. Fraga CG, Motchnik PA, Wyrobek AJ, et al. Smoking and low antioxidant levels increase oxidative damage to sperm DNA. *Mutat Res* 1996; **351**: 199–203.
10. Ollero M, Guzman-Gil E, Lopez MC, et al. Characterization of subsets of human spermatozoa at different stages of maturation: implications in the diagnosis and treatment of male infertility. *Hum Reprod* 2001; **16**: 1912–21.
11. Saleh RA, Agarwal A, Kandirali E, et al. Leukocytospermia is associated with increased reactive oxygen species production by human spermatozoa. *Fert Steril* 2002; **78**: 1215–24.
12. Drevet JR. The antioxidant glutathione peroxidase family and spermatozoa: a complex story. *Mol Cell Endocrinol* 2006; **250**: 70–9.

13. Aitken RJ, Gordon E, Harkiss D, et al. Relative impact of oxidative stress on the functional competence and genomic integrity of human spermatozoa. *Biol Reprod* 1998; **59**: 1037–46.

14. Agarwal A, Makker K, Sharma R. Clinical relevance of oxidative stress in male factor infertility: an update. *Am J Reprod Immunol* 2008; **59**: 2–11.

15. Shekarriz M, Thomas AJ Jr., Agarwal A. Incidence and level of seminal reactive oxygen species in normal men. *Urology* 1995; **45**: 103–7.

16. Allamaneni SSR, Agarwal A, Nallela KP, et al. Characterization of oxidative stress status by a simple clinical test: evaluation of reactive oxygen species levels in whole semen and isolated spermatozoa. *Fertil Steril* 2005; **83**: 800–3.

17. Dresdner RD, Katz DF. Relationships of mammalian sperm motility and morphology to hydrodynamic aspects of cell function. *Biol Reprod* 1981; **25**: 920–30.

18. Mortimer ST. A critical review of the physiological importance and analysis of sperm movement in mammals. *Hum Reprod Update* 1997; **3**: 403–39.

19. Mortimer ST, Swan MA. Variable kinematics of capacitating human spermatozoa. *Hum Reprod* 1995; **10**: 3178–82.

20. ESHRE Andrology Special Interest Group. Guidelines on the application of CASA technology in the analysis of spermatozoa. *Hum Reprod* 1998; **13**: 142–5.

21. Mortimer ST. CASA – practical aspects. *J Androl* 2000; **21**: 515–24.

22. Mortimer D, Kossakowski J, Mortimer ST, Fussell S. Prediction of fertilizing ability by sperm kinematics. Abstract OC-05-043. *J Ass Reprod Genet* 1997; **14**(5) Suppl 52S.

23. Mortimer D, Mortimer ST. Laboratory investigation of the infertile male. In: Brinsden PR, ed. *A Textbook of In-Vitro Fertilization and Assisted Reproduction*. 3rd edn. London: Taylor & Francis Medical Books 2005: 61–91.

24. Cummins JM, Pember SM, Jequier AM, et al. A test of the human sperm acrosome reaction following ionophore challenge: relationship to fertility and other seminal parameters. *J Androl* 1991; **12**: 98–103.

25. Makkar G, Ng EH, Yeung WS, et al. The significance of the ionophore-challenged acrosome reaction in the prediction of successful outcome of controlled ovarian stimulation and intrauterine insemination. *Hum Reprod* 2003; **18**: 534–9.

26. Liu DY, Stewart T, Baker HW. Normal range and variation of the zona pellucida-induced acrosome reaction in fertile men. *Fertil Steril* 2003; **80**: 384–9.

27. Liu DY, Baker HW. Disordered zona pellucida-induced acrosome reaction and failure of in vitro fertilization in patients with unexplained infertility. *Fertil Steril* 2003; **79**: 74–80.

28. Bastiaan HS, Menkveld R, Oehninger S, et al. Zona pellucida induced acrosome reaction, sperm morphology, and sperm-zona binding assessments among subfertile men. *J Assist Reprod Genet* 2002; **19**: 329–34.

29. Bastiaan HS, Windt ML, Menkveld R, et al. Relationship between zona pellucida-induced acrosome reaction, sperm morphology, sperm-zona pellucida binding, and in vitro fertilization. *Fertil Steril* 2003; **79**: 49–55.

30. World Health Organization. *WHO Laboratory Manual for the Analysis of Human Semen and Sperm-Cervical Mucus Interaction*. 4th edn. Cambridge, UK: Cambridge University Press 1999.

31. Mortimer D, Curtis EF, Camenzind AR. Combined use of fluorescent peanut agglutinin lectin and Hoechst 33258 to monitor the acrosomal status and vitality of human spermatozoa. *Hum Reprod* 1990; **5**: 99–103.

32. Cross NL, Morales P, Overstreet JW, Hanson FW. Two simple methods for detecting acrosome-reacted human sperm. *Gamete Res* 1986; **15**: 213–26.

33. Talbot P, Chacon R. A new procedure for rapidly scoring acrosome reactions of human sperm. *Gamete Res* 1980; **3**: 211–6.

34. Mortimer D. *Practical Laboratory Andrology*. New York: Oxford University Press 1994.

35. Burkman LJ, Coddington CC, Franken DR, et al. The hemizona assay (HZA): development of a diagnostic test for binding of human spermatozoa to the human zona pellucida to predict fertilization potential. *Fertil Steril* 1988; **49**: 688–93.

36. Franken DR, Oehninger S, Burkman LJ, *et al.* The hemizona assays (HZA): a predictor of human sperm fertilizing potential in in vitro fertilization (IVF) treatment. *J in Vitro Fertil Embryo Transf* 1989; **6**: 44–9.

37. Liu DY, Lopata A, Johnston WIH, Baker HWG. A human sperm-zona pellucida binding test using oocytes that failed to fertilize in vitro. *Fertil Steril* 1988; **50**: 782–8.

38. Franken DR, Kruger TF, Menkveld R, *et al.* Hemizona assay and teratozoospermia: increasing sperm insemination concentrations to enhance zona pellucida binding. *Fertil Steril* 1990; **54**: 497–503.

39. Menkveld R, Franken DR, Kruger TF, *et al.* Sperm selection capacity of the human zona pellucida. *Mol Reprod Dev* 1991; **30**: 346–52.

40. Franken DR, Oehninger S. The clinical significance of sperm-zona pellucida binding: 17 years later. *Front Biosci* 2006; **1**: 1227–33.

41. Oehninger S, Franken DR, Sayed E, *et al.* Sperm function assays and their predictive value for fertilization outcome in IVF therapy: a meta-analysis. *Hum Reprod Update* 2000; **6**: 160–8.

42. Rubes J, Selevan SG, Sram RJ, *et al.* GSTM1 genotype influences the susceptibility of men to sperm DNA damage associated with exposure to air pollution. *Mutat Res* 2007; **625**: 20–8.

43. Steele EK, McClure N, Maxwell RJ, Lewis SE. A comparison of DNA damage in testicular and proximal epididymal spermatozoa in obstructive azoospermia. *Mol Hum Reprod* 1999; **5**: 831–5.

44. Lewis SEM, O'Connell M, Stevenson M, *et al.* An algorithm to predict pregnancy in assisted conception. *Mol Hum Reprod* 2004; **19**: 1385–90.

45. Greco E, Scarselli F, Iacobelli M, *et al.* Efficient treatment of infertility due to sperm DNA damage by ICSI with testicular spermatozoa. *Hum Reprod* 2005; **20**: 226–30.

46. Ollero M, Gil-Guzman E, Lopez MC, *et al.* Characterization of subsets of human spermatozoa at different stages of maturation: implications in the diagnosis and treatment of male infertility. *Hum Reprod* 2001; **16**: 1912–21.

47. Suganuma R, Yanagimachi R, Meistricht M. Decline in fertility of mouse sperm with abnormal chromatin during epididymal passage as revealed by ICSI. *Hum Reprod* 2005; **20**: 3101–8.

48. Cui J, Holmes EH, Greene TG, Liu PK. Oxidative DNA damage precedes DNA fragmentation after experimental stroke in rat brain. *FASEB J* 2000; **14**: 955–67.

49. Sergerie M, Laforest G, Bujan L, *et al.* Sperm DNA fragmentation: threshold value in male fertility. *Hum Reprod* 2005; **20**: 3446–51.

50. Evenson DP, Jost LK, Marshall D, *et al.* Utility of the sperm chromatin structure assay as a diagnostic and prognostic tool in the human fertility clinic. *Hum Reprod* 1999; **14**: 1039–49.

51. Fernandez JL, Vazquez-Gundin F, Delgado A, *et al.* DNA breakage detection-FISH (DBD-FISH) in human spermatozoa: technical variants evidence different structural features. *Mutat Res* 2000; **453**: 77–82.

52. Fernandez JL, Muriel L, Rivero MT, *et al.* The sperm chromatin dispersion test: a simple method for the determination of sperm DNA fragmentation. *J Androl* 2003; **24**: 59–66.

53. Manicardi GC, Bianchi PG, Pantano S, *et al.* Presence of endogenous nicks in DNA of ejaculated human spermatozoa and its relationship to chromomycin A3 accessibility. *Biol Reprod* 1995; **52**: 864–7.

54. Singh N, MacCoy M, Tice R, *et al.* A simple technique for the quantification of low levels of DNA damage in individual cells. *Exp Cell Res* 1998; **15**: 1338–44.

55. Singh N, Danner D, Tice R, *et al.* Abundant alkali-sensitive sites in DNA of human and mouse sperm. *Exp Cell Res* 1989; **184**: 461–70.

56. Gorczyca W, Gong J, Darzynkiewicz Z. Detection of DNA strand breaks in individual apoptotic cells by the in situ terminal deoxynucleotidyl transferase and nick translation assays. *Cancer Res* 1993; **53**: 945–51.

57. Duran EH, Morshedi M, Taylor S, Oehninger S. Sperm DNA quality predicts intrauterine insemination outcome: a prospective cohort study. *Hum Reprod* 2002; **17**: 3122–8.

58. Alvarez JG. Efficient treatment of infertility due to sperm DNA damage by ICSI with testicular spermatozoa. *Hum Reprod* 2005; **20**: 2031–2.

59. Borini A, Tarozzi N, Bizarro D, *et al.* Sperm DNA fragmentation: paternal effect on early post-implantation embryo development in ART. *Hum Reprod* 2006; **21**: 2876–81.

60. Muriel L, Meseguer M, Fernandez JL, *et al.* Value of the sperm chromatin dispersion test in predicting pregnancy outcome in intrauterine insemination: a blind prospective study. *Hum Reprod* 2006; **21**: 738–44.

61. Negoescu A, Guillermet C, Lorimier P, *et al.* Importance of DNA fragmentation in apoptosis with regard to TUNEL specificity. *Biomed Pharmacother* 1998; **52**: 252–8.

62. Evenson DP, Wixon R. Data analysis of two in vivo fertility studies using Sperm Chromatin Structure Assay-derived DNA fragmentation index vs. pregnancy outcome. *Fertil Steril* 2008; **90**: 1229–31.

63. Wyrobek AJ, Eskenazi B, Young S, *et al.* Advancing age has differential effects on DNA damage, chromatin integrity, gene mutations, and aneuploidies in sperm. *Proc Natl Acad Sci* 2006; **103**: 9601–6.

64. Alvarez JG, Ollero M, Larson-Cook KL, Evenson DP. Selecting cryopreserved semen for assisted reproductive techniques based on the level of sperm nuclear DNA fragmentation resulted in pregnancy. *Fertil Steril* 2004; **81**: 712–3.

65. Werthman P, Wixon R, Kasperson K, Evenson DP. Significant decrease in sperm deoxyribonucleic acid fragmentation after varicocelectomy. *Fertil Steril* 2008; **90**: 1800–4.

66. De Jonge CJ, Centola GM, Reed ML, *et al.* Human sperm survival assay as a bioassay for the assisted reproductive technologies laboratory. *J Androl* 2003; **24**: 16–8.

67. Claassens OE, Wehr JB, Harrsion KL. Optimizing sensitivity of the human sperm motility assay for embryo toxicity testing. *Hum Reprod* 2000; **15**: 1586–91.

68. Coccia ME, Becattini C, Criscuoli L, *et al.* A sperm survival test and in-vitro fertilization outcome in the presence of male factor infertility. *Hum Reprod* 1997; **12**: 1969–73.

69. Mortimer D, Curtis EF, Camenzind AR, Tanaka S. The spontaneous acrosome reaction of human spermatozoa incubated in vitro. *Hum Reprod* 1989; **4**: 57–62.

Tests of sperm–cervical mucus interaction

For natural conception *in vivo*, spermatozoa must be deposited at the site of insemination around the external cervical os during the peri-ovulatory period, when the cervical mucus is receptive to penetration by spermatozoa. The penetration of spermatozoa into the cervical mucus, followed by their migration through the mucus column contained within the cervical canal, are the essential first steps in the complex series of events by which spermatozoa traverse the female tract and reach the site of site of fertilization in the ampulla of the oviduct [1,2]. Assessment of sperm–cervical mucus interaction is, therefore, an integral part of the diagnostic work-up of an infertile couple [3], and the most commonly used techniques are described below.

The in-vivo test of sperm–mucus interaction is the "post-coital test" (PCT), which requires sampling the cervical mucus several hours after intercourse performed during the peri-ovulatory period, and examining it for the presence of spermatozoa. While the clinical value of the PCT has long been questioned, it can provide information of predictive value for fertility [4,5].

In-vitro tests of sperm–mucus interaction are derived from two basic techniques: "slide tests" using apposed drops of semen and mucus under coverslips; and "tube" (or "Kremer") tests, where mucus-filled capillary tubes are placed with one end in contact with liquefied semen. Penetration in either system is assessed by counting motile spermatozoa at various distances from the semen–mucus interface at certain times after establishment of this contact [3,4,6].

For physiological and clinical relevance, tests must be performed during the peri-ovulatory period, when the estrogenic mucus is receptive to penetration by spermatozoa. Experimental evidence has demonstrated that results obtained in estrogen-treated women can provide reliable indications of normal mucus receptivity to sperm penetration [7], but the integration of such therapy into the routine management of infertile couples is uncommon in the era of assisted conception treatment.

Mucus must be sampled from within the cervical canal; receptive intracervical mucus will have an Insler score of ≥10/15 and a pH ≥7.0. Three days of sexual abstinence should be observed prior to the test (either an in-vivo PCT or an in-vitro test), both to provide optimum semen characteristics, and to minimize any "contamination" of the mucus with spermatozoa from a previous insemination. A complete semen analysis should be performed on the ejaculate used for the test. If the abstinence is not for three days then some tests may need to be repeated because of abnormal findings of uncertain origin.

As with all tests of sperm function, sperm–mucus interaction tests (SMITs) must be commenced as quickly as possible after ejaculation. Normal semen samples are liquefied within 30 minutes, making it an ideal standard starting time. If liquefaction is retarded then, while tests can be delayed, mucus-penetrating ability might be reduced by the longer exposure of spermatozoa to seminal plasma [8,9]. Although seminal plasma is important for sperm penetration into cervical mucus, sperm motility and vitality both decline markedly with prolonged exposure.

Sampling cervical mucus

Scheduling

The mucus secretion of the cervix is under endocrine control and shows cyclic variations during the menstrual cycle. Around the fertile period, the mucus is being secreted under estrogenic control; it is an abundant, clear, watery secretion (when compared to the mucus produced during the luteal and early follicular phases), and is receptive to penetration by spermatozoa.

Cervical mucus receptivity to sperm penetration increases over a period of about four days before ovulation and decreases rapidly (within 2 days) after. Most cycle length variation occurs in the follicular phase, with the day of ovulation being equivalent to Day 14 of a "standard" 28-day cycle (Day 1 being the first day of menstruation). A simple method for scheduling cervical mucus assessments is, therefore, to book the women for 14 days before the next expected onset of menstruation [10], although this is not always the day of maximum receptivity [11], and could lead to false diagnoses of cervical hostility. Abnormal test results must therefore be confirmed by repeat testing in at least one subsequent cycle.

To ensure optimum mucus quality, women can be treated with estradiol for several days before sampling, e.g. 80 µg ethinyl estradiol per day for seven days [7]. This ensures optimum mucus for the tests, the results of which are predictive of fertility, but it might conceal an underlying endocrine disorder that would affect the chances of in-vivo conception.

Equipment

- Sterile speculum

Disposable materials

- Sterile mucus aspiration device (e.g. Aspiglaire, CryoBioSystem or *Aspirette*®, Cooper Surgical)
- Sterile disposable syringe (e.g. 1 ml or 3 ml)
- Clean microscope slides, 3″ × 1″
- Coverslips, 22 × 22 mm, #1½ or #2 thickness
- Indicator test strips to measure mucus pH, e.g. EMD Merck *colorpHast*® test strips (Merck KGaA Cat. No. 9583–3 for pH 6.5–10.0 and 9582–3 for pH 4.0–7.0)

Reagents

- Coverslip support material (see section on the "Post-coital test," below)

Procedure

1. Insert a warmed speculum into the vagina and examine the cervix for the dilation and appearance of the external os, including the amount of mucus present there.
2. Gently wipe the external os clean using a sterile, dry gauze swab.

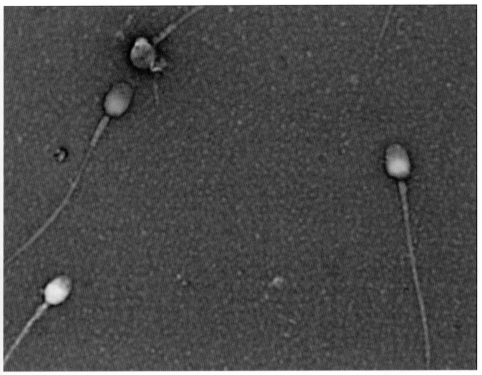

Figure 3.6 A sperm vitality preparation using the one-step eosin-nigrosin stain seen under bright field optics (Köhler illumination) showing three dead (red) spermatozoa and one live (white) spermatozoon with a "leaky neck."

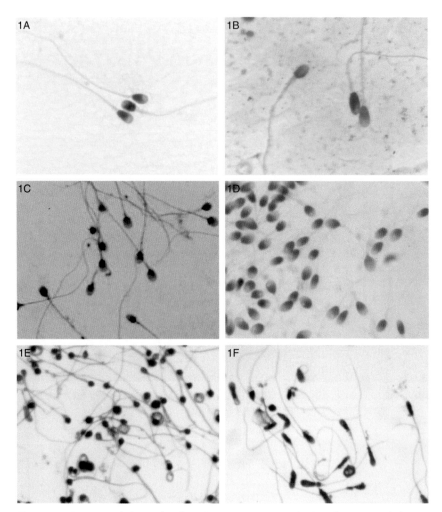

Figure 3.8 Sperm morphology color plates. (1) Sperm staining methods and sperm morphology patterns. (1A) Papanicolaou staining – elongated spermatozoa. (1B) Hemacolor® (Merck) rapid staining. Same patient as in 1A. Note slight swelling of spermatozoa, leading to rounder and larger forms, as well as background staining. (1C) Spermac staining®. Acrosomes and tail stain green and nucleus stains red. (1D) Normal morphology pattern of spermatozoa bound to the zona pellucida of a hemizona assay. (1E) Globozoospermia. Spermac staining®. Note small round heads only with red staining, indicating the absence of the acrosomes. (1F) Stress pattern. All the spermatozoa are elongated. This condition can return to normal if cause of stress can be removed. Spermac staining®.

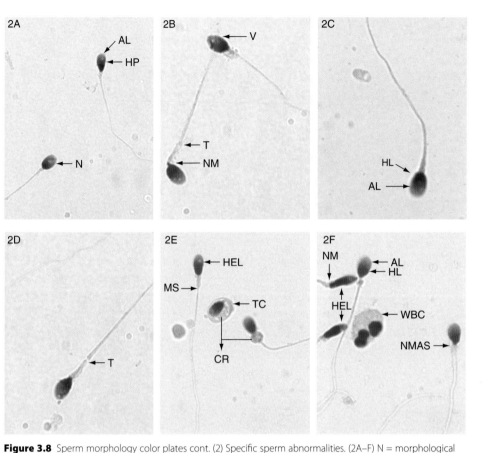

Figure 3.8 Sperm morphology color plates cont. (2) Specific sperm abnormalities. (2A–F) N = morphological ideal or normal spermatozoon; NM = neck/midpiece defect; T = tail defect; CR = cytoplasmic residue defect; V = vacuole(s). (2A) AL = large acrosome; HP = pyriform head. (2C) HL = head large (2E) MS = mitochondria shift to wards head; TC = coiled tail (DAG defect after a bull called DAG, where this abnormality was first diagnosed). (2F) HEL = head medium elongated; WBC = polymorphonuclear white blood cell; NMAS = asymmetrical implantation of the neck.

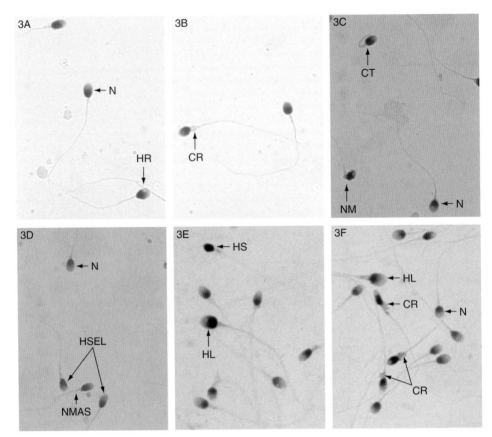

Figure 3.8 Sperm morphology color plates cont. (3) Specific sperm abnormities – continued. (3A–F) N = morphological ideal or normal spermatozoon; NM = neck/midpiece defect; T = tail defect; CR = cytoplasmic residue defect. (3A) HR = round head. (3C) CT = coiled tail. (3D) HSEL = slightly elongated head; NMAS = asymmetric implantation of the neck. (3E) Heterogeneous picture with small- and large-headed spermatozoa. HS = small head; HL = large head. (3F) HL = large head.

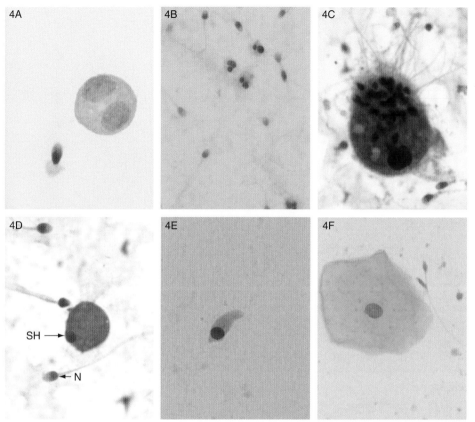

Figure 3.8 Sperm morphology color plates cont. (4) Semen cytology – non-spermatozoal cells possible in semen. (4A) Secondary spermatocyte. (4B) Polymorphonuclear white blood cells. (4C) Macrophage with phagocytosed spermatozoa. (4D) Monocyte with phagocytosed sperm head (SH). (4E) Prostate cell. (4F) Epithelium cell.

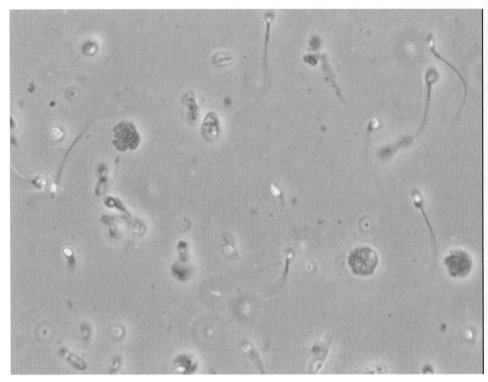

Figure 3.9 Appearance of brown-stained peroxidase-positive cell (inflammatory cell) in semen under phase contrast optics (40× objective).

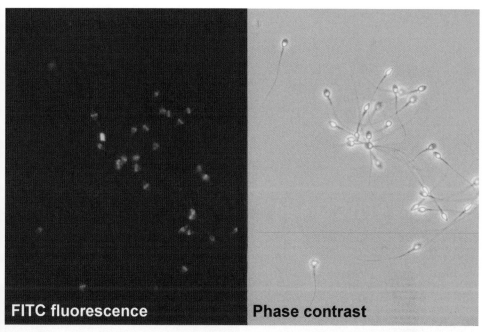

Figure 5.3 Photomicrographs of the same field of spermatozoa following agonist treatment to induce the acrosome reaction under either phase contrast optics (right panel) or epifluorescence for FITC-labelled PNA lectin (left panel). Note the fluorescent labelling over the equatorial segment of the acrosome denoting the acrosome-reacted status.

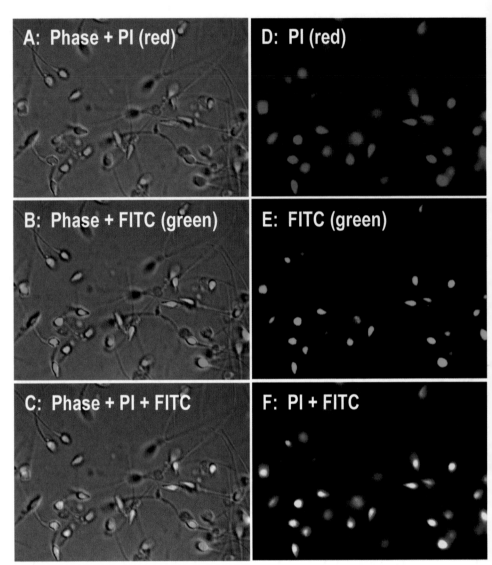

Figure 5.6 Sperm chromatin assessment by TUNEL using fluorescence microscopy. All images are of the same field of spermatozoa: matching images of propidium iodide ("PI" as a general DNA stain; red), FITC (green), and PI+FITC fluorescence, with and without concurrent phase contrast optics, are shown in the left and right hand columns respectively. See text for further explanation of the TUNEL assay. However, it is clear that some spermatozoa are not labelled by either fluorochrome, indicating the origin of possible artefact in this test. (Images courtesy of Madelaine From Björk, Andrology Laboratory, Karolinska University Hospital, Huddinge, Sweden.)

3. Insert the sampling device about 1 cm into the cervical canal and gently pull back on the plunger to draw mucus into the catheter. Maintain gentle suction, and slowly withdraw the catheter from the cervix. If the mucus is very elastic (i.e. high spinnbarkeit), use a pair of forceps to close off the open end of the collection catheter to prevent the mucus from pulling back out of the catheter as it is withdrawn from the vagina.

   Note: Collecting mucus into a syringe (e.g. 1-ml tuberculin type) is acceptable for PCTs, but disrupts the mucus ultrastructure, and should not be used when collecting mucus for in-vitro sperm–mucus interaction testing.

4. Expel the mucus from the catheter onto a clean glass microscope slide.

5. Measure the pH of the mucus.

The Insler Score

This semi-quantitative score is used to assess the quantity and quality of cervical mucus. The original score proposed by Insler and colleagues [12] has since been modified to include mucus cellularity as a fifth parameter and the criteria have been simplified for more practical application [3,4,13]. Each parameter is scored, assigning a value between 0 and 3, based on the criteria shown in Table 6.1.

Table 6.1 Criteria for assigning component values for the Insler score [3,4,12,13].

Criterion			Score
Appearance of the cervical os			
Tightly closed, same pink color as the surrounding tissue			0
Beginning to open and redden			1
Intermediate between grades 1 and 3			2
Maximally dilated (ca. 6 mm diameter)			3
Mucus quantity			
None visible at the external os, and none aspirated		(WHO: 0.0 ml)	0
None visible at the external os, but some aspirated		(WHO: 0.1 ml)	1
Visible at the external os and can be aspirated		(WHO: 0.2 ml)	2
Definite cascade visible at the external os		(WHO: ≥0.3 ml)	3
Spinnbarkeit			
Will not stretch at all			0
Stretches for 1–4 cm before breaking			1
Stretches for 5–8 cm before breaking			2
Stretches for >8 cm before breaking			3
Ferning			
None visible anywhere on the slide			0
Less than half the mucus is starting to fern			1
More than half shows good ferning (1° and 2° stem ferning)			2
All the mucus shows good ferning, with 3° and 4° stem ferning			3
Mucus cellularity (leukocytes)			
Mucus is full of leukocytes:	>20 per 40× field	>1000/mm^3	0
Many leukocytes:	11–20 per 40× field	501–1000/mm^3	1
Few leukocytes:	1–10 per 40× field	1–500/mm^3	2
No leukocytes at all			3

Note: See the section on the post-coital test for an explanation of the relationship between cells/40× field and cells/mm^3 (see also [12]).

Appearance of the cervical os considers the degree of dilation and hyperemia of the external cervical os.

Mucus quantity is assessed at the same time as the cervical appearance, and is based on a combination of whether mucus can be seen at the external os, and how much can be aspirated.

Spinnbarkeit considers the stretchability or elasticity of the mucus, and is best measured by placing a small drop of mucus (about 5 mm diameter) on a clean slide. Place a second slide across the first in the form of a "+" sign and spread the mucus evenly between them. Then gently pull the slides apart and measure the length of the mucus thread.

Ferning is then assessed on the same mucus as used for the spinnbarkeit determination. Spread the mucus evenly on the slide, and allow it to dry before assessing the presence and degree of ferning (crystallization pattern). Detailed counting of the numbers of side branches in the crystallization pattern is unnecessary; it is more important to ensure that the degree of ferning is assessed over the entire preparation rather than concentrating upon a small area which shows, or does not show, ferning.

Mucus cellularity considers the number of leukocytes (not erythrocytes or epithelial cells), and is assessed as an inverse score.

Calculating the Insler Score

The five component scores are added together to give a total Insler Score out of 15. A score of 12 or more is considered to indicate good ovulatory cervical mucus, and scores of 10 or 11 indicate adequate ovulatory cervical mucus.

Cervical mucus pH

Peri-ovulatory cervical mucus is usually pH 8.0–8.4. The optimum pH range for sperm migration and survival is between 7.0 and 8.5; sperm progression is impaired below pH 6.8, and pH 6.0 is incompatible with sperm vitality. Consequently, acidic mucus may be at least a partial explanation for poor sperm–mucus interaction.

Storage of cervical mucus

Many workers have reported that frozen cervical mucus can be unreliable and unsatisfactory for use in in-vitro testing procedures. Consequently, cervical mucus should only be stored for a few days at +4°C. Seal the ends of the collection catheter with an inert material such as hematocrit tube sealant (*Plasticine* is spermotoxic). Stored mucus must be allowed to re-equilibrate to ambient temperature, and its pH and Insler score should be re-assessed before use.

Post-coital test (PCT)

Background

The post-coital test (PCT) allows the assessment of sperm–cervical mucus interaction during the peri-ovulatory period under in-vivo conditions [14]. Aspirated intracervical mucus is examined under a phase contrast microscope and motile spermatozoa are counted in randomly selected fields. While the PCT evaluates the penetration of spermatozoa from liquefied semen into cervical mucus, and their survival within that environment, debate continues as to the true clinical value and significance of the PCT. In cases with suspected sexual dysfunction, a positive PCT can be taken as evidence of an adequate coital technique. Although antisperm antibodies in cervical mucus can cause poor PCTs, technical problems might also be responsible, and caution must be used before attributing a poor PCT to immunologically hostile mucus. Notwithstanding these issues, many gynecologists still consider the PCT to be an essential part of an infertile couple's work-up [5], and full-service, infertility diagnostic laboratories should be able to offer the procedure.

Principle(s)

The post-coital test (PCT) consists of sampling the cervical mucus several hours after intercourse and examining it for the presence of spermatozoa. A PCT must be performed during the peri-ovulatory period, and three days of sexual abstinence prior to the "test intercourse" is strongly recommended to provide optimum semen characteristics, and to minimize any "contamination" of the mucus with spermatozoa from a previous insemination. Although the use of condoms during the follicular phase of the test cycle can facilitate interpretation of the findings, it is unlikely to be practiced by infertility patients.

Specimen(s)

- Intracervical mucus is obtained, ideally within 12 hours after intercourse. Its pH is measured and its quality assessed as described in the section on the Insler Score (see above)

Equipment (see also Appendix 2)

- Microscope configured for andrology with phase contrast optics (10×, 20× and 40× objectives)
- Tally counter

Disposable materials

- As for semen collection and analysis
- As for cervical mucus collection and assessment
- Coverslip support material (see "Reagents," below)

Reagents

- *Coverslip support material:* A mixture of glass beads in silicone grease is used to make the 100 μm fixed-depth preparations [15] although experience has shown that when this material is being prepared for relatively short-term diagnostic use only (up to 3 months) the preparation protocol can be greatly simplified to merely mixing the pre-washed glass beads (Sigma G4649, 106 μm diameter and finer) with high-vacuum silicone grease (e.g. Dow Corning) in approximate 1 : 5 proportions. To create a dispenser for the material, remove the plunger from a 5-ml plastic syringe and, using a weighing spatula, fill the syringe barrel with the glass beads/silicone grease mixture. Replace the plunger and expel as much air as possible from the syringe and fit the syringe with a blunt needle (e.g. Monoject™ 202, 18G × 1″, see www.kendallhq.com).

Calibration

Although older reports describe results in terms of cells per high power field or "HPF" (i.e. a 40× objective), proper quantitative performance of this test requires that the microscope field be calibrated so that numbers of spermatozoa per field can be converted to numbers per unit area (i.e. per mm^2 ≡ per 10^6 μm^2), and that glass beads are used to standardize the preparation depth, allowing sperm numbers to be expressed per unit volume (i.e. per mm^3 ≡ per μl: see below). For a 100-μm-deep preparation, the field volume for a modern microscope using a 40× objective (numerical aperture or "NA" 0.65) and wide-field oculars will be approximately 0.02 mm^3, so that a traditional count of 10 cells/HPF (non-wide-field oculars) will be equivalent to 500 cells/mm^3 [3,13].

The field area of a given combination of objective, intermediate magnification and oculars can be readily calibrated using a micrometer slide to measure the field diameter, and then applying simple geometry. For a "typical" field volume of 0.02 mm^3, with no intermediate magnification, the factor to correct a number of cells per field to per unit volume is ×50. If intermediate magnification is used, then to convert from 1.0× (i.e. no intermediate magnification) to 1.25×, multiply by an additional 1.55; to convert from 1.0× to 1.5×, multiply by an additional 2.23.

If there are very large numbers of spermatozoa in a field, then an eyepiece fitted with a graticule may be used to delimit small areas of the field. An additional factor is then used to correct for the proportion of the whole field area represented by the fraction of the grid in which the cells were counted; see Figure 6.1 for an illustration of this calculation [3].

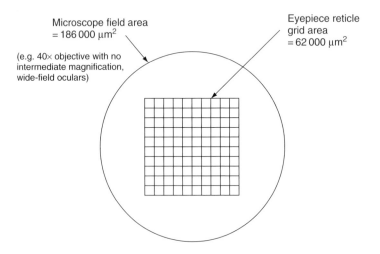

Microscope field area
= 186 000 μm^2

(e.g. 40× objective with no intermediate magnification, wide-field oculars)

Eyepiece reticle grid area
= 62 000 μm^2

Figure 6.1 Explanation of how to use an eyepiece graticule (or reticle) to subdivide for easier counting of a microscope field of view containing many cells.

To convert cells per 100 squares (entire grid), multiply by 3 (i.e. 186 000 ÷ 62 000)

Hence: for cells per 20 grid squares (two rows), multiply by 15
  for cells per 10 grid squares (one row), multiply by 30
  for cells per 4 grid squares, multiply by 75

Quality control

This is a straightforward observational procedure, but its objective assessment does require the prior calibration of the microscope field size. Quality control aspects relating to the mucus quality assessment are dealt with in the section on "The Insler Score" (see above).

Procedure

1. Prepare a cleaned microscope slide with four "posts" of the glass beads/silicone grease mixture arranged in a square pattern with sides of about 20 mm (see Figure 6.2).

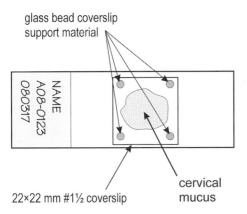

Figure 6.2 The post-coital test.

glass bead coverslip
support material

NAME
A08-0123
080317

22×22 mm #1½ coverslip

cervical mucus

2. Place a drop (*ca.* 3 mm diameter) of endocervical mucus in the center of this square and cover it with a 22 × 22 mm coverslip. Press down gently on the coverslip so that the "posts" are flattened and the coverslip is fixed with a single layer of beads between it and the slide. The mucus drop will spread towards the edges of the coverslip; if it extrudes from under the coverslip, another preparation must be made using less mucus.

3. Microscopic screening of the mucus is performed under a 40× objective using phase-contrast optics. Briefly scan the slide to check that the sperm distribution in the mucus sample is more or less uniform.

4. In each of 10 randomly selected fields away from the coverslip edge (fields with air bubbles or large patches of epithelium can be rejected), count the number of spermatozoa according to their motility:

   a. Count the number of progressively motile spermatozoa.

   b. Count all the other spermatozoa present in the same field of view, classifying each one as immotile, non-progressively motile, or "shaking" (see also the SCMC test, below).

   Note: If there are very large numbers of spermatozoa per field, then a part of the field, delimited by an eyepiece graticule, may be used. Ensure that the microscope calibration factor allows for the reduced sample area.

Calculations and results

1. a. Calculate the average number per field of each type of spermatozoa over the ten fields.

   b. Use the appropriate microscope field correction factor to convert these averages to numbers per unit volume (see "Calibration," above).

2. Some gynecologists still disagree with the objective assessment criteria described below, but they are based upon recalculation from historic clinical series allowing for modern microscope optics and quantitative laboratory methods.

3. According to the average numbers of progressively motile spermatozoa per unit volume, grade the test as shown in Table 6.2.

Note: If ≥20% of the spermatozoa are shaking, this should be noted on the report. If >50% of the spermatozoa show shaking, then a PCT will always be classified as "Poor."

Table 6.2 Assigning results to the "post-coital test" (PCT) [3,13].

No. of spermatozoa per unit volume (per µl)	Test result
None at all	Negative
Present, but <500	Poor
500–999	Average
1000–2500	Good
>2500	Excellent

Notes and interpretation guidelines

1. An Insler Score of <10 can be considered at least a partial explanation of a poor PCT.

2. Cervical mucus is normally between pH 8.0 and 8.5; acidic mucus (especially if <7.0) can be at least a partial explanation of a poor PCT.

3. Sperm motility decreases with increasing time *post-coitum*. Therefore, a PCT performed after a long post-coital delay that shows many non-progressive spermatozoa (as distinct from shaking spermatozoa) might have been attributed a better result than the number of progressive spermatozoa alone would indicate had it been performed after a shorter delay.

4. Interpretation of the clinical significance of a PCT must be the responsibility of the physician requesting the test. Such interpretation should always take into account the mucus quality and partner's semen characteristics (and adequacy of coital technique) since low sperm count and particularly poor sperm motility (especially in conjunction with poor sperm morphology) will significantly reduce the quantitative penetration of spermatozoa into mucus.

Kurzrok–Miller test (K–M test)

Principle

The Kurzrok–Miller (or "K–M") test is the oldest in-vitro test of sperm–mucus interaction [16]. It consists simply of establishing an interface between a drop of endocervical mucus and fresh liquefied semen under a coverslip.

Specimen(s)

- Cervical mucus and semen samples are required (see Kremer test below for details)

Equipment (see also Appendix 2)

- Phase-contrast compound microscope configured for andrology (10×, 20× and 40× objectives)
- Tally counter
- Air incubator
- Humid chamber

Disposable materials

- As for semen collection and analysis
- As for cervical mucus collection and assessment
- Coverslip support material (see "Reagents," below)
- 2″ × 2″ sterile gauze swabs

Reagents

- *Coverslip support material:* A mixture of glass beads in silicone grease is used to make the 100 μm fixed-depth preparations [15]; see "Post-coital test" (above) for details.
- *Water:* Sterile water for injection.

Calibration

None required as this test is only interpreted subjectively.

Quality control

The K–M test is an observational technique subject to uncontrollable factors such as the geometry of the semen–mucus interface. If results are reported as described below then the test will have achieved its maximum practicable standardization.

Procedure

1. Prepare a cleaned microscope slide with four "posts" of the glass beads/silicone grease mixture arranged in a square pattern with sides of about 20 mm (see Figure 6.2, above).

2. Place a drop (*ca.* 3 mm diameter) of endocervical mucus in the center of this square and cover it with a 22 × 22 mm coverslip. Press down gently on the coverslip so that the "posts" are flattened and the coverslip is fixed with a single layer of beads between it and the slide. The mucus drop will spread towards the edges of the coverslip; if it extrudes from under the coverslip another preparation must be made using less mucus.

3. Place a drop (about 10 μl) of semen next to the edge of the coverslip. The semen will flow under the coverslip and establish a contact interface with the mucus (see Figure 6.3).

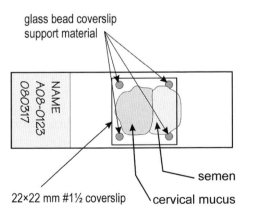

glass bead coverslip
support material

22×22 mm #1½ coverslip

cervical mucus

semen

Figure 6.3 The Kurzrok–Miller test.

155

4. Incubate the test in a humidified chamber at 37°C for 20–30 min.

5. Examine the preparation at a magnification of 200× to 250× using phase-contrast optics (i.e. using a 20× or 25× objective).

Calculations and results

Because of the great problems of standardizing the semen–mucus interface, some laboratories only use the K–M test as a qualitative assessment of sperm–mucus interaction. The test is reported according to the following observational criteria:

Normal result:	Spermatozoa penetrate into the mucus phase, and the great majority (>90%) are motile with definite progression.
Poor result:	Although spermatozoa penetrate into the mucus phase, most do not progress further than 0.5 mm (i.e. about 10 sperm lengths) from the semen–mucus interface.
Abnormal result:	Spermatozoa penetrate into the mucus phase, but rapidly become either immotile or show the "shaking" pattern of movement.
Negative test:	Spermatozoa congregate along the semen side of the interface but none penetrate through the semen–mucus interface; phalanges may or may not be formed.

Notes and interpretation guidelines

1. An Insler Score of <10 can be considered at least a partial explanation of a poor K–M test.

2. Cervical mucus is normally between pH 8.0 and 8.5; acidic mucus (especially if <7.0) can be at least a partial explanation of a poor K–M test.

3. A prior 3-day period of sexual abstinence is advisable as samples produced outside the range of 2–4 days of abstinence might show impaired mucus-penetrating capacity.

4. Since the exposure of spermatozoa to seminal plasma rapidly impairs their mucus-penetrating ability, tests should be set up by 30 minutes post-ejaculation (see the introduction to this chapter). All variations from the normal condition should be noted and reported.

Kremer capillary tube "sperm penetration" test

Principle

The Kremer sperm penetration test is an in-vitro test of sperm–mucus interaction, in which a glass capillary tube is filled with cervical mucus and its open end placed in contact with a reservoir of semen [6,8]. Penetration of motile spermatozoa into and along the mucus column is assessed by counting their numbers at various distances from the semen–mucus interface.

The outcome of the test is strongly influenced by the concentration of progressively motile spermatozoa at the semen–mucus interface (i.e. in the semen sample) and has been considered as a test of the proportion of successful collisions between spermatozoa capable of mucus penetration and the interface [17]. Consequently, oligozoospermic samples will most likely produce average to poor results, while oligoasthenozoospermic samples will usually produce abnormal test results. However, such generalizations cannot substitute for performing the test in any but the most extreme male factor cases.

The glass "sperm penetration meter" devices developed by Dr Jan Kremer, the inventor of this test in the 1960s [6,8], are no longer commercially available. Also, in the method described below the original round cross-section capillaries have been replaced by rectangular cross-section glass capillaries for easier examination under the microscope. Finally, Kremer's original scoring method, which is rather complicated and hard to standardize, has been replaced by a technique more amenable to routine standardized application [10]; descriptions of Kremer's original assessment scheme are readily available elsewhere [3].

Specimen(s)

- *Mucus:* The test must be performed using peri-ovulatory mucus. Intracervical mucus is collected and assessed in terms of its Insler Score and pH (see above); if the pH is <7.0 then it can adversely affect the outcome of the test.

- *Semen:* A 50-µl aliquot of liquefied semen is required for each test. It must be taken from a well-mixed ejaculate specimen within one hour of collection, and preferably at a standard time such as 30 min. For details, see Chapter 3.

Equipment (see also Appendix 2)

- Microscope configured for andrology with phase contrast optics (10×, 20× and 40× objectives)

- Tally counter

- Air incubator operating at 37°C

- Stainless steel iris scissors, sterile

- Rack for the semen reservoir tube (e.g. BEEM capsules or 0.5-ml Eppendorf tubes)

Disposable materials

- As for semen collection and analysis

- As for cervical mucus collection and assessment

- Glass capillary tubes with rectangular cross-section: 100 × 3 × 0.3 mm rectangular Vitrotubes™ (used to be called "Microslide" capillaries: VitroCom)

- Tube for use as a semen reservoir, e.g. BEEM electron microscopy No.00 embedding capsule, or 0.5-ml Eppendorf tubes

Reagents

- *DTT solution:* A 10 mg/ml solution of dithiothreitol (Sigma D0632) in sterile water. Prepare fresh daily, and maintain at ambient temperature. Discard any unused portion.

Calibration

Fully objective performance of this test requires that microscope objective fields be calibrated so that numbers of spermatozoa per field may be converted to numbers per unit area (i.e. per mm^2, or per 10^6 µm^2; as described for the PCT, see above). Although there is no dependable method for determining sperm numbers per unit volume within capillary tubes, if the same magnification objective is always used then the third dimension will be constant; for this test a 20× objective is preferred due to its greater depth of focus.

The field area of a given combination of objective, intermediate magnification and oculars can be readily calibrated using a micrometer slide to measure the field diameter and then applying simple geometry.

For a modern microscope using a 20× objective (numerical aperture or "NA" 0.46) and wide-field oculars (with no intermediate magnification) the field area will be approximately 0.75 mm^2, so the factor to correct a number of cells per field to per unit area is ×1.33. If intermediate magnification is used, then to convert from 1.0× (i.e. no intermediate magnification) to 1.25×, multiply by an additional 1.55; to convert from 1.0× to 1.5×, multiply by an additional 2.23.

If there are very large numbers of spermatozoa in a field, then an eyepiece fitted with a graticule may be used to delimit small areas of the field. An additional factor is then used to correct for the proportion of the whole field area represented by the fraction of the grid in which the cells were counted (see the section of this chapter on the PCT for further explanation).

Quality control

This is a straightforward observational procedure. Quality control aspects relating to the semen analysis and mucus quality assessment are dealt with under the appropriate tests.

The field area of each combination of microscope objective, intermediate magnification, and oculars must be calibrated to allow calculation of sperm numbers per unit area (see "Calibration," above).

Due to the marked influence of temperature upon sperm progression, these tests must be run at 37°C. Because changing the incubation time and/or temperature will alter sperm migration along the mucus column, Kremer tests must be run at 37°C for the expected 60 minutes; shorter times will require completely re-defined criteria for determining the result.

Procedure

1. a. Mark a flat capillary tube at 10-mm intervals using a fine-pointed indelible (spirit-based) marker pen.

    b. Prepare the semen reservoir by making a slit or hole in its cap (e.g. using a punch plier) sufficient to allow the glass capillary to pass through quite easily.

2. Expel the mucus from the collection catheter onto a clean glass slide; cut trailing mucus using iris scissors. Mucus from the proximal 20 mm of the collection catheter (corresponding more or less to mucus from the endocervical level of the canal) should be used.

3. Aspirate mucus from the slide into the capillary tube using a syringe and tubing manifold. The mucus meniscus should be 20–30 mm from the top of the tube, creating a mucus column of 70–80 mm (exact length is noted to the nearest mm). Mucus trailing from the lower end of the tube is cut with iris scissors after the loading manifold has been removed. Seal the upper end of the tube with hematocrit tube

sealant. After sealing the mucus should protrude slightly from the open end of the tube.

4. Before setting up the test, the mucus-filled capillary tube is checked under the microscope (phase-contrast optics, same magnification as will be used for scoring the test) for the presence of spermatozoa. If any spermatozoa are seen, the number in 10 random fields along the length of the mucus column are counted (including classification of their motility) so that the average "contamination" per field can be used to correct the sperm penetration scores (see "Calculations," below).

5. At 30 min post-ejaculation, a 50-μl aliquot of the mixed liquefied semen is transferred into the bottom of the semen reservoir tube, which is held upright in a rack, and the cap of the tube closed.
Note: A complete semen analysis is performed on ejaculate.

6. The open end of the mucus-filled capillary tube is inserted through the slit in the lid of the semen reservoir until its corners rest on the tapered base of the tube. The mucus interface will be immersed 1–2 mm into the semen (see Figure 6.4).

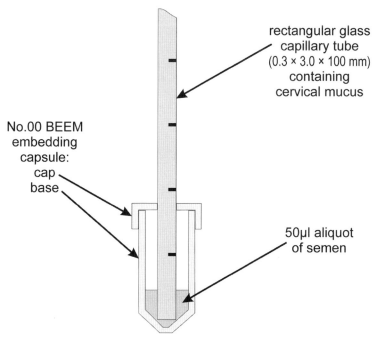

rectangular glass capillary tube (0.3 × 3.0 × 100 mm) containing cervical mucus

No.00 BEEM embedding capsule: cap base

50μl aliquot of semen

Figure 6.4 Diagrammatic illustration of the use of a BEEM No. 00 electron microscopy embedding capsule as the semen reservoir in a Kremer test.

7. Replace the test in the rack and incubate at 37°C for 60 min.

8. After incubation, remove the capillary tube, and rinse its open end thoroughly with a freshly prepared solution of DTT to remove residual spermatozoa from the mucus interface and surface of the capillary. Stand the open end of the tube in the DTT solution for 30–60 s to ensure complete removal of any contaminating semen.

9. Assess the depth and degree of sperm penetration into the mucus column under the microscope (phase contrast optics, 20× objective). Count the number of in-focus spermatozoa present in each of three microscope fields at the 10, 40, and 70 mm marks along

the tube. Select fields that are mid-way between the upper and lower walls of the capillary, and do not adjust the microscope focus to find additional spermatozoa.

10. Determine the farthest distance travelled along the mucus column by the "vanguard" spermatozoon.

Calculations and results

1. For each of the 10, 40, and 70 mm distances along the tube:
   a. calculate the average number of spermatozoa present per field;
   b. correct the average number of spermatozoa per field for any "contaminating" spermatozoa that were present in the mucus at the start of the test; and
   c. convert the corrected number into per unit area (see above) using the appropriate microscope calibration factor.

2. Use these values to calculate the "sperm penetration test" or "SPT" score, an empirically derived scheme used to create a semi-quantitative score for this test [10], as shown in Table 6.3.

Table 6.3 Criteria for calculating the "sperm penetration test" (SPT) score [10].

Spermatozoa/mm^2	Score	Vanguard spermatozoa (mm)
0	0	<30
1–30	1	30–39
31–60	2	40–49
61–120	3	50–59
121–200	4	61–69
>200	5	>70

3. Derive the test result from the calculated total SPT score according to the criteria shown in Table 6.4.

Table 6.4 Criteria for deriving the result of the "sperm penetration test" (SPT) [10].

Total SPT score	Test result
0	Negative
1–8	Poor
9–11	Average
12–15	Good
16–20	Excellent

Notes and interpretation guidelines

1. An Insler Score of <10 can be considered at least a partial explanation of a poor Kremer test.

2. Cervical mucus is normally between pH 8.0 and 8.5; acidic mucus (especially if <7.0) can be at least a partial explanation of a poor Kremer test.

3. A prior 3-day period of sexual abstinence is advisable, as samples produced outside the range of 2–4 days of abstinence might show impaired mucus-penetrating capacity.

4. Since the exposure of spermatozoa to seminal plasma rapidly impairs their mucus-penetrating ability, tests should be set up by 30 min post-ejaculation (see the introduction to this chapter). All variations from the normal condition should be noted and reported.

Sperm–cervical mucus contact (SCMC) test

Principle

The sperm–cervical mucus contact (SCMC) test is a slide test whereby spermatozoa and cervical mucus are mixed to establish the presence of any sperm-immobilizing antisperm antibodies in either the seminal plasma or the cervical mucus [18]. This test is performed by mixing drops of mucus and semen (see Figure 6.5, below).

Specimens

- *Semen:* A 50-µl aliquot of liquefied semen is required for each test. It must be taken from a well-mixed ejaculate specimen within one hour of collection, and preferably at a standard time such as 30 min. For details see Chapter 3.
- *Mucus:* The test must be performed using peri-ovulatory mucus. Intracervical mucus is collected and assessed in terms of its Insler Score and pH (see above); if the pH is <7.0 then it can adversely affect the outcome of the test.

Equipment (see also Appendix 2)

- Microscope configured for andrology with phase contrast optics (10×, 20× and 40× objectives)
- Tally counter

Disposable materials

- As for semen collection and analysis
- As for cervical mucus collection and assessment

Reagents

- None required

Calibration

None required.

Quality control

This is a simple, subjective, observational test. Provided that the results are reported as noted in "Results" then the test will have achieved its maximum practicable standardization.

Procedure

1. Place a 3- to 5-mm diameter drop of endocervical mucus and a drop (about 25 µl) of liquefied semen side by side on a clean microscope slide and mix gently using a disposable plastic stirring rod or disposable pipettor tip (see Figure 6.5).

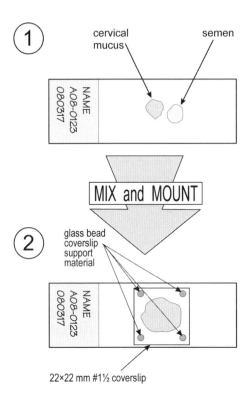

Figure 6.5 The sperm–cervical mucus contact (SCMC) test.

2. Cover with a 22 × 22 mm coverslip and press gently to spread the preparation to the edges of the coverslip.

3. Examine immediately under phase-contrast optics (200–500× magnification) for a period of 5–10 min. Note the development of any "shaking" pattern of the movement of motile spermatozoa. Shaking describes a specific pattern of movement whereby the spermatozoa are actively motile but non-progressive; they appear to be stuck to some invisible structure inside the mucus.

4. Count at least 100 actively motile spermatozoa to determine the percentage of shaking spermatozoa.

Calculations and results

The SCMC test is reported according to criteria shown in Table 6.5.

Table 6.5 Criteria for assigning the result of the "sperm–cervical mucus contact" (SCMC) test.

Shaking sperm	Test result	
0–25	Negative	(–)
26–50	Positive	(+)
51–75	Positive	(++)
76–100	Highly positive	(+++)

Notes and interpretation guidelines

1. Acidic cervical mucus can kill spermatozoa quickly, preventing an SCMC test from being read.

Crossed-hostility testing

Principle(s)

When the result from a homologous sperm–mucus interaction test has been average or worse then a crossed-hostility test (XHT) should be performed in a subsequent cycle to simultaneously verify the previous cycle's finding, and also evaluate the origin of the problem, i.e. semen or mucus (see Figure 6.6).

However, given the difficulty in obtaining donor mucus, and the current expense of donor semen, XHT format testing is nowadays quite rare.

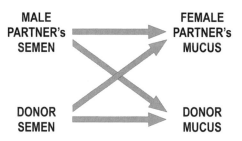

MALE PARTNER's SEMEN → **FEMALE PARTNER's MUCUS**

DONOR SEMEN → **DONOR MUCUS**

Figure 6.6 The crossed hostility test (XHT) format.

Specimens

Patient mucus and semen: These are obtained as for the Kremer test.

Donor mucus: Obtained from a patient receiving artificial insemination (AI) treatment. Mucus samples are taken and assessed as per standard procedures (see "Insler Score," above) and, to be suitable for this test, must have an Insler score of $\geq 12/15$ and a pH ≥ 7.0. Donor mucus may be stored at $+4°C$ for up to 4 days before being used; ensure that stored mucus has re-equilibrated to ambient temperature before use.

Donor semen: Usually cryopreserved donor semen (or fresh "control donor" semen) with known good mucus-penetrating ability.

Equipment, disposable materials and reagents

- All as for the component Kremer and SCMC tests (see above)

Calibration and quality control

As for the component Kremer and SCMC tests (see above).

Procedure

- Whenever sufficient material is available, the Kremer test method should be used as the basic test. However, if only a limited amount of the patient's mucus is available, then the K-M test may be used instead.

- An SCMC test (see above) should also be performed on at least the homologous (i.e. patients') sperm–mucus interaction, mucus quantity permitting. If at all possible SCMC tests should be performed on all four combinations.

Calculations and results

The results of each component test are derived according to the procedures described for those tests.

Notes and interpretation guidelines

While the physician requesting the XHT procedure is solely responsible for interpreting the results of the component tests, the following general guidelines can be established when the interaction of the donor materials was normal.

- If the man's spermatozoa penetrate neither his partner's mucus, nor the donor mucus then there is probably a male factor problem (e.g. abnormal sperm motility, antisperm antibodies on the sperm surface).
- If neither the man's, nor the donor's spermatozoa penetrate the patient's mucus then there is probably a female factor problem (e.g. abnormal mucus quality, antisperm antibodies in the mucus).
- In some cases, both the above problems may be seen simultaneously. This indicates the likely presence of both male and female factors.

Complementary tests

The need for donor semen and cervical mucus often makes the routine implementation of crossed-hostility format testing rather impractical. Additional tests can provide essentially similar information to that obtainable from studying the interactions of a man's spermatozoa with donor mucus, and of donor spermatozoa with his partner's mucus. Such protocols can obviate the need for donor mucus and/or donor sperm, making a comprehensive assessment of the interaction between a man's spermatozoa and his partner's cervical mucus more practicable in a full-service diagnostic andrology laboratory in the "modern age" of assisted conception treatment.

Testing for antisperm antibodies

Including a direct test for antisperm antibodies on the man's spermatozoa and an indirect IBT on his partner's mucus will greatly facilitate the interpretation of abnormal XHT findings (see Chapter 4 for further information).

Sperm kinematics

Kinematic analysis of sperm movement using CASA might also help understand the possible origin of a male factor problem (see Chapter 4 for further information) [2].

Cervical mucus substitutes

Although there was early interest in the use of bovine cervical mucus as a surrogate medium for human sperm testing, commercial products such as Serono Diagnostics' *Penetrak*® disappeared some years ago.

The ability of spermatozoa to penetrate into, and migrate along, a capillary tube filled with a synthetic medium containing high-molecular-weight sodium hyaluronate was found to be dependent upon very similar sperm characteristics to those required for human peri-ovulatory cervical mucus [19,20,21]. However, due to the unavailability of a commercial product that can be used in such tests, the "hyaluronate migration test" never entered routine practice.

References

1. Mortimer D. Sperm transport in the female genital tract. In: Grudzinskas JG, Yovich JL, eds. *Cambridge Reviews in Human Reproduction. Volume 2: Gametes – The Spermatozoon.* Cambridge: Cambridge University Press 1995; 157–74.

2. Mortimer ST. A critical review of the physiological importance and analysis of sperm movement in mammals. *Hum Reprod Update* 1997; **3**: 403–39.

3. World Health Organization. *WHO Laboratory Manual for the Analysis of Human Semen and Sperm-Cervical Mucus Interaction.* 4th edn. Cambridge: Cambridge University Press 1999.

4. Mortimer D. *Practical Laboratory Andrology.* New York: Oxford University Press 1994.

5. Hunault CC, Habbema JD, Eijkemans MJ, et al. Two new prediction rules for spontaneous pregnancy leading to live birth among subfertile couples, based on the synthesis of three previous models. *Hum Reprod* 2004; **19**: 2019–26.

6. Kremer, J. A simple sperm penetration test. *Int J Fertil* 1965; **10**: 209–14.

7. Eggert-Kruse W, Leinhos G, Gerhard, I, et al. Prognostic value of in vitro sperm penetration into hormonally standardized human cervical mucus. *Fertil Steril* 1989; **51**: 317–23.

8. Kremer J. The in vitro spermatozoal penetration test in fertility investigations. MD thesis. Groningen, Rijksuniversiteit te Groningen, 1968.

9. Kremer J, Jager S, van Slochteren-Draaisma T. The "unexplained" poor post-coital test. *Int J Fertil* 1978; **23**: 277–81.

10. Pandya IJ, Mortimer D, Sawers RS. A standardized approach for evaluating the penetration of human spermatozoa into cervical mucus in vitro. *Fertil Steril* 1986; **45**: 357–65.

11. Makler A. A new method for evaluating cervical penetrability using daily aspirated and stored cervical mucus. *Fertil Steril* 1976; **27**: 533–40.

12. Insler V, Melmed H, Eichenbrenner I, et al. The cervical score: a simple quantitative method for monitoring of the menstrual cycle. *Int J Gynaecol Obstet* 1972; **10**: 223–8.

13. World Health Organization. *WHO Laboratory Manual for the Analysis of Human Semen and Sperm-Cervical Mucus Interaction.* 3rd edn. Cambridge: Cambridge University Press 1992.

14. Moghissi KS. Postcoital test: physiologic basis, technique and interpretation. *Fertil Steril* 1976; **27**: 117–29.

15. Drobnis EZ, Yudin AL, Cherr GN, Katz DF. Hamster sperm penetration of the zona pellucida: kinematic analysis and mechanical implications. *Devel Biol* 1988; **130**: 311–23.

16. Kurzrok R, Miller EG. Biochemical studies of human semen and its relation to mucus of the cervix uteri. *Am J Obstet Gynecol* 1928; **15**: 56–72.

17. Katz DF, Overstreet, JW, Hanson FW. A new quantitative test for sperm penetration into cervical mucus. *Fertil Steril* 1980; **33**: 179–86.

18. Kremer J, Jager S. The sperm-cervical mucus contact test. A preliminary report. *Fertil Steril* 1976; **27**: 335–40.

19. Mortimer D, Mortimer ST, Shu MA, Swart R. A simplified approach to sperm-cervical mucus interaction using a hyaluronate migration test. *Hum Reprod* 1990; **5**: 835–41.

20. Aitken RJ, Bowie H, Buckingham D, *et al.* Sperm penetration into a hyaluronic acid polymer as a means of monitoring functional competence. *J Androl* 1992; **13**: 44–54.

21. Neuwinger J, Cooper TG, Knuth UA, Nieschlag E. Hyaluronic acid as a medium for human sperm migration tests. *Hum Reprod* 1991; **6**: 396–400.

Chapter 7

Sperm preparation

Background

Spermatozoa in the ejaculate are prevented from undergoing capacitation by decapacitation factor(s) (DF) present in the seminal plasma. Seminal plasma also contains one or more factors prolonged exposure to which adversely affects sperm function, including the ability to penetrate cervical mucus, undergo the acrosome reaction *in vitro* and the fertilization process generally [1,2]. Exposure to seminal plasma for more than 30 minutes after ejaculation permanently diminishes the fertilizing capacity of human spermatozoa *in vitro* [3], and contamination of prepared sperm populations with only trace amounts of seminal plasma (0.01% v/v ≡ 1-in-10 000) can decrease their fertilizing capacity [4] (see Figure 7.1).

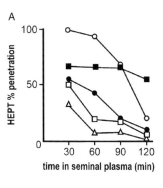

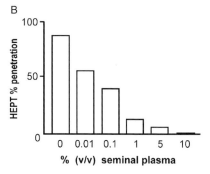

Figure 7.1 Influence of (A) prolonged exposure to seminal plasma and (B) seminal plasma contamination during sperm capacitation on the fertilizing ability of human spermatozoa, as assessed using the zone pellucida-free "hamster egg penetration test" (HEPT). Figures redrawn from [3,4].

Because capacitation is essential for fertilization both *in vivo* and *in vitro*, spermatozoa for clinical procedures such as IUI or IVF (and also for laboratory tests of sperm fertilizing ability) must be separated from the seminal plasma environment, not only as soon as possible after ejaculation (allowing for the required wait for liquefaction) but also as efficiently as possible to eliminate DF, and the spermatozoa must then be suspended in a culture medium capable of supporting capacitation. Consequently, these essential prerequisites for capacitation dictate the requirements for manipulating spermatozoa to be used for clinical IVF [1,2].

Because the area of sperm preparation methods has been reviewed extensively elsewhere [2,5,6], only an overview of the four basic approaches for sperm preparation is provided here as background to the established "safe" methods in common current usage:

1. Simple dilution and washing to separate spermatozoa from semen.
2. Methods based on sperm migration to separate motile spermatozoa.

3. Adherence-based methods to eliminate dead spermatozoa and debris.

4. "Selective" washing methods using density gradients to separate motile spermatozoa.

Simple washing

Simple dilution of semen with a relatively large volume (typically 5 to 10×) of culture medium and separation of the spermatozoa by centrifugation, is the simplest method for washing spermatozoa. Repeated centrifugation (usually 2 or 3 times) is often used to ensure removal of contaminating seminal plasma, although it is essential to avoid forces greater than 800 g [7]. This procedure has the great disadvantage that all the spermatozoa, including the dead, moribund and abnormal ones, present in the original semen remain in the final sperm population, as well as all other cells that were present in the semen, including germ line cells that were sloughed from the seminiferous epithelium and leukocytes of various types.

The presence of large numbers of non-functional gametes in the final preparation could be detrimental by inhibiting capacitation and has been reported to increase the risk of developing antisperm antibodies if inseminated into the uterine cavity at IUI [8]. Furthermore, it has been known for two decades that if "whole" semen is centrifuged, the functional potential of the motile cells, even when isolated later, is impaired [9,10,11]. Centrifuging human ejaculates causes the production of ROS within the resulting pellet, causing irreversible damage to the spermatozoa via peroxidation of sperm plasma membrane phospholipids and via oxidative damage to the sperm chromatin. Indeed, ROS can cause substantial degradation of the sperm DNA while not necessarily affecting their fertilizing ability [12,13].

Consequently, the practice of washing spermatozoa by centrifuging unselected sperm populations is potentially hazardous, and it has been recommended, since 1991, that it should be abandoned in favor of known "safe" practices such as direct swim-up from semen and DGC techniques [14].

Migration-based techniques

In vivo, the potentially functional sperm population is separated from liquefied semen by virtue of their migration into cervical mucus. Sperm migration into a culture medium layer is therefore considered functionally equivalent to the process whereby human spermatozoa escape from the ejaculate and colonize the cervical mucus [15,16,17], although some differences do exist due to the different rheological characteristics between the culture medium and mid-cycle cervical mucus.

In the original "swim-up" technique, liquefied semen is layered beneath culture medium (or culture medium is layered over the semen, but the former provides a much cleaner interface). During a subsequent incubation period (15–60 min depending on the application) the progressively motile spermatozoa migrate from the semen into the culture medium.

A combined migration–sedimentation technique, designed originally for asthenozoospermic samples, combined swim-up from semen with gravitational settling of spermatozoa from the upper medium layer using special "Tea-Jondet" tubes [18]. While the method was an interesting approach for dealing with male factor semen samples with very sluggish motility (direct swim-up from semen being preferable for samples with average or better progression), it is rarely used nowadays.

"Direct swim-up from semen" (DSUS): Aliquots of semen are taken as soon as the sample is liquefied and placed in a series of tubes underneath layers of culture medium. Round-bottomed, not conical, tubes are used to maximize the surface area of the interface between the semen layer and the culture medium, and multiple tubes containing relatively small volumes of semen will increase the total interface area (e.g. sufficient semen to bring the interface to the point of maximum diameter of the tube under 600 μl of culture medium) and hence maximize the yield (Figure 7.2). Tubes can be incubated at an angle of 45° to increase the interface area, but they must then be kept at that angle until after harvesting so as not to risk contaminating the medium layer with seminal plasma as the tube is returned to the vertical. After an appropriate incubation period at 37°C – longer incubations give greater yields (although this should not exceed 60 min) – most of the upper culture medium layer (typically 2/3 or 3/4) is removed, taking great care not to aspirate from the interface. This sperm population is then usually washed once by centrifugation and resuspended into fresh culture medium at the desired concentration of motile spermatozoa. Keeping a small aliquot of the preparation back while the majority is being centrifuged allows sperm concentration and motility counts to be completed during the centrifugation.

Direct swim-up from semen

Figure 7.2 The "direct swim-up from semen" (DSUS) sperm preparation procedure.

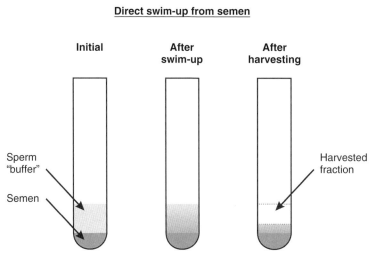

"Swim-up from a washed pellet or sperm suspension": While these methods have been used successfully in many clinical IVF programs, especially with non-male factor cases, the established risk of adversely affecting the fertilizing ability of many men's spermatozoa makes it a poor choice in the modern era where IVF is frequently used for couples where there is a significant male factor, and whose chances of successful IVF could be compromised. Responsible laboratory management should preclude the continued use of a technique incorporating steps known to cause irrevocable damage to spermatozoa prejudicial to a desired functional endpoint.

Adherence-based methods

These methods are based on the fact that dead and moribund spermatozoa are extremely "sticky" and will attach to glass surfaces even in the presence of relatively high concentrations of protein (the "sticking-to-glass" phenomenon). Techniques using glass wool columns were quite common in the 1980s, but reports that glass wool could induce damage to the sperm plasma membrane and acrosome [19], and the danger of glass wool fragments in the final sperm population, led to their abandonment, especially for preparing sperm populations to be used for intrauterine insemination (IUI). Methods based on glass beads, while used widely for preparing rodent spermatozoa, saw little use with human spermatozoa. Selective filtration using Sephadex columns was also described, but only limited studies comparing the functional competence of these sperm preparations with techniques such as direct swim-up from semen and density gradients were reported.

Selective washing using density gradient centrifugation (DGC)

These methods separate cells based upon their density or specific gravity (i.e. mass per unit volume), and result in cells being distributed throughout a gradient column according to the location in the gradient that matches their density, i.e. at their isopycnic points. Although density gradients can be either continuous, where the density of the material comprising the gradient changes in a smooth manner from its minimum at the top of the gradient to its maximum at the bottom, or discontinuous, where a series of layers of decreasing density are placed one on top of another, the latter have been used almost exclusively for clinical applications with human spermatozoa.

In discontinuous gradients the interfaces separating the layers create step-wise changes in densities and can become clogged by cells or other materials, retarding – or even preventing – the passage of more dense cells down the gradient. DGC methods were popularized in the early 1980s following the commercialization of colloidal silica that had been coated with polyvinylpyrrolidone – Percoll® (Pharmacia Biotech, Uppsala, Sweden), which dominated clinical human sperm preparation until its withdrawal from clinical use by its manufacturer in 1996 [2]. Density gradients for human sperm preparation were also described using other products such as Nycodenz® [20], OptiPrep™ and Accudenz® (all from Nycomed Pharma, Oslo, Norway [21,22]), although the osmotic activity of these molecules required special media for their optimal use.

Mature, morphologically normal human spermatozoa have a density (specific gravity) above 1.12 g/ml, whereas immature, and many abnormal spermatozoa have densities between 1.06 and 1.09 g/ml [23]. The specific gravity of colloidal silica preparations equivalent to 40% and 80% of the original Percoll® product is about 1.06 and 1.10 g/ml respectively, therefore only the most mature, normal spermatozoa can penetrate the lower layer of an appropriately formulated density gradient (Figure 7.3).

Several intrinsic properties of colloidal silica make it an ideal density gradient material for sperm preparation. Being a mineral, it allows the preparation of high-density preparation media, but makes no osmotic contribution to the media and, because it is a colloid rather than a solution, it has low viscosity and so does not retard sperm cell sedimentation. The toxic effect of pure colloidal silica is eliminated by coating the particles with a suitable

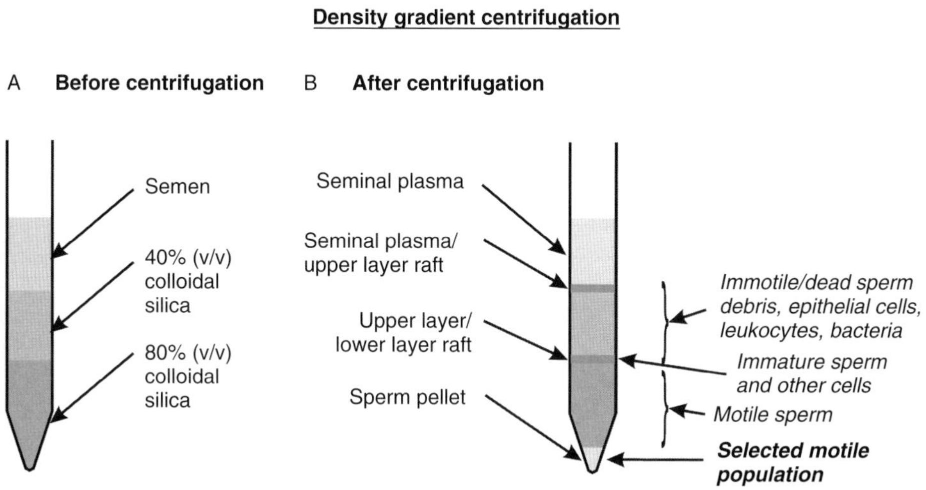

Density gradient centrifugation

A   **Before centrifugation**   B   **After centrifugation**

Figure 7.3 The "density gradient centrifugation" (DGC) method of sperm preparation. Panel A shows the loaded gradient before centrifugation, while panel B shows the same tube after centrifugation in a swing-out rotor.

material (e.g. PVP as in Percoll®, or covalently bound silane molecules ["silanized silica"], as in current human sperm preparation products such as PureSperm®, ISolate® or Sil-Select™; see Appendix 3 for manufacturers and their contact details). The physical characteristics of these new colloids are equivalent to Percoll® preparations, and their clinical utility is at least as good, if not better [2]. The only real difference is that whereas Percoll® was sold as colloidal silica in a weak inorganic buffer solution (requiring it to be used in conjunction with a 10× buffer to make "isotonic" 90% v/v Percoll® colloid), the silanized silica-based products are prepared in an isotonic culture medium ready-to-use.

Unfortunately, this has given rise to a crucial difference between modern DGC products that can affect their performance unless used carefully, as in the erroneous comparison in the 4th edition of the WHO laboratory manual [24]. While PureSperm® was formulated as a direct equivalent of 100% stock Percoll® colloid as supplied from the manufacturer, ISolate® is produced as an equivalent to "isotonic" 90% v/v Percoll® colloid. Hence comparing a 90% ISolate® lower layer with 90% PureSperm® would result in PureSperm® giving a lower yield – but only because it was actually a 90% colloid-equivalent layer, instead of the 81% colloid in the ISolate® lower layer. Likewise, an 80% ISolate® lower layer (i.e. 72% colloid-equivalent) would give an even higher yield, but only by allowing less good spermatozoa into the pellet – i.e. ones with a higher ROS-generating capacity [10]. Consequently, proper use of modern DGC products with human spermatozoa requires that manufacturers state the actual colloid concentration, so that a lower layer of 1.10 g/ml can be employed. The protocol provided below is based on upper and lower layers of correct 40% and 80% colloid respectively, e.g. 40%/80% PureSperm® or 45%/90% ISolate®.

A variety of physical and practical factors affect the optimization of human sperm preparation using colloidal silica-based DGC methods [2,5,6].

Tube shape and size, and rotor type

A more discrete pellet is obtained when a tube is centrifuged in a swing-out rotor rather than a fixed-angle rotor, making it easier to recover the entire pellet when harvesting the gradient.

Tube shape affects the area of the bottom of the tube where the pellet is located, hence a more discrete pellet will be formed in a conical tube, again making it easier to recover the entire pellet (Figure 7.4). Cross-sectional area of the tube, i.e. the area of the interface between the layers, will reduce the rate of formation of the "rafts" that block the gradient, allowing more spermatozoa to reach their isopycnic point – giving higher yields when using larger diameter tubes.

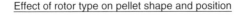

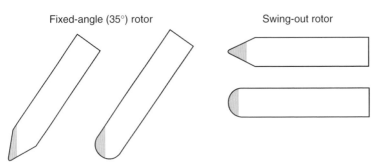

Effect of rotor type on pellet shape and position

Fixed-angle (35°) rotor   Swing-out rotor

Figure 7.4 The effect of tube shape and centrifuge rotor type on the location and shape of the pellet.

Layer number and volume

Longer column layers (i.e. larger volume layers) also result in higher yields (Figure 7.5), but there is no general benefit to using more than two layers (40% and 80% colloid-equivalent) in routine practice. Very occasionally for extremely dirty specimens a third, intermediate layer of 60% colloid can be helpful by slowing/reducing the formation of the "rafts" at the interfaces between layers, but routinely using three layers unnecessarily increases technical complexity as well as both materials and labor costs.

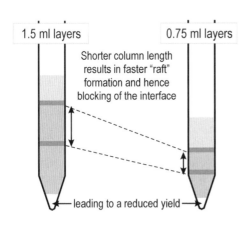

1.5 ml layers   0.75 ml layers

Shorter column length results in faster "raft" formation and hence blocking of the interface

leading to a reduced yield

Figure 7.5 Influence of gradient layer volume on the yield obtained using the density gradient centrifugation method of sperm preparation.

Centrifugation time and speed

Since the earliest work with Percoll® gradients have been centrifuged at 300 g_{max}, it having been found empirically to provide optimum sperm recovery. Various studies during the past

10–15 years have shown no systematic benefit to changing either the centrifugation speed or time for this step. Slower centrifugation speeds (i.e. lower *g*-force) only serve to reduce the yield, they do not improve sperm quality, and faster speeds do not increase the yield since the method is a true isopycnic separation (by 20 min all the spermatozoa have reached their isopycnic points).

Harvesting technique

Although early Percoll® gradient methods described the recovery of the pellet by passing a glass Pasteur pipette straight through the entire gradient, these studies were conducted mostly on research donors or normal fertile men, whose semen samples were reasonably "clean." When using DGC with poor quality patient specimens the "rafts" that build up at the interfaces can be dragged down with the pipette tip, contaminating the pellet. The standard recommended method is to aspirate downwards from the meniscus, stopping once the raft between the 40% and 80% layers has been removed leaving a clear 80% colloid layer. Then, using a clean (sterile) Pasteur pipette, the pellet is recovered through the remaining part of the 80% layer, ensuring that it is not contaminated by any of the seminal plasma and raft material that is slowly running down the inside wall of the tube and collecting on the meniscus of the residual 80% layer (Figure 7.6). Pellets are then transferred to clean centrifuge tubes for washing.

Harvesting the pellet

Figure 7.6 The density gradient centrifugation (DGC) method of sperm preparation: correct harvesting procedure.

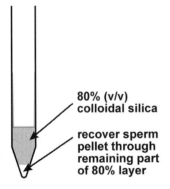

80% (v/v) colloidal silica

recover sperm pellet through remaining part of 80% layer

The following incorrect actions will result in contamination of the pellet to a greater or lesser degree, and should not be employed:

1. Removing all of the bottom gradient layer to reveal the pellet for recovery (mild risk of contamination).

2. Recovering the pellet using the same pipette as was used to remove the upper layers (moderate contamination).

3. Resuspending the pellet in the gradient tube (certain high level contamination).

Such incorrect techniques were used in several published studies, and readers should be aware that results reported from such studies may have been compromised, even to the extent of having no practical relevance.

Washing

The second "wash" centrifugation step needs to be sufficient to recover the great majority of the spermatozoa without exposing them to excessive centrifugal force. For this, the combination of 500 g_{max} × 10 min has been found to be optimal; lower speeds increase the risk of discarding spermatozoa in the supernatant, and neither higher speed nor longer time provides any significant benefit, while speeds higher than 800 g_{max} should be avoided [7]. More than one "wash" step has not been shown to have any measurable benefit in terms of IVF fertilization rate or embryo quality: additional washing is inadvisable. To reduce exposure to unnecessary centrifugation and to avoid the loss of spermatozoa that occurs during each wash step, and hence optimize efficiency and cost-effectiveness, only one "wash" step is advisable.

Post-gradient swim-up

Performing a "swim-out" or "sperm-rise" migration step following the post-gradient wash step in an attempt to eliminate all remaining immotile spermatozoa from the final preparation is ill-advised because:

1. A few immotile spermatozoa in the inseminate have no detectable adverse effects on either fertilization rate or embryo quality; hence a few such spermatozoa are not biologically – or clinically – relevant.

2. The time taken for this step greatly increases the overall time for sperm preparation, decreasing laboratory efficiency and increasing costs.

3. The vast majority of sperm preparations should have >90% progressively motile spermatozoa in the final preparation (typically >95%) if the technique was done properly. So, in the absence of technical error, a sperm preparation with <85% motility must be seen as an indication of some sperm pathology.

"Safe" methods for sperm preparation

Although discontinuous DGC using silane-coated colloidal silica is the current "gold standard" method for human sperm preparation, direct swim-up from semen with one wash step can also be used safely for semen samples showing good sperm progression. Both these methods can provide sperm populations with selected morphology, and also spermatozoa with fewer DNA nicks and better chromatin stability, although DGC seems to be better overall [2,25,26]. A particular importance of this is that, while many ART laboratories prepare their IVF spermatozoa using density gradients, many continue to use simple washing for their ICSI spermatozoa, since the attendant risk of ROS-induced sperm dysfunction is considered unimportant. However, men who need ICSI have high levels of abnormal spermatozoa, and are hence most susceptible to ROS-induced sperm DNA damage. Moreover, since it is well-established that ROS can cause substantial degradation of the sperm DNA that does not necessarily affect their fertilizing ability [12,13], spermatozoa prepared by simple washing will have an increased risk of contributing a defective genome to the embryo. Indeed, this might underlie the increased developmental failure of ICSI-derived embryos after the 8-cell stage when the embryonic genome is activated [27].

Given that the fundamental principle of medical care is *primum non nocere* (first, do no harm), clinical scientists participating in the management of ART programs are obligated to avoid techniques that have known hazards if other, safer techniques are available. To this end, the following sections provide detailed procedures for human sperm preparation using direct swim-up from semen and DGC techniques.

Which type of medium should be used for sperm preparation?

Because centrifugation is usually performed under air, rather than under a CO_2-enriched atmosphere, DGC preparative techniques should use a zwitterion-buffered medium (e.g. HEPES), often referred to as a "sperm wash buffer" rather than a bicarbonate-based medium (this is regardless of whatever suggestion might be made by the embryo culture medium company). Swim-up techniques should also be performed in a "sperm buffer" (and incubated either in an air incubator or else in tightly-capped tubes in a CO_2 incubator) as this will prevent premature capacitation. Because sperm capacitation requires the presence of significant concentrations of bicarbonate ions, the final resuspension of sperm populations that are to undergo in-vitro capacitation must be into a bicarbonate-buffered "sperm wash medium" otherwise their fertilizing capacity will be compromised.

For IUI preparations, a "sperm buffer" can be employed as it will be greatly diluted after insemination, and also because if the spermatozoa undergo capacitation *in vitro* during prolonged incubation prior to insemination their hyperactivated motility might compromise their ability to traverse the utero-tubal junction [17,28]; although if insemination is to be performed soon after sperm preparation then a "medium" can be used safely. Spermatozoa being prepared for ICSI can be processed and resuspended in a "sperm buffer" since capacitation is irrelevant for fertilization using ICSI.

Sperm preparation using direct swim-up from semen (DSUS)

Principle

Sperm migration into a layer of culture medium mimics the process whereby human spermatozoa escape from the liquefied ejaculate and colonize the cervical mucus. Seminal plasma contains decapacitation factors(s) that prevent spermatozoa from undergoing capacitation [2]. Exposure to seminal plasma for more than 30 minutes after ejaculation can permanently diminish human sperm fertilizing ability [3], and only trace amounts of seminal plasma contaminating prepared sperm populations can decrease their fertilizing capacity [4]. Consequently, spermatozoa for clinical procedures such as IUI or IVF (as well as for laboratory tests of sperm fertilizing ability) must be separated from the seminal plasma environment, not only as soon as possible after ejaculation (allowing for the required wait for liquefaction), but also as efficiently as possible. Depending on their intended use, the spermatozoa are then suspended in culture media either capable of supporting in-vitro capacitation (e.g. for IVF), or not (e.g. for IUI or ICSI).

Specimen

Liquefied, homogeneous human semen, ideally within 30 minutes of ejaculation. Longer post-ejaculatory delays, incomplete liquefaction and increased viscosity must be noted on the laboratory and report forms. For other types of specimens and abnormal semen samples, see the section on "Dealing with atypical specimens" later in this chapter.

Equipment (see also Appendix 2)

- Microscope configured for andrology with phase contrast optics (10×, 20× and 40× objectives)
- Air incubator operating at 37°C
- Centrifuge
- Tally counter
- Syringe + tubing adapter to permit volumetric control of glass Pasteur pipettes
- Rubber bulbs to control glass Pasteur pipettes
- Counting chamber (e.g. Makler chamber)

Disposable materials

- Semen collection container*
- Sterile serological pipette*
- Round-bottom polystyrene 7-ml culture tubes* (e.g. Falcon #2003 or #2058)
- Round-bottom polystyrene 14-ml culture tubes* (e.g. Falcon #2001 or #2057)
- Conical-bottom polystyrene 15-ml centrifuge tubes* (e.g. Falcon #2095)
- Glass Pasteur pipettes*

*All disposables that will come into contact with spermatozoa that are to be used for either therapeutic or critical testing purposes should be either pre-tested for sperm toxicity or else obtained from a trusted manufacturer, e.g. if a sterile plastic syringe is used during processing then it must be of a brand known not to have any deleterious effects upon spermatozoa [29].

Reagents

- "Sperm buffer" culture medium (HEPES- or MOPS-buffered) containing at least 10 mg/ml human serum albumin[†]
- Sperm washing medium (bicarbonate-buffered culture medium) containing at least 10 mg/ml human serum albumin[†]
- IVF medium (bicarbonate-buffered) containing at least 10 mg/ml human serum albumin[†]

[†]All reagents that are to be used in preparing human spermatozoa for therapeutic purposes must be CE-marked (or equivalent) and certified as pyrogen-free and not having any sperm toxicity. Reagents for IVF and ICSI applications should also be certified as not being embryotoxic.

Calibration

Centrifugation speeds must not be described using rpm values as these are highly dependent upon the rotational radius of the centrifuge rotor. Also, the g forces are expressed as g_{max} values, calculated for what the spermatozoa would experience at the bottom of the centrifuge tube (not the bottom of the centrifuge bucket). The formula describing the relationship between rotation speed, rotational radius and g-force is:

$$g = 0.0000112 \times r \times N^2 \qquad \text{OR} \qquad N = \sqrt{[g/(0.0000112 \times r)]}$$

where:

> g = the maximum g-force achieved at the bottom of the tube
> r = the rotational radius (in centimeters)
> N = the rotational speed (rpm)

Quality control

All specimen containers and processing/preparation tubes must be labeled with two identifiers, e.g. the man's name and the specimen's laboratory reference or ID number. Temporary analytical preparations (e.g. sperm motility slides) can be identified using the specimen's laboratory reference or ID number only.

Procedure

1. Label the following tubes with the man's name and specimen ID number:

   a. 2 × round-bottom 14-ml culture tubes (more tubes can be prepared if a higher yield is required);

   b. 1 × conical-bottom 15-ml centrifuge tube; and

   c. 1 × round-bottom 7-ml culture tube (this will be for the final sperm preparation).

2. Using aseptic technique, place 0.6 ml of "sperm buffer" into the bottom of each tube and place in the incubator to warm to 37°C before use.

3. Using a sterile glass Pasteur pipette, carefully underlay well-mixed, liquefied semen into the bottom of each tube under the "sperm buffer"; the interface should be sharp and clearly visible (see Figure 7.2). Approximately 300 μl will be required to fill the hemispherical bottom part of the tube; adding more semen than this will not improve the yield.

4. Cap the tube and place upright in the rack (see Note 1). Transfer the rack to the incubator for 20–30 min at 37°C.

5. Using a clean, sterile, glass Pasteur pipette, remove the upper 2/3 of the culture medium layer (*ca.* 400 μl). Take great care not to disturb the medium–semen interface. If the semen layer is disturbed then the preparation should be discarded.

6. Transfer the aspirated upper layer material to the 15-ml centrifuge tube.

7. Repeat steps 5 and 6 for the other tube, transferring the aspirated upper layer material to the same 15-ml centrifuge tube.

8. Add 6 ml of "sperm buffer" to the sperm suspension and mix gently.

9. Cap the tube and centrifuge at 500 g_{max} for 10 min.

10. Using a clean glass Pasteur pipette aspirate the supernatant almost to the pellet.

11. Resuspend the pellet in a suitable volume of the final sperm preparation medium (see Note 2), mixing gently by aspirating in and out of the Pasteur pipette. The volume of medium to use will depend on the size of the pellet and the desired final sperm concentration.

12. Analyze the sperm concentration and motility, e.g. using a Makler chamber (see Note 3).

13. Adjust the sperm concentration, if necessary, by adding more of the final sperm preparation medium. Transfer the final sperm preparation into the 7-ml culture tube.

14. Hold the specimen at the appropriate temperature (see Note 1) until required.

Calculations and results

Use the concentration and sperm motility results to calculate the concentration of progressively motile spermatozoa in the final preparation (see also Note #3) and, using the preparation volume, the total number of such spermatozoa in the final preparation.

Interpretation guidelines

None; this is a preparative technique only (but see sections "Evaluating a sperm preparation method" and "Selecting a sperm preparation method" later in this chapter).

Notes

1. Tubes can be incubated at an angle of 45° to increase the interface area, but they must then be kept at that angle until after harvesting so as not to risk contaminating the medium layer with seminal plasma as the tube is returned to the vertical.

2. Each migration tube should be harvested separately, and the individual preparations combined only after verifying that they contain very high proportions of motile spermatozoa (typically >90–95% motile), and are not contaminated with debris or other cellular elements from the semen fraction.

3. The final sperm preparation medium will vary according to the intended use of the sperm preparation and the likely delay prior to its use. The principle here is to prevent premature sperm capacitation and sperm senescence that will occur when sperm are incubated for prolonged periods at 37°C, especially in a medium that supports sperm capacitation *in vitro*. For example:

   IUI: It is recommended that a "sperm buffer" be employed as it will prevent premature sperm capacitation should there be a prolonged delay before insemination (the zwitterion will be greatly diluted after insemination and have no adverse effect on the spermatozoa). Hold the sperm preparation at ambient temperature (ideally in a styrofoam box to protect it from light and cold drafts). If insemination is to be performed more-or-less immediately after sperm preparation then a bicarbonate-buffered "medium" at 37°C in a CO_2 incubator can be used safely.

   IVF: A bicarbonate-buffered medium capable of supporting sperm capacitation (e.g. IVF medium) should be used. However, if there will be a long delay before IVF insemination then the prepared spermatozoa could be resuspended in a "sperm buffer" and held at ambient temperature until about 2 h beforehand and then washed into fertilization medium and incubated in a CO_2 incubator for the final 90 min before inseminating the oocytes.

   ICSI: Spermatozoa being prepared for ICSI can be processed and resuspended in a "sperm buffer" since capacitation is irrelevant for fertilization using ICSI. Again the preparation should be held at ambient temperature (ideally in a styrofoam box to protect it from light and cold drafts) until the ICSI dish is prepared.

4. If a small, known volume of the resuspended pellet preparation is kept back while the remainder is being washed (e.g. 100 μl from the total specimen), the sperm concentration and motility can be determined during the centrifugation step. The washed pellet could

then be resuspended into a specific volume to give the desired concentration of progressively motile spermatozoa.

Also see the section on "Dealing with atypical specimens" later in this chapter for information relevant to this part of the standard operating procedure (SOP).

Sperm preparation using density gradient centrifugation (DGC)

Background

Seminal plasma contains decapacitation factors(s) that prevent spermatozoa from undergoing capacitation [2]. Exposure to seminal plasma for more than 30 minutes after ejaculation can permanently diminish human sperm fertilizing ability [3], and only trace amounts of seminal plasma contaminating prepared sperm populations can decrease their fertilizing capacity [4]. Consequently, spermatozoa for clinical procedures such as IUI or IVF (as well as for laboratory tests of sperm fertilizing ability) must be separated from the seminal plasma environment not only as soon as possible after ejaculation (allowing for the required wait for liquefaction), but also as efficiently as possible. Depending on their intended use, the spermatozoa are then suspended in culture media either capable of supporting in-vitro capacitation (e.g. for IVF) or not (e.g. for IUI or ICSI).

Principle

Mature, morphologically normal human spermatozoa have a density (specific gravity) above 1.12 g/ml, whereas immature and many abnormal spermatozoa have densities between 1.06 and 1.09 g/ml [22]. Therefore, if they are centrifuged on a density gradient whose bottom layer has specific gravity of 1.10 g/ml (equivalent to 80% of the original Percoll® colloidal silica product), only the most mature, normal spermatozoa will penetrate this layer and form a pellet.

Specimen

Liquefied, homogeneous human semen, ideally within 30 minutes of ejaculation. Longer post-ejaculatory delays, incomplete liquefaction, and increased viscosity must be noted on the laboratory and report forms. For other types of specimens and abnormal semen samples, see the section on "Dealing with atypical specimens" later in this chapter.

Equipment (see also Appendix 2)

- Microscope configured for andrology with phase contrast optics (10×, 20× and 40× objectives)
- Air incubator operating at 37°C
- Centrifuge
- Tally counter
- Syringe + tubing adapter to permit volumetric control of glass Pasteur pipettes
- Rubber bulbs to control glass Pasteur pipettes

Disposable materials
- Semen collection container*
- Sterile serological pipette*
- Round-bottom polystyrene 7-ml culture tubes* (e.g. Falcon #2003 or #2058)
- Conical-bottom polystyrene 15-ml centrifuge tubes* (e.g. Falcon #2095)
- Conical-bottom polystyrene 50-ml centrifuge tubes* (e.g. Falcon #2074) – for retrograde urine
- Glass Pasteur pipettes*
- Counting chamber (e.g. Makler chamber)

    *All disposables that will come into contact with spermatozoa that are to be used for either therapeutic or critical testing purposes should be either pre-tested for sperm toxicity or else obtained from a trusted, reliable manufacturer, e.g. if a sterile plastic syringe is used during processing then it must be of a brand known not to have any deleterious effects upon spermatozoa [29].

Reagents
- Density gradient colloid† (silane-coated colloidal silica). See the discussion (above) regarding the correct colloid concentrations to be used for different manufacturers' products (also Note 1)
- "Sperm Buffer" medium for diluting a 100% density gradient colloid†
- Sperm washing medium†

    †All reagents that are to be used in preparing human spermatozoa for therapeutic purposes must be CE-marked (or equivalent) and certified as pyrogen-free and not having any sperm toxicity. Reagents for IVF and ICSI applications should also be certified as not having any embryo toxicity.

- *Upper layer*: 40% v/v colloid diluted using Sperm Buffer, either prepared by mixing 20 ml of stock 100% colloid and 30 ml of Sperm Buffer, or purchased as a ready-made product (see Note 1).
- *Lower layer*: 80% v/v colloid diluted using Sperm Buffer, either prepared by mixing 40 ml of stock 100% colloid and 10 ml of Sperm Buffer, or purchased as a ready-made product (see Note 1).

Calibration
Centrifugation speeds must not be described using rpm values as these are highly dependent upon the rotational radius of the centrifuge rotor. Also, the g forces are expressed as g_{max} values, calculated for what the spermatozoa would experience at the bottom of the centrifuge tube (not the bottom of the centrifuge bucket). The formula describing the relationship between rotation speed, rotational radius and g-force is:

$$g = 0.0000112 \times r \times N^2 \qquad \text{OR} \qquad N = \sqrt{[g/(0.0000112 \times r)]}$$

where:

   g = the maximum g-force achieved at the bottom of the tube
   r = the rotational radius (in centimeters)
   N = the rotational speed (rpm)

Quality control

All specimen containers and processing/preparation tubes must be labeled with two identifiers, e.g. the man's name and the specimen's laboratory reference or ID number. Temporary analytical preparations (e.g. sperm motility slides) can be identified using the specimen's laboratory reference or ID number only.

Procedure

1. Label the following tubes with the man's name and specimen ID number:

   a. 3 × conical-bottom 15-ml centrifuge tubes (2 for the gradients, 1 for the wash); and

   b. 1 × round-bottom 7-ml culture tube.

2. Using a sterile Pasteur pipette place the upper layer (1.5 ml or 2.0 ml) into each of the 15-ml conical tubes. Then, carefully add the lower layers underneath the upper layers. A clear interface should be visible between the two layers. See Figure 7.3A "Before centrifugation."

   Alternatively, the lower layer can be placed in a tube first and the upper layer added on top, but this approach often results in a less sharp interface between the two layers than using the under-layering method.

3. Carefully overlay liquefied semen onto each (maximum volume is the same as the volume of the upper gradient layer). Cap the tubes tightly.

4. Centrifuge at 300 g_{max} for 20 min in a swing-out rotor with sealed buckets.

5. a. For each gradient, using a sterile glass Pasteur pipette carefully aspirate from the meniscus downwards to remove the seminal plasma, upper interface "raft," upper (40%) layer and the lower interface "raft"; leave most of the lower (80%) layer in place. Discard the aspirated material. See Figure 7.3B "After centrifugation."

   b. Using another clean, sterile glass Pasteur pipette, remove the soft pellet from the bottom of the gradient by direct aspiration (maximum 0.5 ml) from the bottom of the tube beneath the lower (80%) layer. See Figure 7.6.

   c. Transfer the pellet to a single clean conical tube.

   d. Repeat steps 5a–c for the other gradient.

6. Resuspend the pellets in 5–10 ml of Sperm Buffer and mix gently. Cap the tube.

7. Centrifuge at 500 g_{max} for 10 min.

8. Aspirate the supernatant with a sterile Pasteur pipette and resuspend the pellet in 1–3 ml of fresh Sperm Buffer or IVF medium. Transfer to a small round-bottom culture tube, then:

   a. For IUI or DI (sperm resuspended in Sperm Buffer) leave the sample at ambient temperature in a styrofoam box on the bench until it is collected by the nurse for insemination; or

   b. For IVF (sperm resuspended in IVF Medium) equilibrate the loose-capped tube in a CO_2 incubator for 30 min then cap it tightly and place it in the dark at room temperature (i.e. in a cupboard in the Embryology Laboratory); or

   c. For ICSI, cap the tube tightly and place in a 37°C incubator.

9. Assess the concentration and motility of the washed sperm preparation using a Makler chamber (if available, computer-aided sperm analysis "CASA" can be used).

a. Even though there will be some (perhaps even 10%) immotile or dead spermatozoa in the final preparation, this is not a problem and there is no need to perform any further preparation (e.g. swim-up) as it will have no benefit and could compromise sperm function or survival.

b. On occasions, a washed sperm preparation in culture medium might contain a high proportion of hyperactivated cells that, although very vigorous, may present little progression. In such cases the motility report should state the percentages of progressive and hyperactivated cells, as well as the total motility.

Calculations and results

Use the concentration and sperm motility results to calculate the concentration of progressively motile spermatozoa in the final preparation (see Note 2) and, using the preparation volume, the total number of such spermatozoa in the final preparation.

Interpretation guidelines

Typically, none, as this is a preparative technique only (but see sections "Evaluating a sperm preparation method" and "Evaluating a sperm preparation method" later in this chapter). However, if an IUI or IVF sperm preparation shows such reduced motility, serious consideration should be given to switching the treatment modality to ICSI, and almost certainly switching if there is <80% motility. Obviously this is best established during a pre-treatment "diagnostic" sperm preparation or "trial wash," rather than discovering it on the day of treatment – although an aberrant preparation might arise due to an intervening problem with the man (e.g. a bout of febrile illness).

Notes

1. An optimum density gradient for separating mature, normal human spermatozoa requires that the bottom gradient layer have a density of 1.10 g/ml, equivalent to 80% v/v of the original Percoll® colloid product. Consequently, products for which the manufacturer does not state the actual colloid concentration might not be able to be employed reliably for optimal sperm preparation.

2. If a small, known volume of the resuspended pellet preparation is kept back while the remainder is being washed (e.g. 100 µl from the total specimen), the sperm concentration and motility can be determined during the centrifugation step. The washed pellet could then be resuspended into a specific volume to give the desired concentration of progressively motile spermatozoa.

Also see the section on "Dealing with atypical specimens" later in this chapter for information relevant to this part of the SOP.

Evaluating a sperm preparation method

The usefulness or applicability of a sperm preparation technique should be considered in terms of both the quantity and quality of the spermatozoa obtained in the final preparation.

Quantitative aspects

Here we are usually only concerned with spermatozoa showing progressive motility, since non-progressive spermatozoa have negligible functional competence under any circumstances other than ICSI.

Relative yield

Relative yield is the proportion of progressively motile spermatozoa submitted to a preparative procedure that are present in the final preparation:

$$\text{Yield} = (v \times c \times pm\%)/(V \times C \times PM\%) \times 100\%$$

where:

v	= final preparation volume
c	= sperm concentration in the final preparation
pm%	= prepared sperm population progressive motility
V	= volume of semen used
C	= sperm concentration in the semen
PM%	= progressive motility in the semen

Absolute yield

Absolute yield is the total number of progressively motile spermatozoa that could be obtained were the whole ejaculate to be used (an allowance usually being made for losing an aliquot of semen used for semen analysis purposes, e.g. 0.3 ml). Note that the progressive motility and yield are each divided by 100 to convert the percentage values back into fractions.

$$\text{Absolute yield} = (V - 0.3) \times (PM\%/100) \times (\text{Yield}/100)$$

Qualitative aspects

The quality of the prepared sperm population is also of vital importance, especially when creating embryos, and includes considerations not only of both sperm fertilizing ability and sperm DNA integrity, but also the yield purity (e.g. the reduction or elimination of infectious microorganisms such as bacteria and viruses) [2].

Dealing with atypical semen specimens

Highly viscous samples

It can be extremely difficult to obtain good yields of motile spermatozoa from highly viscous samples, but do not "needle" viscous semen through a 19G or 22G needle as the high shear forces exerted upon the spermatozoa can damage them [30]. Instead, dilute the semen with a 1–2× volume of "sperm buffer" (i.e. a medium that is not based on a bicarbonate buffer, so that it can be used safely under an air atmosphere) and mix gently using a sterile Pasteur pipette before loading onto the gradient. If the sample does not disperse within 2 minutes of pipetting, incubate at 37°C for 10 minutes and then mix further. Once the sample has been successfully diluted it can be loaded onto the gradients as usual. Alternatively, the man could collect into chymotrypsin-coated MARQ™ Liquefaction Cups (Embryotech Laboratories).

"Dirty" specimens

With semen samples that are heavily contaminated with particulate debris or contain high numbers of other cells, the "rafts" at the interfaces between either the seminal plasma and 40% layer or the 40 and 80% layers might form too quickly, and/or be too dense, and block the gradient, drastically reducing the sperm yield. To avoid this problem:

a. only process part of the ejaculate; and/or

b. load less semen onto each gradient, perhaps dividing the sample over four gradients instead of two; and/or

c. use longer columns of colloid, e.g. 3 ml per layer; and/or

d. when loading the semen onto the gradient, mix it gently with the upper one-fifth of the upper layer; and/or

e. prepare a three-step gradient using layers of 40%, 60%, and 80% colloid (but do not use a lower layer of >80% colloid as it will reduce the sperm yield).

Cryopreserved specimens

Cryopreserved spermatozoa are in a highly hypertonic medium (due to the cryoprotectant medium) and hence will suffer extreme osmotic shock upon entering the upper layer of a density gradient, and hence decrease their specific gravity – causing them to be too buoyant to pass through the density gradient (and also causing impaired sperm function). Therefore, cryopreserved sperm specimens must be diluted with a relatively large volume of "isotonic" medium prior to loading onto the gradients. For spermatozoa cryopreserved using a traditional TEST-yolk-glycerol (TYG) cryoprotectant medium a 10× dilution works well, but with many egg yolk-free cryoprotectant media a 5× dilution is sufficient. The thawed specimen should be diluted slowly (drop-wise) with constant gentle mixing over a period of at least 10 min. Now, the maximum volume that can be loaded onto a single gradient is based on the original semen component, i.e. if semen was diluted 1 : 1 with a cryoprotectant medium, and then diluted 5× after thawing, 1 ml of the original semen is now contained in 12 ml of diluted material, making it very hard to overload a gradient. If the total volume exceeds the maximum volume that can be loaded onto a pair of gradients, the diluted post-thaw material can be centrifuged at 500 g_{max} for 10 min and, after removing and discarding the supernatant, the pellet resuspended in 1–2 ml of fresh medium (still, ideally, Sperm Buffer), and then loaded onto a pair of gradients. This procedure is sub-optimal, but relatively safe because the cells that generate ROS during centrifugation do not survive the freezing and thawing process.

Poor quality specimens

An increased yield can be obtained from most samples, but especially low concentration ones, and ones with low sperm motility, if slightly less dense layers are used, e.g. 72% and 36% colloid. However, this is only achieved by recovering less dense, and hence less good quality, spermatozoa and should only be used as a last resort. Whatever spermatozoa can be recovered from a standard 40/80 gradient will always be the best available from the specimen.

Retrograde ejaculate urine specimens

In the case of retrograde ejaculation, the semen does not pass out to the exterior through the urethra ("antegrade ejaculation") but passes back into the bladder. Various protocols exist for managing these cases, but after the retrograde ejaculate urine specimen has been concentrated by centrifugation (e.g. 500 g_{max} × 10 min in one or more 50-ml polystyrene conical tubes) and resuspended into a small volume of a "sperm buffer," the material is layered over one or several 2-step (40%/80%) density gradients and processed as though it were a normal semen sample.

Surgically retrieved sperm specimens

In the case of sperm suspensions obtained from the epididymis (or after homogenization of testicular tissue), it might be necessary to separate all the spermatozoa from the other cells, etc. This can be most easily achieved by centrifuging the material through a single column of 40% colloid, using the standard conditions of 300 g_{max} × 20 min. After carefully removing most (e.g. 3/4) of the supernatant, the pellet is recovered through the remaining 1/4 of the layer using a clean, sterile glass Pasteur pipette. See also Chapter 9.

Selecting a sperm preparation method

Selecting an appropriate sperm preparation method requires consideration of the following perspectives:

1. Relative simplicity and rapidity of a method, for reasons of laboratory efficiency.

2. Cost of the materials (and equipment) required for the method.

3. Any risk of iatrogenic damage inherent in the method, balanced against the level of protection from iatrogenic damage that the method affords.

4. General applicability of a method, i.e. the range of semen qualities relative to what is seen by the laboratory for which the method will provide adequate yields of motile spermatozoa for the intended form of treatment.

Defining "acceptable yield" relates to the ultimate use of the prepared sperm population: e.g. IUI requires 5×10^6 motile spermatozoa in a 100-µl volume for insemination, whereas IVF uses only about 80 000 motile spermatozoa per oocyte or per well if oocytes are inseminated as a group. "Heavy insemination" as a form of IVF for men with moderate male factor (up to 500 000/ml [31]) has largely been replaced by ICSI as a more reliable way to ensure a good fertilization rate.

Because of the risks of potentially severe detrimental effects upon the spermatozoa, methods involving any centrifugal washing of semen that result in the pelleting of unselected spermatozoa (e.g. "swim-out" or "sperm-rise") have been contraindicated since the late 1980s [9,10,14].

Direct swim-up from semen (DSUS) remains the simplest technique for obtaining populations of highly motile spermatozoa, and has been recommended by the WHO for >20 years. It can be a very rapid procedure when working with normal semen samples but the most widely applicable and practical method for preparing motile sperm populations from both normal and abnormal semen samples is DGC. Although the results can be disappointing with asthenozoospermic samples, whatever population of spermatozoa is obtained does represent the good quality spermatozoa that were present in the ejaculate.

Processing multiple samples

Risk management purists assert that only a single semen specimen should be processed by a scientist at any one time, always using a separate centrifuge and workstation for each specimen. However, in a busy clinical laboratory this is frequently not just impracticable but impossible as it would require unrealistic numbers of staff and centrifuges. Due process analysis reveals that proper observance of a carefully designed process (in conjunction with a formal risk assessment) can permit the "safe" processing of more than one sample at once provided that the following are ensured:

1. Each specimen is allocated to a separate tube rack (see Figure 7.7).

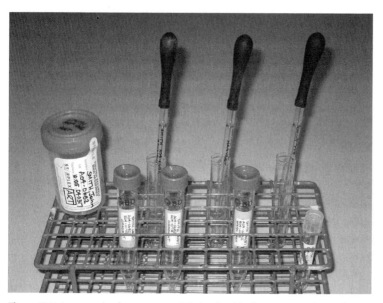

Figure 7.7 An example of a system to minimize the risk of cross-contamination between sperm specimens being processed in parallel. All the tubes, etc., for a given specimen are placed in a single rack, so that even if two specimens are being centrifuged together, they are each harvested and resuspended separately. Note that the semen collection jar is labeled with the man's name and the andrology lab reference number (A04–0682), as well as the date and time of collection. Each tube and pipette are labeled with the name, plus both the andrology lab number and the oocyte retrieval case number (R04–0179) as identifiers, along with the date and the purpose of each item. There is no label on the rack because it is the identity of each of the individual items that must be verified at each stage of the process; if there was a large label on the rack, there might be a tendency to read only that when going to work on a sample. Reproduced from [32] with permission.

2. All disposable materials are labeled using at least two unique identifiers, one of which must be a number (since the human brain innately "completes" sequences of letters as words), and perhaps also using a color-coding scheme.

3. All the disposable materials to be used for a specimen are held together in a defined working area, such as a plastic box or tray.

4. Racks and trays are *never* labeled, only tubes, so as to ensure their proper re-identification at every step.

5. Pipettes should be labeled for each specimen, and organized in such a way that they cannot be confused between specimens being processed in parallel; e.g. they can be held in a second rack in the tray alongside the tube rack.

6. Only one specimen is actually worked on at any point in time, i.e. only one rack or tray is in a scientist's "active" work area at a time, and a scientist *never* has tubes from more than one sample open at a time.

7. Multiple samples may be centrifuged at the same time so long as there is an established procedure for verification of each tube's identity afterwards, before it is opened.

8. Each re-identification step should be documented and, if possible, witnessed.

References

1. Yanagimachi R. Mammalian fertilization. In: Knobil E, Neill JD, eds. *The Physiology of Reproduction.* 2nd edn. New York: Raven Press 1994: 189–317.

2. Mortimer D. Sperm preparation methods. *J Androl* 2000; **21**: 357–66.

3. Rogers BJ, Perreault SD, Bentwood BJ, *et al.* Variability in the human-hamster in vitro assay for fertility evaluation. *Fertil Steril* 1983; **39**: 204–11.

4. Kanwar KC, Yanagimachi R, Lopata A. Effects of human seminal plasma on fertilizing capacity of human spermatozoa. *Fertil Steril* 1979; **31**: 321–7.

5. Mortimer, D. Sperm recovery techniques to maximize fertilizing capacity. *Reprod Fertil Devel* 1994; **6**: 25–31.

6. Mortimer D. *Practical Laboratory Andrology.* New York: Oxford University Press 1995.

7. Jeulin C, Serres C, Jouannet P. The effects of centrifugation, various synthetic media and temperature on the motility and vitality of human spermatozoa. *Reprod Nutr Dévélop* 1982; **22**: 81–91.

8. Friedman AJ, Juneau-Norcross M, Sedensky B. Antisperm antibody production following intrauterine insemination. *Hum Reprod* 1991; **6**: 1125–8.

9. Aitken RJ, Clarkson JS. Cellular basis of defective sperm function and its association with the genesis of reactive oxygen species by human spermatozoa. *J Reprod Fertil* 1987; **81**: 459–69.

10. Aitken RJ, Clarkson JS. Significance of reactive oxygen species and antioxidants in defining the efficacy of sperm preparation techniques. *J Androl* 1988; **9**: 367–76.

11. Selley ML, Lacey MJ, Bartlett MR, *et al.* Content of significant amounts of a cytotoxic end-product of lipid peroxidation in human semen. *J Reprod Fertil* 1991; **92**: 291–8.

12. Aitken RJ, Gordon E, Harkiss D, *et al.* Relative impact of oxidative stress on the functional competence and genomic integrity of human spermatozoa. *Biol Reprod* 1998; **59**: 1037–46.

13. Aitken RJ. Free radicals, lipid peroxidation and sperm function. *Reprod Fertil Devel* 1995; **7**: 659–68.

14. Mortimer D. Sperm preparation techniques and iatrogenic failures of in-vitro fertilization. *Hum Reprod* 1991; **6**: 173–6.

15. Katz DF, Morales P, Samuels SJ, Overstreet JW. Mechanisms of filtration of morphologically abnormal human sperm by cervical mucus. *Fertil Steril* 1990; **54**: 513–6.

16. Mortimer, D. Sperm transport in the female genital tract. In: Grudzinskas JG, Yovich JL, eds. *Cambridge Reviews in Human Reproduction. Volume 2: Gametes – The Spermatozoon.* Cambridge (UK): Cambridge University Press 1995: 157–74.

17. Mortimer ST. A critical review of the physiological importance and analysis of sperm movement in mammals. *Hum Reprod Update* 1997; **3**: 403–39.

18. Tea NT, Jondet M, Scholler R. A 'migration-gravity sedimentation' method for collecting motile spermatozoa from human semen. In: Harrison RF, Bonnar J, Thompson W, eds. *In Vitro Fertilization, Embryo Transfer and Early Pregnancy.* Lancaster (UK): MTP Press Ltd. 1984: 117–20.

19. Sherman JK, Paulson JD, Liu KC. Effect of glass wool filtration on ultrastructure of human spermatozoa. *Fertil Steril* 1981; **36**: 643–7.

20. Gellert-Mortimer ST, Clarke GN, Baker HWG, *et al.* Evaluation of Nycodenz and Percoll density gradients for the selection of motile human spermatozoa. *Fertil Steril* 1988; **49**: 335–41.

21. Sbracia M, Sayme N, Grasso J, *et al.* Sperm function and choice of preparation media: comparison of Percoll and Accudenz

discontinuous density gradients. *J Androl* 1996; **17**: 61–7.

22. Smith TT, Byers M, Kaftani D, Whitford W. The use of iodixanol as a density gradient material for separating human sperm from semen. *Arch Androl* 1997; **38**: 223–30.

23. Oshio S, Kaneko S, Iizuka R, Mohri H. Effects of gradient centrifugation on human sperm. *Arch Androl* 1987; **17**: 85–93.

24. World Health Organization. *WHO Laboratory Manual for the Analysis of Human Semen and Sperm-Cervical Mucus Interaction.* 4th edn. Cambridge (UK): Cambridge University Press 1999.

25. Sakkas D, Manicardi GC, Tomlinson M, *et al.* The use of two density gradient centrifugation techniques and the swim-up method to separate spermatozoa with chromatin and nuclear DNA anomalies. *Hum Reprod* 2000; **15**: 1112–6.

26. Tomlinson MJ, Moffatt O, Manicardi GC, *et al.* Interrelationships between seminal parameters and sperm nuclear DNA damage before and after density gradient centrifugation: implications for assisted conception. *Hum Reprod* 2001; **16**: 2160–5.

27. Shoukir Y, Chardonnens D, Campana A, Sakkas D. Blastocyst development from supernumerary embryos after intracytoplasmic sperm injection: a paternal influence? *Hum Reprod* 1998; **13**: 1632–7.

28. Shalgi R, Smith TT, Yanagimachi R. A quantitative comparison of the passage of capacitated and uncapacitated hamster spermatozoa through the uterotubal junction. *Biol Reprod* 1992; **46**: 419–24.

29. de Ziegler D, Cedars MI, Hamilton F, *et al.* Factors influencing maintenance of sperm motility during in vitro processing. *Fertil Steril* 1987; **48**: 816–20.

30. Knuth UA, Neuwinger J, Nieschlag E. Bias to routine semen analysis by uncontrolled changes in laboratory environment – detection by long-term sampling of monthly means for quality control. *Int J Androl* 1989; **12**: 375–83.

31. Wolf DP, Byrd W, Dandekar P, Quigley MM. Sperm concentration and the fertilization of human eggs in vitro. *Biol Reprod* 1984; **31**: 837–48.

32. Mortimer D, Mortimer ST. *Quality and Risk Management in the IVF Laboratory.* Cambridge (UK): Cambridge University Press 2005.

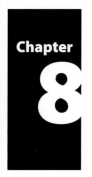

Sperm cryobanking

Fundamentals of cryobiology

The main objective of cryopreservation of cells is to maintain their viability and functionality over extended periods of subzero storage. Cryopreserved cells are stored at −196°C (in liquid nitrogen). At this temperature, neither the phenomenon of diffusion, nor sufficient latent thermal energy exist for chemical reactions to occur. Therefore, the difficulties of freezing do not arise from exposure to low temperatures but rather from the freezing and thawing processes.

Cellular responses to freezing and thawing

Cold shock or chilling damage (from 37°C to >0°C)

Cold shock is the damage to cells caused by their sensitivity to the cooling rate, and it results from lipid phase transition effects and ionic imbalances such as calcium loading. Chilling sensitivity is damage arising from cells' sensitivity to a specific temperature or temperature range. Lipids can exist in an ordered rigid state (gel) or in a more flexible and relatively disordered state (fluid). The transition from one state to another takes place over a certain temperature range. This temperature depends on the composition of the fatty acids that compose the membrane. Most membranes of eukaryotic cells have a melting temperature between 0°C and 15°C. The transition phase of a plasma membrane does not occur simultaneously in all of its phospholipids and therefore there is a coexistence of domains in both fluid and gel states during the transition. This situation produces defects in the packing of membranes (mechanical shearing) and conformational changes in membrane topography that give rise to non-linear kinetic responses in some enzymes. These changes are associated with a greater permeability of solutes through the membrane [1].

Ice formation (<0°C to −130°C)

The existence of solutes in the water produces a decrease in the freezing (cryoscopic) point to between −10°C and −15°C and, as a result, the crystallization of water occurs at lower temperatures than the freezing point of pure water (0°C). When temperatures are this low the sample is supercooled. In this situation, the onset of ice formation is random. To avoid this problem, in many protocols ice formation is provoked in the extracellular medium by means of an abrupt reduction in temperature ("seeding") – thus the system is guaranteed to be in phase change, and ice is present. Ice formation can be induced in many ways, but typically by touching the specimen with a small object that is at a lower temperature than that of the phase change. Seeding is important because, during the crystallization process, a sample releases sufficient heat (latent heat of fusion) to cause a sharp increase in temperature, and consequently the sample temperature does not decrease in tandem with the fall in the chamber temperature. In fact, the sample temperature can remain static for two to three minutes before resuming its decrease [2].

The formation of ice in the extracellular medium removes water from this compartment, and this triggers a solvent flow across the semi-permeable membrane towards the region with a higher concentration of solutes. As a result, formation of ice in the extracellular medium provokes cellular dehydration [3].

Thawing

During the thawing process, the osmotic changes that take place are the opposite of what occurred during freezing: as frozen water changes state (solid to liquid) the concentration of solutes in the extracellular medium is progressively reduced and the cell hydrates in order to compensate for the difference in concentration between the extracellular and intracellular compartments. Fast rewarming rates are required for optimal cell recovery due to the formation and growth of small intracellular ice crystals while the cell is between the transition point of water (about –132°C) and the melting point. In addition, as the post-thaw temperature increases the lipids and proteins of the plasma membrane undergo structural rearrangements.

Cryodamage

When cell survival is plotted as a function of the cooling rate, the curve produced is a characteristic inverted U-shape (Figure 8.1). In order to clarify this effect of cooling on survival rates, the "2-factor" hypothesis proposes two different mechanisms to account for cellular damage during the cryopreservation process: ice production and osmotic stress.

Intracellular ice formation

Once extracellular ice formation has begun, along with the corresponding cellular dehydration, events in the intracellular space depend on the cooling rate. If freezing occurs too quickly, the cell will not be able to dehydrate efficiently, and the remaining water will form intracellular ice – and the more ice formed within the cell, the lower the chance of cellular survival [4].

Osmotic stress

Osmotic stress is active at low cooling rates, and is related to the mechanical cellular deformation caused by the reduction in size originating from the intense process of dehydration, and by prolonged cellular exposure to high concentrations of electrolytes. This mechanism is known as the "solution effect" [3]. Two complementary theories exist to explain the phenomenon of osmotic stress during the cryopreservation process:

1. The hypothesis of high ion concentrations attributes the cause to the interaction between the high ion concentrations in the extracellular medium and the membrane proteins [1].
2. The hypothesis of minimum cellular volume relates the effect of dehydration caused during the concentration of solutes and cellular death, with the return of isotonic conditions after the freezing process (osmotic shock). As the cell volume decreases during freezing (by dehydration) the compression of the cytoplasmic contents increases the resistance of the cell to further loss of volume, and when this physical resistance is exceeded an irreversible change in permeability is caused [5].

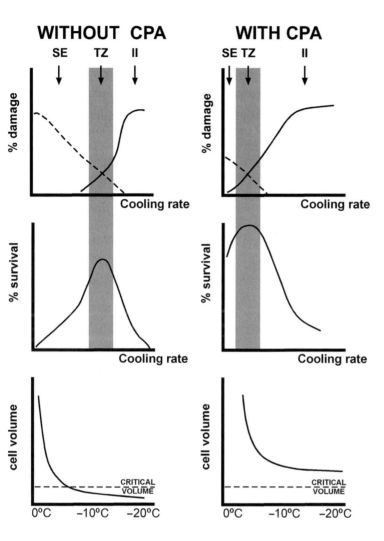

Figure 8.1
Cryodamage, survival, and cell volume changes during cryopreservation with and without CPA. SE = solution effect; TZ = transition zone; II = intracellular ice.

In summary, when lower cooling rates are used cellular damage is caused by high extracellular solute concentrations and by high cooling rates causing intracellular ice formation. There is an optimal cooling range for each cell, referred to as the "transition zone," in which these damaging conditions are minimized, and hence when there will be maximum probability of cell cryosurvival (Figure 8.1). Although the universal validity of this principle has been verified, each cell type requires its own optimized cryopreservation protocol, based on the cell's biophysical properties [6].

Recrystallization

All biological material must be stored below the glass transition temperature of water (about −132°C) in order to stop all biological activity. At higher temperatures, longevity is reduced to a matter of weeks or months. Glass transition of an already frozen aqueous solution does not occur suddenly at −132°C; it is a progressive phenomenon between this temperature and −90°C. Therefore, at −80°C there is a great risk of substantial change having occurred. At this temperature, warming energy is returned to the system, permitting molecules to resume their natural orientation, and very small ice crystals are formed.

Cryoprotective agents (CPAs)

In addition to achieving suitable cooling rates, optimizing cellular viability requires alteration of the physicochemical behavior of the aqueous environment in which cryopreservation takes place. For this reason, CPAs are added to the cryopreservation medium – substances that are very hydro-soluble and low in cytotoxicity, and which lower the eutectic point (i.e. the freezing/melting point) of the solution. Cryoprotectants can be divided into permeating and non-permeating agents, depending on their permeability through the cell membrane.

Permeating CPAs

CPAs are low-molecular-weight molecules which pass through the cell membrane, most commonly glycerol, 1,2-propanediol, dimethyl sulfoxide and ethylene glycol. Although the cell is permeable to these agents, their permeabilities are not of the same magnitude as that of water.

Non-permeating CPAs

Non-permeating CPAs are substances of much higher molecular weight than permeating CPAs, and are most effective when employed in a high-speed freezing process. Since these molecules do not penetrate the cell they are not actually cryoprotectants themselves, but act as such by promoting fast cellular dehydration, and are usually used in association with permeating CPAs. The most commonly used non-permeating CPAs are sucrose, glucose, dextrose, polyvinylpyrrolidone (PVP), raffinose, trehalose, lactose, and hydroxyethyl starch.

CPAs can be added or removed either in a single step, which reduces the time of cellular exposure to the CPA, or step-wise, so as to gradually increase/decrease the concentration of the CPA in the medium, which reduces the osmotic stress on the cell to be frozen or thawed and can avoid exceeding the cells' critical volume limits [7,8]. The optimal approach is usually determined empirically.

Benefits of CPAs

Although CPAs are commonly used in cryopreservation, their protection mechanisms are not completely known, but the following physical mechanisms certainly act to promote cellular survival: dilution of electrolytes, decreasing water concentration, increasing viscosity, "salt buffering" effect, and stabilization of the cell membrane by means of electrostatic interactions [1].

Harmful aspects of CPAs

There are two main harmful effects of CPAs:

1. Toxicity: Permeating CPAs are chemical substances that are not normally found in the cell, and are effectively poisoning the cell [2]. However, as cell metabolism slows the toxic effects are markedly diminished, unless very high concentrations are used at relatively high temperatures (around 0°C).

2. Osmosis: Addition of CPAs exerts osmotic stress on the cell caused by the increased osmolarity of the medium. The cells initially dehydrate to compensate for the osmotic pressure (cell shrinkage) but then, as the permeating CPA enters the cells, the cells return to their original isotonic volume. Upon removal of the permeating CPA by dilution of the post-thaw specimen, water enters the cells quickly, due to the osmotic gradient, and the CPA leaves the cells more slowly; hence, the cells swell before equilibrium is restored. These cell volume excursions (shrinkage and swelling) can be extensive enough to cause irreversible cell damage if the cell exceeds either or both of its critical volume limits (Figure 8.2) [5].

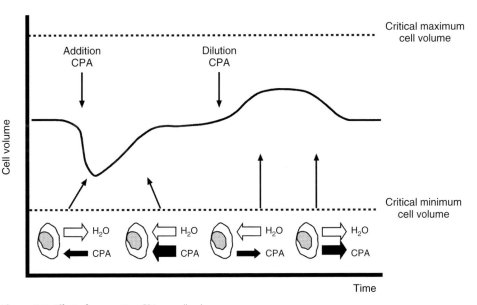

Figure 8.2 Effect of permeating CPA on cell volume.

Vitrification

Vitrification is the solidification of a solution into a solid, glass-like state without crystallization or expansion, hence intracellular water undergoes an extreme increase in viscosity without intracellular ice formation. This process is achieved by increasing both the rate of freezing and the concentration of the cryoprotectant solution. Generally speaking, vitrification involves extremely high cooling and warming rates to prevent intracellular ice formation. Even when a 0.25-ml straw is directly plunged into liquid nitrogen or warmed by immersion in water (where cooling and warming rates can be as high as 2500°C/min between –25°C and –175°C), intracellular ice crystals can still form leading to cellular damage. Using other devices such as an electron microscopy grid, open-pulled straw, cryoloop, cryotop and cryotip, cooling and warming rates can be increased to 22 500°C/min and intracellular ice formation can be avoided. However, in order to obtain these high rates it is necessary for the volume in which the cells are contained to be very small, meaning that very few cells can be vitrified [2].

Cryopreservation methods

Background

Although human semen cryobanking can be generally divided into the two broad areas of autoconservation and donor banking, there are many permutations for their clinical application (Table 8.1). Enabling human spermatozoa to survive cryopreservation depends on various factors (Table 8.2). Although the bibliography on the subject is vast [6,9], there is no universally accepted method, as many are capable of achieving at least satisfactory results. Moreover, given the high degree of variability between men, in sperm cryosurvival rates, it is difficult to compare studies and identify the best method of cryopreservation [10,11,12].

Table 8.1 Sperm bank users.

Area of activity	Applications
Donor spermatozoa	• To prevent the transmission of hereditary or infectious disease in a hetero-sexual couple.
	• Insemination for single women.
	• Insemination for lesbian women.
Autoconservation	• Pre-vasectomy (fertility "insurance").
	• Fertility preservation: before chemotherapy, radiotherapy, or orchidectomy, e.g. cancer, autoimmune diseases.
	• Testicular biopsy/epididymis.
	• Washed semen from men carrying infectious diseases.
	• Difficulty in the collection of semen, e.g. retrograde ejaculation, erectile dysfunction, psychological problems.
	• Unavailability of the male on the day of the ART.
	• Patients with progressive loss of the seminal quality, e.g. Y-chromosome microdeletions, transient azoospermia.
	• Occupational hazards, sports, death risk (e.g. military).
	• Post-mortem storage, e.g. desire of the family in case of unexpected death of the male (epididymal aspirations or testicular biopsy specimens).
Research	• Clinical research.
	• Basic biology research.
	• Fundamental cryobiology research.

At present, apart from purely biological and technical aspects, other practical factors affect the choice of protocol to be applied in freezing spermatozoa. For example, government regulations require, if possible, the use of a commercially available cryopreservation medium (CPM) and supplements that conform to pharmaceutical standards. In addition, there must be traceability regarding all laboratory activities affecting cryopreserved cells, including the temperature at which the cells are kept, which means that freezing systems must be fitted with temperature monitoring and recording equipment.

Table 8.2 Factors affecting the optimization of human sperm preservation.

Biological factors	Within-subject variability:
	• Sexual abstinence
	• Season
	Between–subject variability:
	• Genetic factors
	• Seminal fluid quality
	• Seminal quality
Technical factors	Cryopreservation medium
	Addition/removal cryoprotectants
	Cooling rate
	Packaging
	Storage
	Thawing

Biological factors affecting sperm cryopreservation

Various biological factors have been related to within- and between-male variability of sperm cryopreservation, including sexual abstinence, seasonality, composition of the seminal fluid and genetic factors. Also, although there is a relationship between pre-freeze and post-thaw sperm motility, it is not possible to predict exactly the survival rates of spermatozoa after thawing from the standard semen parameters. Subfertile sperm samples are more susceptible to freezing and thawing injuries than are fertile samples, and epididymal and testicular spermatozoa are more susceptible to cryopreservation injury than are ejaculated spermatozoa [6,13].

Technical factors affecting sperm cryopreservation

The protocols for adding and later eliminating cryoprotective agents consist of one or more stages in which the cells are immersed in a medium containing cryoprotectants of a given composition, for a given period of time, at a given temperature – each of which must be specified at each stage of the process. Consequently, the number of permutations in a method for a particular cell will preclude empirical evaluation of all possible protocols, making the use of theoretical models fundamental to the development of a freezing protocol – notwithstanding the effect of biological variability that can lead to conflicting results [2].

Cryopreservation medium

The permeating CPA most commonly used in sperm cryopreservation is glycerol, although experimental models have shown that higher sperm survival rates can be achieved using ethylene glycol [7,8]. Sucrose and glucose are the non-permeating CPAs most often used. Sperm cryopreservation media may also contain the following components:

1. Agents that interact with the plasma membrane: Various substances have been shown to be capable of changing lipidic composition of the cellular membrane, improving its

195

fluidity: lecithin, egg yolk, milk and albumin. Other substances with lipophilic properties, such as methyl-β-cyclodextrin (a derivative of a cyclic oligomer of glucose) and amphipathic compounds such as glycine, betaine, proline and trehalose, are thought to interact directly with membrane lipids and proteins, altering their phase transition behavior and hydration state [14].

2. Chelaters (EDTA, citrate): During cryopreservation, there is poor control of the intracellular concentration of calcium, hence the inclusion of EDTA and citrate in semen diluents could exert beneficial effects via chelating calcium and decreasing its concentration gradient across the sperm-plasma membrane. However, EDTA and other metallic ion chelaters might also act by inhibiting lipid peroxidation.

3. Agents that prevent lipid peroxidation: Butylated hydroxytoluene, glutathione and dithiothreitol have been reported to provide protection against peroxidation during cryopreservation, with improvements in post-thaw motility and acrosomal integrity.

4. Buffers: Many CPMs include glycine, sodium citrate, TRIS, or zwitterionic buffers such as HEPES or TES. Media based on PBS are not recommended because they provide very poor pH buffering at lower temperatures and because of the "solute effect" involving the transport of a large quantity of sodium ions across the cell membrane [11].

CPM formulations

Since research into sperm CPMs began, many combinations of components in cryopreservation media have been used, including: glycerol-egg yolk-citrate (GEYC); HEPES-Tyrode's medium with glycerol and sucrose, glucose, glycine and HSA (HSPM); zwitterion-combination TES-TRIS-sodium citrate-egg yolk-glycerol (TESTCY); and a combination TES-TRIS-egg yolk-glycerol (TYG) [9]. Table 8.3 shows several commercial sperm CPMs.

Table 8.3 Composition of different CE-marked (or equivalent) commercial cryopreservation media.

	Egg yolk	HSA	Glycerol	Other sugar	Buffer	Other components	Dilution (sperm+ medium)
Sperm cryopreservation buffer (Cook Medical)	–	+	+	Glucose, sucrose	HEPES	Gentamicin	1 + 2
Ackerman medium (Cryobiosystem)	+ 20%	–	+12%	Anhydrous glucose	Citrate	Penicillin, streptomycin	1 + 1
Tardigrade medium (Cryobiosystem)	–	+	+24%	Glucose, sucrose	HEPES	–	NDA
Spermstore (Gynemed)	–	+ 0.4%	+15%	–	HEPES	–	1 + 0.7
Freezing medium-TYB (Irvine®)	+ 20%	–	+12%	Fructose	TES–TRIS	Gentamicin sulfate	1 + 1
Sperm maintenance medium (Irvine)	–	+ 2%	+28%	Sucrose, glucose	HEPES	–	3 + 1
Sperm freezing medium (Life Global)	–	+	+15%	Glucose, sucrose	HEPES	–	NDA

Table 8.3 (cont.)

	Egg yolk	HSA	Glycerol	Other sugar	Buffer	Other components	Dilution (sperm+ medium)
Cryosperm (Medicult)	–	–	+	Glucose, raffinose	HEPES	Penicillin, streptomycin	1 + 1
Sperm freezing medium (Medicult)	–	+	+	Glucose, sucrose	HEPES	Penicillin, streptomycin	1 + 1
Sperm cryoprotec (Nidacom)	–	+	+	Glucose	HEPES	–	3 + 1

NDA: No data available.

Which cryopreservation medium should be used?

In the modern era, in which quality and traceability are the cornerstones of "good laboratory practice" (GLP), "good manufacturing practice" (GMP) standards must be applied to the preparation of all cryopreservation media. Consequently, GMP documentation and product validation requirements will clearly preclude in-house media preparation, except under the most rigorous conditions. Moreover, the components used to make in-house media are usually classified as "for *in vitro* use only" and freshly prepared media should be checked periodically with known donor spermatozoa, so both preparation and quality control testing time must be taken into account [15].

As already noted, it is very difficult to establish which CPM is the best, although zwitterion buffers are superior to other buffer systems such as citrate, glycine, or phosphate [11]. While CPMs with egg yolk seem to achieve higher survival rates than media without [11,16], egg yolk is of animal origin and therefore could introduce microbial agents, such as avian influenza or other, as-yet-unknown, infectious diseases. For this reason, CPMs without egg yolk are to be preferred in the modern andrology laboratory [15].

Whenever spermatozoa are to be cryopreserved, it might be necessary to try various CPMs in order to establish which is best-suited for the individual case. Even then, some men, despite having apparently normal pre-freeze and post-thaw sperm quality (and even when their fresh semen is of proven fertility), fail to achieve pregnancies when their cryopreserved spermatozoa are used for insemination [9].

Addition/removal of CPM

It is important to take human sperm sensitivity to shrinkage and swelling into account in cryopreservation techniques in order to increase cryosurvival rates. The human spermatozoon can swell to only 110% of its original isosmotic volume, while it can shrink to 75% of this value and still retain ≥90% of its original motility [7,8]. Consequently, one of the most important aspects is slow CPA addition and removal [17], and most protocols involve a drop-wise addition, with continual mixing for several minutes when adding CPA (freezing) or culture media (thawing) when frozen spermatozoa are to be washed. Rapid dilution can severely damage cryopreserved spermatozoa.

After dilution with the CPM, semen should be packaged and cooled immediately, as the exposure of human spermatozoa to cryoprotectant prior to freezing should be less than 10 minutes in order to achieve optimal cryosurvival rates. The deleterious effects appear to be greater when HSPM is used rather than TEST-yolk medium [18].

Control of cooling and warming rates in cryopreservation

Diverse methods for freezing can be defined, but which temperature control system is best remains an open question [9,17]. Nonetheless, it is crucial to ensure the fulfillment of the intended freezing rate, and so a sensor with a data logger and software to monitor the cooling rate, if not already incorporated into the system, is strongly recommended.

Programmable freezing systems

This type of freezing system allows cells to be frozen gradually, without abrupt temperature changes, providing more time for the cells to become dehydrated and so reducing the damage caused by the formation of intracellular crystals. Such systems also make it possible to carry out seeding at a given temperature, although seeding during normozoospermic semen cryopreservation has not been shown to confer any significant improvement in cryosurvival rates [17,19].

Static vapor phase cooling

In this method a stable temperature gradient is established in the vapor phase above a quantity of liquid nitrogen, held within an insulated container, usually a large cylindrical stainless steel dewar. Straws are placed at predetermined heights above the liquid phase for predetermined periods to achieve the necessary cooling curve. Problems with this method include the abrupt rate of temperature decrease, poor reproducibility of cooling rates, and increased the variability between the straws from the same semen sample. Accordingly, this method is no longer recommended from a cryobiological standpoint [18,20].

Mechanically assisted vapor phase cooling

These cooling machines cause liquid nitrogen vapor to flow around the samples at a controlled rate, so that the desired cooling rate can be achieved. Freezing protocols must be established empirically; for example, the Nicool LM-10 (Cryogenic Material, Marne La Vallée Cedex, France) unit holds 25 0.5-ml straws in the freezing chamber and a variable-speed fan pulls liquid nitrogen vapor past the straws at empirically determined rates to achieve the desired cooling curve. If fewer than 25 straws are to be frozen, the difference must be made up using "ballast", i.e. straws containing only CPM.

Flash-freeze technique (ultra-rapid freezing)

In this method, the straw is inserted directly into the liquid nitrogen. Cooling rates can exceed 2500°C/min for 0.25-ml straws, but nevertheless these rates are not sufficient to prevent intracellular ice formation, and the results achieved are not satisfactory.

Vitrification

Human spermatozoa have been shown to be capable of recovery with vitrification techniques, in which very high cooling rates are applied (>20 000°C/min) [21]. The method is quick and simple, taking only a few seconds, and does not require special freezing equipment. However, to obtain the high cooling rates needed for vitrification, the volume in which the cells are contained must be very small (only a few microliters), which greatly limits the number of spermatozoa that can be vitrified. Therefore, this technique is not suitable for freezing sperm to be used for artificial insemination or IVF, but rather only for ICSI.

Thawing

In general, it is considered that fast warming rates are required for optimal sperm recovery. This has been attributed to the possibility that small intracellular ice crystals formed in some cells during freezing can grow during a slow re-warming process, producing the somewhat counter-intuitive concept of freezing during warming. Only when warming is so fast (e.g. in a water bath at 30°C or 37°C) as to prevent the growth of such ice crystals, can this phenomenon be avoided [20].

Packaging alternatives

Over the years, four main types of packaging containers have been used for human spermatozoa:

1. Glass ampoules – although these have been strongly discouraged for many years for reasons of safety due to their fragility.
2. Plastic screw-top "cryovials," primarily the NUNC™ CryoTube® range of products (Nunc A/S, Roskilde, Denmark, and Nalge Nunc International, Naperville, IL, USA). These are made from polypropylene with either polypropylene or polyethylene screw caps. Different types have either external or internal screw threads, so that the cap screws either into or onto the outside of the cryovial respectively. Tightening the cap compresses a silicone O-ring seal that is supposed to make the cryovial air- and water-tight.
3. Plastic straws or "paillettes" were invented by Cassou [22] and commercialized by his company, "Instruments de Medecine Veterinaire" (IMV: L'Aigle, France). Although originally made from polyvinyl chloride (PVC), they were replaced by straws made from polyethylene terephthalate glycol (PETG) in 1998 because PVC straws could not be sterilized by irradiation without compromising their mechanical integrity. Since Cassou's patent expired, plastic straws have also become available from other companies, e.g. Minitüb (Tiefenbach, Germany).
4. Most recently, straws have been made from an ionomeric resin that confers substantial advantages in terms of mechanical strength at cryogenic temperatures and impermeability to viruses. These are the CBS "High Security Straws" commonly referred to as "CBS straws," from CryoBioSystem (Paris, France) [23]. When used in conjunction with their thermal welding device, the SYMS sealer, they are guaranteed leakproof, and the seals secure up to pressures of 150 kg/cm^2. These straws also use a special filling nozzle to prevent contamination of the outside of the straw with the specimen (a major source of contamination in cryotanks, see [24]) and have both internal and external secure identification options [17].

Straws are widely used for packaging human semen, especially in Europe, although plastic cryovials are also used in many laboratories, especially in the USA. Beyond some clinicians' desire (perceived need?) for larger volume specimens, there are significant technical aspects to the "straws vs. cryovials" debate, which include issues concerning the cooling and warming rates, as well as biocontainment; issues that are tightly interconnected because both are governed by the physical characteristics of the packaging systems. The major points are summarized below, but for more extensive discussions on issues in the straws vs. cryovials debate, readers are referred to the review by Mortimer [17].

Fecundity rates post-thaw

Although there have been no reliable prospective trials comparing the relative fertility of human spermatozoa frozen in straws vs. cryovials, it has been argued that there might be as much as a 6- to 8-fold higher post-thaw fecundity for sperm frozen in straws [17].

Achievement of intended cooling/warming rates

Simple physics dictates that the larger radius of cryovials will impede heat transfer, resulting in uneven heat exchange throughout the sample, but nevertheless in a substantial lag between the programed rate in the controlled-rate freezer and the actual cooling rate achieved inside a cryovial [19]. Similarly, the contents of a cryovial will thaw more slowly and less uniformly when removed from cryostorage than those of a straw, even if immersed in a 30°C water bath. This poses a significant problem, since rapid thawing is required for optimum cryosurvival [17,20]. Figure 8.3A shows that while specimens packaged in all sizes of straws (IMV 0.5 and 0.25 ml and CBS 0.5 ml High Security Straws) experience very similar cooling curves, material packaged in Nunc 1.8-ml cryovials will experience cooling that is considerably delayed behind the programed curve. Figure 8.3B reveals magnified differences between straws and cryovials when warming at 37°C – but this rapid warming rate of straws does require caution when handling specimens outside the cryogenic storage tank for brief periods (e.g. during cryobank audits): a 0.25-ml straw will warm to –80°C within 15 s in air at room temperature [25].

Effective sealing

There are very serious concerns regarding leakage of liquid nitrogen into cryovials [26,27], and Nunc documentation [28] clearly states that storing cryovials immersed in LN_2 is not advised. This liquid nitrogen represents not only a risk of specimen contamination, but can also cause the container to explode when it expands rapidly – by a factor of almost 700× – upon warming when removed from the cryogenic storage tank. For storage under such "extreme" conditions, CryoTube® vials must be correctly sealed in Nunc CryoFlex™ tubing – but cryobanks rarely do this as the CryoFlex tubing hinders attachment of cryovials to canes [29]. Poor sealing can also affect PVC or PETG straws unless great care is paid to ensuring that an air space is left in the straw to allow for the expansion of the specimen as it cools, and that a proper seal has been achieved [17]. However, the thermal soldering technique employed with the CBS ionomeric resin straws does ensure a secure seal.

Fragility at –196°C

PVC and PETG straws are very fragile at –196°C and are easily broken if lateral force is exerted upon them (e.g. attempted bending as a straw is placed into or removed from a storage unit). The CBS High Security Straws cannot be broken, even at cryogenic temperatures, without extreme bending.

Risk of cross-contamination

The isolated report in 1995 of a cluster of six cases of acute hepatitis B virus (HBV) infections among patients undergoing cytotoxic treatment [30] – even though it was later established as

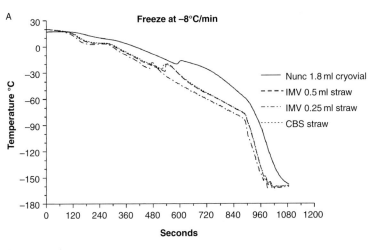

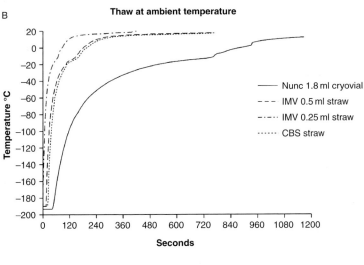

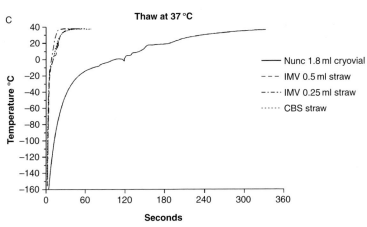

Figure 8.3 Cooling (panel A) and warming (panels B & C) profiles measured by thermocouple inside various packaging systems. Note the much slower warming rate at ambient temperature compared to 37°C. Data generously supplied by Agnés Camus (Cryo Bio System, Paris, France); reproduced from ref. 17 with permission.

having been due to the use of a low-quality type of blood bag packaging – gave rise to extensive concern over the risk of cross-contamination of specimens during cryostorage. There has since been much debate regarding this issue and, while the risk of cross-contamination cannot be ignored as being "theoretical," it is certainly unquantifiable [31], precluding robust risk analysis of its real likelihood. Consequently anyone working in human sperm cryobanking needs to understand its basis and be able to take all practical steps to minimize the risk of its occurring, with CBS High Security Straws (properly sealed using the SYMS device) being the safest packaging method for ensuring biocontainment of cryo-banked specimens [17,32,33].

Cryopreservation procedure

Principles

Large changes in one or more of the technical factors discussed above (temperature, CPA concentration, etc.) would significantly affect the cryosurvival rate, but even small variations could influence the final result, and so it is necessary to take meticulous care in following sperm cryopreservation protocols. In donor sperm banks, what is important is not just the sperm survival rate, but also the homogeneity between different aliquots of sperm, so that a given concentration of mobile spermatozoa per vial can be ensured; small differences in several factors may be responsible for non-uniformity between aliquots from the same ejaculate [18].

This example protocol employs "CBS straws" from CryoBioSystem (Paris, France) since they are the most secure form of packaging currently available.

Equipment (see also Appendix 2)

- Freezing system: Either a controlled-rate freezer (programmable) or mechanically assisted vapor phase freezer [9]
  System for filling and sealing straws (e.g. SYMS, CryoBioSystem, Paris, France)
- Water bath
- Dry bath (block warmer)
- Air incubator operating at 37°C
- Microscope configured for andrology with phase contrast optics (10×, 20× and 40× objectives)
- Cryogenic storage tanks
- Straw handling forceps (Rocket Medical, Watford, UK)
- Label printer
- Liquid nitrogen supply vessel
- Counting chamber (e.g. Makler chamber)

Disposable materials

- Straws, visotubes, goblets, canes, flags
- Self-adhesive labels

- Semen collection container*
- Glass Pasteur pipettes*
- Round-bottom, polystyrene 14-ml culture tubes* (e.g. Falcon #2001 or #2057)
- Aspiration methods and filling nozzle
- Sterile gauze
- Instrument to cut straw: Suture scissors (e.g. Cat.No. R50.000 from Rocket Medical, Watford, UK)

*All disposables that will come into contact with spermatozoa that are to be used for either therapeutic, or critical testing purposes should be either pre-tested for sperm toxicity, or else obtained from a trusted manufacturer, e.g. if a sterile plastic syringe is used during processing then it must be of a brand known not to have any deleterious effects upon spermatozoa.

Reagents

- CPM
- Hypochlorite solution
- Sterile water
- Liquid nitrogen

All CPM that are to be used in cryopreservation of human spermatozoa for therapeutic purposes must be CE-marked (or equivalent) and certified as pyrogen-free and not having any sperm toxicity.

Calibration

Scheduled examinations of controlled-rate freezers must be performed by qualified individuals or companies who can certify that the unit is functioning according to specification, and who can provide service, repairs and parts authorized by the unit's manufacturer. A reference thermometer should be annually (or otherwise, as per manufacturer's recommendation) calibrated by an accredited calibration laboratory (e.g. the National Institute of Standards and Technology in the USA).

Quality control
Sample identification

All specimen containers and processing/preparation tubes must be labeled with two identifiers, e.g. the man's name and the specimen's laboratory reference or ID number. Temporary analytical preparations (e.g. sperm motility slides) can be identified using the specimen's laboratory reference or ID number only. Each straw must be identified individually using a unique straw code.

Cross-contamination

Potentially contaminated parts of the controlled-rate freezer and workstation can be cleaned with ethanol or non-corrosive decontamination fluids.

Temperature

Room temperature sensor, water bath, refrigerators, freezers for storage reagents, and temperature sensors for the freezing system and tank should be checked quarterly using a calibrated thermometer. All results and calibration dates must be recorded. Freezers for reagent storage and cryotanks, if possible, should be equipped with a continuous automatic recording system (data logger) and with alarms set to respond when temperatures rise; the alarm system should sound during regular working hours and be attached to a telephone notification system outside normal working hours. The temperature curve for each sperm cryopreservation run must be stored for purposes of traceability. Shipping tanks should be fitted with a temperature data logger.

Water baths

Water baths should be filled with distilled water and cleaned with a disinfectant solution (e.g. 70% alcohol or 10% sodium hypochlorite solution) weekly [34].

Reagents

CPM must be stored as per manufacturer's recommendations and used before its expiry date. This date should be checked before each use of the CPM. Quality control performed by, or on behalf of, the manufacturer will usually be summarized in a Certificate of Analysis for each batch of CPM that will record biological (bioassay), chemical and physical test data; these certificates must be kept on file (hard copy or electronic as PDF files) [15].

Internal quality control (IQC)

Sample of known donor semen should be frozen and thawed to test equipment function, or to test any new material or commercial cryopreservation medium. New methods should be evaluated using known donor semen specimens. For internal QC semen analysis see the section on "Quality control" in Chapter 10.

External quality control (EQC) of the sperm donor

High variability among sperm banks has been described [35]. There are three components to EQA in a sperm bank: (a) one laboratory can arrange a cross-over proficiency testing (PT) program with another sperm bank, so that straws of frozen semen can be tested by both laboratories; (b) general EQA programs for semen analysis; and (c) an EQA program for bioassay (see the section on "EQA schemes" in Chapter 10).

Homogeneity among straws from the same donor

Within-individual variability in sperm cryopreservation means it is necessary to check every specimen cryopreserved for a given donor. In a commercial sperm bank it is also very important to guarantee homogeneity among the straws from a sperm donor. A possible strategy is to test the sperm concentration in the test thaw sample; this must be within ±10% of half the original semen sperm concentration (assuming a 1 + 1 CPM dilution); otherwise, it would suggest poor mixing of the semen and cryoprotectant. Batches where this condition is not met can show substantial variability in sperm cryosurvival among straws [9]. Another strategy is to randomly test a certain number of straws before starting the delivery of samples from a sperm donor, in order to ensure the required homogeneity (acceptance sampling plan) [36]. If donors do not meet the requisites of the proposed acceptance sampling plan, they should not be included in the distribution schedule. Nevertheless, if they could be used within the same sperm bank at the assisted reproduction center, any poor quality straws found could be replaced immediately.

Specimen

Liquefied, homogeneous human semen, ideally within 30 minutes of ejaculation. Longer post-ejaculatory delays, incomplete liquefaction, and increased viscosity should be noted on the laboratory and report form. For other types of specimens and abnormal semen samples, see the section on "Dealing with atypical semen specimens" in Chapter 7.

As well as the standard procedure for freezing sperm, it is also possible to freeze prepared sperm samples (as described in Chapter 7 "Sperm preparation") using a cryopreservation medium that does not contain egg yolk; these may be used for insemination directly after freezing, with no need for further processing (IUI-ready) [17]. Although IUI-ready samples are regularly prepared as part of sperm sample freezing procedures in sperm banks, this could also be done when preparing samples from patients who will carry out AIH cycles and who for professional or other reasons cannot be present when the insemination is performed, or from patients who have an infectious disease, due to a delayed virological study, or for safety reasons. There is no generalized view as to the technique that should be used for processing IUI-ready samples before freezing [37] or whether this processing prior to freezing has an effect on cryosurvival rates [38].

Testicular/epididymal samples are cryopreserved using the standard semen protocols. When mature spermatozoa are identified after dissecting testicular tissue or in the epididymal aspirate, the homogenate or the aspirate are diluted with the CPM. When there are very few spermatozoa, proceed as later in this chapter ("See Note 5").

Procedures

Note: For safety reasons, whenever liquid nitrogen is being handled, full cryogenic protective equipment must be worn (see Appendices 2 and 8).

A. Freezing phase

1. Ask the patient or donor to collect the semen sample in a sterile, labeled container (preferably by masturbation).

2. While the sample liquefies (no longer than 30 min), prepare the programmable freezer (check the freezing ramps and transfer liquid nitrogen to the system) and allow the CPM to warm to room temperature.

3. As soon as the ejaculate is liquefied, perform a basic semen analysis, either manually or using computer-assisted sperm analysis (see Chapters 3 and 4, as appropriate).

4. Measure out the volume of semen sample to be cryopreserved (e.g. using a wide-necked sterile pipette) and transfer it to the bottom of a clean container.

5. Calculate the number of straws that will be required, taking into account the dilution with CPM recommended by the manufacturer (e.g. 1 + 1 or 3 + 1) (Table 8.3).

6. Label the straws and storage units (e.g. visotubes) by the appropriate identification code(s). Choose an appropriate color (visotube, straw, flag, etc.) and attach self-adhesive labels with the identification code.

Note: Straws must be identified individually. In this way, if two insemination doses are removed from the bank and thawed at the same time, there is no chance of their being confused. The classic bar code method using lines drawn on each straw using a fine-pointed marker is not recommended.

7. Add the cryopreservation medium slowly, drop-wise, with continuous gentle swirling to ensure complete mixing. This step should take 2–5 min (so that an efficient osmotic balance may be achieved with no abrupt alterations in cellular osmolarity).

8. When the mixture is homogeneous, the straws can be filled. Each straw is connected to a suction device (e.g. a 1-ml syringe or a vacuum pump) and the semen–cryopreservation medium mixture is drawn up the straw, leaving a 1-cm air space at the entry (filling) end. The outside of the straw must not be allowed to come into contact with either the semen or the sides of the container, e.g. fill using a filling nozzle.

9. Seal the ends of each straw by thermal pulse sealing (SYMS, Cryo Bio System, Paris, France).

10. Disinfect the outside of each straw using hypochlorite solution, followed by rinsing with sterile water and drying.

11. Transfer the straws into the freezer racking system of the programmable freezing system and start the programed freezer cycle. The following generic cooling curve without seeding is provided as an example:

    a. Ramp 1: Reduce the temperature from room temperature (*ca.* 22°C) to +4°C at a moderate cooling rate of –5°C/min. The sperms become dehydrated but the time is very limited.

    b. Ramp 2: Reduce the temperature from +4°C to –80°C at a rapid cooling rate of –10°C/min. In this ramp, there is no seeding and the spermatozoa solution begins to solidify.

    c. Ramp 3: "Free fall" from –80°C to –160°C. "Free fall" denotes uncontrolled cooling, i.e. a cooling rate as fast as the system being used can achieve. The freezing protocol must cool to below –160°C to minimize the risk of recrystallization damage during transfer from the freezing machine into liquid nitrogen.

    d. Ramp 4: Finally, reduce the temperature from –160°C to –196°C by plunging the straws into liquid nitrogen. This must be done very rapidly.

12. Immerse the previously identified visotube into liquid nitrogen in a transfer dewar until the bubbling stops.

13. Using forceps, rapidly transfer the straws of frozen semen into the visotube (which is full of liquid nitrogen).

14. To check cryosurvival, set aside one straw for assessment of post-thaw sperm motility (either immediately or later).

15. Place the visotube of straws in the appropriate storage location (tank and canister number, container level) in the bank.

16. Make out an index card for the straw identification codes, semen sample identification code (ID number), date of freezing, storage location and the semen analysis laboratory reference number.

17. Record all information in a log book, or using specialized software.

B. Checking post-thaw motility

18. Thaw out the test straw by transferring it into a water bath at 37°C for 10 min.

19. Sanitize the outside of the straw so that the straw can be opened without risk of contamination. Wipe the semen end of the straw with sterile hypochlorite solution, rinse with sterile water, and dry with sterile gauze. Cut the air-bubble end of the straw, insert it into a tube, and then cut the other end (just below the filter) and allow the contents of the straw to run out into the tube. The ends of the straw must be cut with a sterile device, e.g. disposable suture scissors (scalpel blades are not recommended as there is a significant risk of injury). Note: Upon thawing, the outside of all straws or cryotubes will be contaminated with whatever organisms were present in the liquid nitrogen, even if vapor storage was used. Therefore all cryostorage units should be disinfected after thawing before opening.

20. Assess the quantitative and qualitative sperm motility and determine the total sperm concentration.

C. Thawing phase, for insemination or other purposes

21. Identify the location of the desired straws in the cryobank and confirm against the laboratory records and patient/donor records. Record how many straws are to be thawed and how many remain.

22. Remove the straws from the visotube and thaw quickly by placing in 37°C water bath for 10 min.

23. Sanitize and open without risk of contamination (see step 19).

24. Evaluate the qualitative and quantitative aspects of sperm concentration and motility.

25. Process the thawed sample as described in Chapter 7 "Sperm preparation – Dealing with atypical semen specimens – Cryopreserved specimens." "IUI-ready" samples can be used directly with no need for pre-processing.

Cryopreservation results

The adequacy of semen cryopreservation can be evaluated in several ways [9].

1. Cryosurvival factor (CSF), which is calculated as:

$$\text{CSF} = \frac{\%\ \text{motile spermatozoa post-thaw}}{\%\ \text{motile spermatozoa post-freeze}} \times 100$$

2. Concentration and number of progressively motile spermatozoa per straw post-thaw: Use the post-thaw sperm concentration and motility to calculate the concentration of progressively motile spermatozoa post-thaw per straw and, using the straw volume, the total number of such spermatozoa in the straw post-thaw. The number of motile sperm required is dependent on the intended use of the contents of the straw, ranging from donor intracervical insemination (ICI), to patient ICSI. This parameter is used to classify the straw and to guarantee homogeneity among the different samples from the same donor (see section on "Quality control," below).

3. Suitability for use after thawing: Based on the CSF and motility, a CSF value $\geq$50%, together with a sperm motility of $\geq$30% motile, with $\geq$25% progressively motile after thawing is considered optimum [39]. To determine the minimum number of progressively motile spermatozoa after thawing, per straw, it should be borne in mind that the greater the concentration of sperm, the lower the proportion of motile sperm that will be necessary to achieve the minimum motile count per straw (although lower motility can indicate lower overall sperm quality). A method to relate the concentration and motility observed in a straw after thawing, taking analytical variation into account, has been described previously [36].

Autocryopreservation

As the quality of cryopreserved semen stored by patients before cancer treatment is often poor the only therapeutic option might be assisted fertilization. In this case, straws containing just a few motile spermatozoa are often sufficient to give acceptable fertilization rates using ICSI. As very few spermatozoa are required for assisted conception, it is wise to freeze only a small number per straw (e.g. 40 000), so as to maximize the number of fertilization attempts per semen sample [17].

Donor sperm

A minimum number of progressively motile spermatozoa post-thaw must be determined for each sperm donor bank in order to decide whether cryopreservation is feasible.

1. Straws for intracervical insemination (ICI): Although ICI achieves a lower rate of pregnancies than does intrauterine insemination (IUI), the multiple pregnancy rates are much lower. Therefore, it has been proposed that for some women it might be appropriate to perform six cycles of ICI and then IUI [40]. Some studies have recommended a minimum of 4–5 $\times$ 10^6 progressively motile spermatozoa per straw post-thaw [12,13,40].

2. Straws for IUI: A straw containing less than the generally accepted minimum of 4 $\times$ 10^6 motile spermatozoa can be used for IUI as this process involves the removal of seminal plasma and the concentration of spermatozoa prior to insemination.

3. Straws for IVF: The number of motile spermatozoa per straw of cryopreserved donor semen does not correlate with either fertilization rates or pregnancy rates in IVF, reflecting the highly selected nature of the spermatozoa stored.

4. Second chance sperm donor: Although the inter-sample variability in a sperm donor is high [11,12], and an aberrant preparation might arise due to an intervening problem with the donor (e.g. a bout of febrile illness), a very small percentage of donors are allowed a second opportunity when the first sperm donor cryopreservation produces borderline unacceptable results [12,36].

Notes

1. Repeat freezing for patients or donor: When freezing subsequent specimens for a patient or donor it is always advisable to review the test-thaw results from previous specimens in order to avoid any past problems affecting the processing of the current specimen.

2. Highly viscous samples: It can be extremely difficult to obtain good mixing of the semen and cryoprotectant. A needle must not be used. Dilute and pipette the sample with sperm buffer in autoconservation; if the sample does not disperse within 2 min

of pipetting, incubate at 37°C for 10 min and then mix further. Collect the sample into chymotrypsin-coated MARQ™ Liquefaction Cups (Embryotech Laboratories, Wilmington, MA, USA).

3. Centrifuging before cryopreservation: Any centrifuging of the sample that involves the formation of a pellet containing all of the spermatozoa in the sample can lead to sperm damage (see section on "Safe methods for sperm preparation" in Chapter 7). Therefore, it is necessary to avoid centrifugation to concentrate high volume/low count specimens in order to obtain the requisite minimum progressively motile spermatozoa (e.g. <60 × 10^6/ml). Techniques of sperm preparation should be used with these samples.

4. Refreezing: Valuable samples (e.g. from cancer patients, testicular sperm) can be refrozen [41].

5. Very few spermatozoa: Different techniques have been described as a vehicle for the storage of very few or single human spermatozoa, including human, mouse or hamster zonae pellucidae [42]. The use of zonae pellucidae implies a potential contamination of the spermatozoa with infectious or foreign genetic material, and the use of human zonae is especially problematic given their limited availability. Consequently, this approach cannot be recommended.

6. Fragility of cryopreserved spermatozoa: Due to the very high osmolarity of cryoprotectant media, and the damage sustained by spermatozoa during freezing and thawing, great care must be taken when handling post-thaw specimens (see also Chapter 7 regarding sperm preparation).

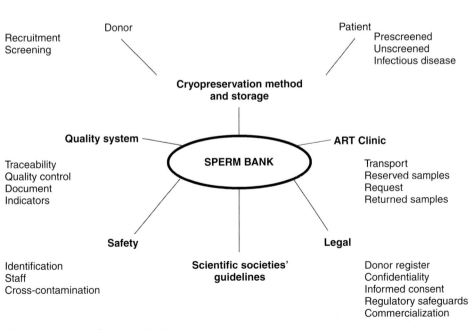

Figure 8.4 Aspects of sperm cryobank organization.

Sperm cryobank organization

Various factors influence the organization of a sperm cryobank (see Figure 8.4).

Sample storage location

For this purpose, various parameters are employed, including the location (each storage tank and canister should be sequentially numbered, e.g. Tank 1, Canister 5), canister level, the shape of the visotube, a combination of colors (e.g. visotube, flag, straw) and a straw code. Radiofrequency identification (RFID) tags and barcodes can also be used.

Canister

This is a cylindrical container that is hung by a rod (its handle) from the mouth of the cryotank such that its contents (goblets) are submerged in the liquid nitrogen. The different canisters (the number depends on the capacity of the nitrogen tank) are numbered to specify the location of cryopreserved specimens.

Canister level

Depending on the tank design, canisters may be short (5″ or 13 cm) or tall (11″ or 28 cm). Visotubes can be placed directly inside the short canisters, but with tall ones the use of plastic goblets allows each canister to be divided into upper (U) and lower (L) levels.

Goblet

This is a large (e.g. 35 or 65 mm) plastic cup into which the visotubes are inserted. Goblets are available in a range of colors.

Visotubes

These are plastic tubes that hold groups of straws. They can be different shapes (round, triangular, hexagonal, polygonal), different diameters (7.1, 9.2, 10, 12, 13 mm, etc.), and are available in a range of colors.

Cryo cassettes

The straws are safely secured inside the cassettes (rectangular or wedge-shaped in cross-section), making it impossible for the straws to float inside the storage bank. Cassettes incorporate a lifter making it fast and easy to remove or insert a straw.

Cryo cane

This is an aluminum rod to which cryovials or visotubes (of straws) can be attached. They have fixed positions and remain firmly in place during storage in liquid nitrogen.

Cryo flex

A heat-shrinkable protective tubing providing extra safety when storing biological samples in cryotubes when immersed in liquid nitrogen.

Storage box

Cardboard storage box for 100 cryotubes.

Flag

Aluminum rods which are wider at the top, for labels or colors. Flags can be inserted into visotubes or goblets.

Samples and tank types

To facilitate cryobank management and reduce the possibility of cross-contamination in a sperm bank, there should be different types of tanks corresponding to the origin of the samples. All patients and donors (Table 8.1) whose semen is going to be frozen should be screened for major viral markers in advance to minimize the risk of potentially infective material (see "Donor screening" below). Semen should not be stored with embryos or oocytes.

Donor tanks

Donor tanks for specimens from all types of semen donors.

Pre-screening patient tanks

Autoconservation for patients who have time for screening, e.g. pre-vasectomy, or patients with repeat screenings.

Unscreened patient tanks

Autoconservation for patients without time for screening, for example cancer.

Infectious disease patient tanks

Autoconservation for patients with an infectious disease. In theory we should have more than seven tanks for infectious disease patients. This number is excessive, but when CBS High Security Straws are used, all of these patients can be stored in the same tank.

Quarantine tank

Quarantine tank for washed semen samples from patients with infectious diseases awaiting the results of the virology laboratory. When the results are negative, they pass to the infectious disease patient tank. In some banks, the *quarantine tank* is used to store semen from donors for six months and wait for all donor samples in a quarantine tank to be *cleared* before allowing any samples to be transferred to the *definitive* donor tank – but if even one sample tests positive for a pathogen then the entire tank contents should be discarded and the tank emptied and sterilized (which, from experience, is rarely actually done). An adequate cost-benefit analysis of this tank should be made in each bank [31]. However, in our opinion such quarantine tanks are not necessary when using CBS straws since they achieve effective biocontainment of all specimens. This should also meet, in principle and effect, the requirement for "separate storage" under Directive 2006/17/EC, e.g. as in Annex III, ¶2.3.

Emergency tanks or cleaning of other tanks

These are used in the case of an accident with one of the other tanks or when other tanks are to be cleaned. A periodic cleaning of the storage tanks should be carried out by allowing the cryotank to warm, wiping with a disinfectant solution and rinsing with distilled water. Allow to dry before re-filling [34]. If CBS High Security Straws are not used cleaning should be carried out annually. However, if these secure straws are used the major source of the material that forms the white *slurry* at the bottom of cryotanks is the *fogging* from room air or the exhaled breath of operators when a cryotank is opened. Consequently, cleaning should only be carried out perhaps every five years.

Reserved samples

A protocol to reserve spermatozoa from a donor for further pregnancies by a patient should exist.

Storage systems

When a sample stored below –132°C warms above this temperature a recrystallization of frozen water molecules takes place. This recrystallization can induce incipient damage to the cryopreserved cells, damage that will not become evident until months or years later when the sample is finally thawed. Moreover, this damage is cumulative; each incident of warming above –132°C will contribute to decreasing the functional survival possibilities of the cryopreserved cells.

There are four types of storage systems for cryogenically frozen samples: liquid phase nitrogen, vapor phase nitrogen, super cold air and mechanical freezers. The factors to keep in mind to decide what type of storage to utilize are: storage temperature, temperature fluctuation during audit, theoretical cross-contamination risks, staff safety, equipment cost, packaging systems, and the size and space of the cryobank [17,27,31,32]. Clearly, the lower the storage temperature, the greater the margin of safety when a specimen is removed briefly to check its identity. The lowest storage temperature is reached with storage in liquid phase nitrogen; the slightly higher theoretical cross-contamination risk in such cryotanks can be minimized using CBS High Security Straws [17].

Inventory control systems

Each sample to be processed by a sperm bank is immediately identified in accordance with the sample identification protocol (e.g. two identifiers system: name and ID number). This identification must be mechanized, whenever possible, for greater clarity of references. The final identification of the straws can be carried out using a double system of barcodes and alphanumeric characters on labels. Straws are generally located by a local inventory code (straw, visotube and flag color, canister, tank). Inventory details must be recorded in a dedicated inventory logbook, and in a password-protected electronic inventory database, with varying levels of access to users. Straw codes should be linked so that key individuals with appropriate access rights can interrogate other relevant datasets, e.g. clinical data, follow-up data. The local inventory code and straw-code can be used in conjunction with a national or international code [43] to ensure straw traceability, and straws issued for use should be accompanied by all relevant documentation. According to the EU Tissues and Cells Directive [43], a single European identifying code shall be allocated to all donated semen specimens, and this European Coding System (not yet finalized) shall incorporate at least information on: donation identification (identification of the tissue establishment and unique identification donation number – ID number) and product identification (product code and split number).

Traceability

A system to ensure the traceability of frozen sperm samples must be established, and this would also make it possible to verify compliance with quality and safety standards. Traceability should operate both from the donor to the recipient and vice versa, and include all products and materials that come into contact with the semen that could have an effect on specimen quality and safety. Traceability should also include the chain of custody: who received a semen sample, who performed the cryopreservation, who audited the frozen straw, etc. [43].

Legal considerations

Sperm banking includes a variety of ethical concerns pertaining to such values as dignity, bodily integrity, autonomy, ownership and privacy. These ethical concerns have been translated into a complex and incoherent apparatus of private, public, national and international standards and provisions. All these norms not only differ with respect to whether they are legally binding, but also reveal that there is no clear national or international consensus on pivotal issues in sperm banking. The framework of norms relating to sperm banking is under permanent reconstruction. The main factors considered in this regard are: commercialization, confidentiality, informed consent, and regulatory safeguards. Information registries concerning donation must be kept for at least 30 years in order to enable the traceability of the donors and to fulfill the possible need for information about the donor [43]. Other legal aspects (air quality) of sperm banks have been analyzed previously [44].

Concerning posthumous reproduction, since one category of people who cryostore their gametes or reproductive tissues are patients affected by serious diseases, there is a real chance that some people will die with their reproductive material in storage. Such a possibility must be raised and talked through in counseling sessions prior to banking material. Posthumous use is regulated in some countries, so a specific procedure is necessary for proper management of these samples [45].

Regarding storage period, while the longest period of cryopreservation that has resulted in a human birth is 21 years [46], in most countries there is a legal limitation on semen storage. Reproductive tissues and gametes should only be stored until the age at which it is considered acceptable for them to be used for the achievement of a pregnancy [45].

Considering the maximum number of children born from a donor, the regulation of live births per donor varies greatly between countries. However, it is generally accepted that the limit on the maximum number of children per donor should be by families created and not by patients treated [40].

Transportation

Dry shippers

To ensure the maximum performance of a shipping tank, its integrity has to be tested periodically. Weigh the shipping tank empty and then after filling (allow it to cool slowly with repeated additions of liquid nitrogen over a period of several hours to ensure maximum performance), and then monitor its static evaporative loss over a few days to verify its integrity [9].

Transport

To achieve safe transportation of biological material, international recommendations for transportation of biological material must be observed. International and national regulatory agencies require that anyone involved in the shipping and packaging of dangerous goods must receive training and certification in the proper regulations that govern the transport, packaging, and labeling of those materials. Consequently, patients should not transport frozen sperm samples themselves.

Returning sperm samples

As a general rule, if returning semen to the provider cryobank (e.g. cancelled insemination cycle), the cryobank can only accept the return of samples when the following three conditions are met: (a) the samples have not been thawed; (b) the integrity of the package can be demonstrated (the seals are intact); and (c) proper storage temperature for the sample has been maintained throughout the transport (and can be demonstrated).

Donor screening

The recruitment of sperm donors is an increasingly difficult process. At most, one out of ten men initially evaluated is accepted as a donor [11,12]. The three principal reasons for this acceptance rate are lack of interest after the initial phone interview or after completing the intake questionnaire, issues arising from the serology testing or medical history, and on the basis of semen quality or post-thaw survival.

Clinical history and physical screening

A complete personal and sexual history should be obtained and an abbreviated version of the donor's personal history should be obtained before each donation, thus highlighting changes that might require a donor to be excluded from the donation program [47]. Semen from donors older than 45 years should not be admitted. Psychological screening is an acceptable part of medical screening, in order to rule out pathology or coercion, and to anticipate stressors for the purpose of counseling. Psychological screening that exceeds these objectives should not be carried out. Sperm donor candidates should undergo a complete physical examination, including tests for urethral discharge, warts and scattered ulcers, disseminated lymphadenopathies, anal injures and venal punctures [47,48]. These physical examinations should be repeated every six months, as long as the donor is participating in the donation program. Routine biochemical and hematological laboratory screening, including tests for blood group and Rh factor, is also recommended.

Genetic screening

A donor's family history up to three generations should be compiled, with the donor being rejected if his antecedents present a significant risk with respect to a specific disease that is deemed to be greater than that of the general population. A karyotype study should be carried out for donations of gametes [48,49]. Genetic screening must also take into account the influence of ethnic groups, since certain hereditary diseases are more or less prevalent depending on the racial/ethnic origin of the donor and their relatives [47].

Serological and microbiological tests

Screening for infectious diseases (HIV-1 and HIV-2, HCV, HBV and syphilis) is essential before the cryopreservation of donated semen, although no method exists to ensure total effectiveness regarding the non-transmission of infectious agents [17]. Laboratory tests used in the screening of semen donors should be approved by the FDA [47], or by the EU [49], or other regulatory bodies as appropriate. Serological tests of semen donors should be performed seven days before the first freezing for treatment purposes, and every six months while they are making donations. There is no need to perform repeat screening for transmissible infectious diseases if every donation is screened using PCR [43].

Tests for anti-HTLV-I and -II antibodies should be performed for all donors who reside in or who come from zones of high incidence of specific diseases, or whose spouse/partner or family come from these zones [43,49] – or where required by regulation. A donor with a non-specific positive test for syphilis should not be rejected if a specific test produces a negative result [43]. Reject donors with active cytomegalovirus (CMV) infections (positive CMV IgM antibodies or a recently positive IgG seroconversion), and use donor semen with negative CMV IgM antibodies and positive CMV IgG (indicative of past infection, and low probability of virus-containing semen) for recipients with the same serological status [47,49]. There remains considerable debate as to the type of test (culture, PCR), specimens (semen, urine and urethral) and testing intervals for *Chlamydia trachomatis, Neisseria gonorrhoeae* and general culture [43,47,48,49,50]. However, these tests must be negative at the initial screening, and again at the end of the donation period. Collaboration with the local Sexually Transmitted Disease (Genito-Urinary Medicine) Clinic concerning the type of screening tests, testing intervals, etc., is often very informative.

Semen analysis

A classical semen analysis must be done on all sperm donor candidates according to the guidelines described in this book (see Chapter 3). To avoid unnecessary freezing of donor specimens, a baseline of acceptable pre-freeze sperm characteristics should be established in order to guarantee a minimum acceptable motile sperm count after thawing (e.g. sperm concentration $>50 \times 10^6$/ml, $\geq 40\%$ progressively motile, and other seminal parameters within reference values). No agreement exists with respect to these parameters between the different authors [9,12,13] due to the high inter-individual variability of sperm cryopreservation [10,11,12]. In consideration of the aforementioned factors, we can only expect to be able to estimate the post-thaw survival rate from the pre-freeze sperm characteristics with a certain probability of error [36].

References

1. Cryo Bio System. *Fundamentals of Cryobiology.* Paris: CryoBioSystem 2006. www.cryobiosystem-imv.com/Cryobiology/ Basesfondamentalesdelacryobiologie/tabid/ 251/Default.aspx (viewed 10/08/2008).

2. Fuller B, Paynter S. Fundamentals of cryobiology in reproductive medicine. *Reprod Biomed Online* 2004; **9**: 680–91.

3. Mazur P, Leibo SP, Farrant J, *et al.* Interactions of cooling rate, warming rate and protective additive on the survival of frozen mammalian cells. In: Wolstenholme GE, O'Connor M, eds. *The Frozen Cell.* London: Churchill Press 1970: 69–88.

4. Nei T. Mechanism of haemolysis of erythrocytes by freezing, with special reference to freezing at near-zero temperatures. In: Wolstenholme GE, O'Connor M, eds. *The Frozen Cell.* London: Churchill Press 1970: 131–47.

5. Merryman HT. The exceeding of a minimum tolerable cell volume in hypertonic suspension as a cause of freezing injury. In: Wolstenholme GE, O'Connor M, eds. *The Frozen Cell.* London: Churchill Press 1970: 565–9.

6. Nijs M, Ombelet W. Cryopreservation of human sperm. *Hum Fertil* 2001; **4**: 158–63.

7. Gao D, Liu J, Liu C, *et al.* Prevention of osmotic injury to human spermatozoa during addition and removal of glycerol. *Hum Reprod* 1995; **10**: 1109–22.

8. Gilmore JA, Liu J, Gao DY, *et al.* Determination of optimal cryoprotectants and procedures for their addition and removal from human spermatozoa. *Hum Reprod* 1997; **12**: 112–8.

9. Mortimer D. *Practical Laboratory Andrology.* Oxford: Oxford University Press 1994: 301–23.

10. Centola GM, Raubertas RF, Mattox JH. Cryopreservation of human semen. Comparison of cryopreservatives, sources of variability, and prediction of post-thaw survival. *J Androl* 1992; **13**: 283–8.

11. Keel BA, Webster BW. Semen cryopreservation methodology and results. In: Barrat CLR, Cooke ID, eds. *Donor insemination.* Cambridge: Cambridge University Press 1993: 96–71.

12. Barrat CL, Clements S, Kessopoulou E. Semen characteristics and fertility tests required for storage of spermatozoa. *Hum Reprod* 1998; 13 Suppl 2: 1–7.

13. Yogev L, Kleiman S, Shabtai E, *et al.* Seasonal variations in pre- and post-thaw donor sperm quality. *Hum Reprod* 2004; **19**: 880–5.

14. Holt WV. Basic aspects of frozen storage of semen. *Anim Reprod Sci*, 2000; **62**: 3–22.

15. Stacey G. Validation of cell culture media components. *Hum Fertil* 2004; 7: 113–8.

16. Nallella KP, Sharma KK, Allamaneni SS, *et al.* Cryopreservation of human spermatozoa: comparison of two cryopreservation methods and three cryoprotectants. *Fertil Steril* 2004; **82**: 913–8.

17. Mortimer D. Current and future concepts and practices in human sperm cryobanking. *Reprod Biomed Online* 2004; **9**: 134–51.

18. Stanic P, Tandara M, Sonicki Z, *et al.* Comparison of protective media and freezing techniques for cryopreservation of human semen. *Eur J Obstet Gynecol Reprod Biol* 2000; **91**: 65–70.

19. Morris J. *Asymptote Cool Guide to Cryopreservation* 2002. Cambridge: Asymptote Ltd.: 49. www.asymptote.co.uk/cryo/CoolGuid.pdf (viewed 06/04/2008).

20. Henry MA, Noiles EE, Gao D, *et al.* Cryopreservation of human spermatozoa. IV. The effects of cooling rate of warming rate on the maintenance of motility, plasma membrane integrity, and mitochondrial function. *Fertil Steril* 1993; **60**: 911–8.

21. Isachenko V, Isachenko E, Katkov II, *et al.* Cryoprotectant-free cryopreservation of human spermatozoa by vitrification and freezing in vapor: effect on motility, DNA integrity, and fertilization ability. *Biol Reprod* 2004; **71**: 1167–73.

22. Cassou R. La méthode des paillettes en plastique adaptée a la généralisation de la congélation. *5th Int Cong Anim Reprod Artif Insem, Trento* 1964; **4**: 540–6.

23. Cryo Bio System. *CBS™ High Security Cryobanking Systems Product Monograph.* Paris: Cryo Bio System 2006. www.cryobiosystem-imv.com/Portals/3/PDF/Monograph.pdf (viewed 10/08/2008).

24. Russell PH, Lyaruu VH, Millar JD, *et al.* The potential transmission of infectious agents by semen packaging during storage for artificial insemination. *Anim Reprod Sci* 1997; **47**: 337–42.

25. Tyler JP, Kime L, Cooke S, *et al.* Temperature change in cryo-containers during short exposure to ambient temperatures. *Hum Reprod* 1996; **11**: 1510–2.

26. Byers KB. Risks associated with liquid nitrogen cryogenic storage systems. *J Am Biol Safety Assoc* 1998; **3**: 143–6.

27. Clarke GN. Sperm cryopreservation: is there a significant risk of cross-contamination? *Hum Reprod* 1999; **14**: 2941–3.

28. Nalge Nunc International. *Cryopreservation Manual.* Rochester: Nalge Nunc International Corporation 1998.

29. Wood MJ. The problems of storing gametes and embryos. *Cryo-Letters* 1999; **20**: 155–8.

30. Tedder RS, Zuckerman MA, Goldstone AH, *et al.* Hepatitis B transmission from contaminated cryopreservation tank. *Lancet* 1995; **346**: 137–40.

31. Tomlinson M, Sakkas D. Is a review of standard procedures for cryopreservation needed? Safe and effective cryopreservation – should sperm banks and fertility centres move towards storage in nitrogen vapour? *Hum Reprod* 2000; **15**: 2460–3.

32. Mortimer D. Setting up risk management systems in IVF laboratories. *Clinical Risk* 2004; **10**: 128–37.

33. Mortimer D, Mortimer ST. *Quality and Risk Management in the IVF Laboratory.* Cambridge: Cambridge University Press 2005.

34. Elder K, Baker D, Ribes J. *Infections, Infertility and Assisted Reproduction.* Cambridge: Cambridge University Press 2005.

35. Carrell DT, Cartmill D, Jones KP, *et al.* Prospective randomized, blinded evaluation of donor semen quality provided by seven commercial sperm banks. *Fertil Steril* 2002; **78**: 16–21.

36. Castilla JA, Sánchez-León M, Garrido A, *et al.* Procedure control and acceptance sampling for donor sperm banks a theoretical study. *Cell Tissue Bank* 2007; **8**: 257–65.

37. Chan CC, Chen IC, Liu JY, *et al.* Comparison of nitric oxide production motion characteristics of sperm after cryopreserved in three different preparations. *Arch Androl* 2004; **50**: 1–3.

38. Grizard G, Chevalier V, Griveau JF, *et al.* Influence of seminal plasma on cryopreservation of human spermatozoa in a biological material-free medium: study of

normal low-quality semen. *Int J Androl* 1999; **22**: 190–6.

39. David G, Czyglik F, Mayaux MJ, *et al.* Artificial insemination with frozen sperm: protocol, method of analysis and results for 1188 women. *Br J Obstet Gynaecol* 1980; **87**: 1022–8.

40. Le Lannou D, Thepot F, Jouannet P. Multicentre approaches to donor insemination in the French CECOS Federation: Nationwide evaluation donor matching, screening for genetic diseases and consanguinity. *Hum Reprod* 1998; **13** Suppl 2: 35–54.

41. Ofeim O, Brown TA, Gilbert BR. Effects of serial thaw-refreeze cycles on human sperm motility and viability. *Fertil Steril* 2001; **75**: 1242–3.

42. Cohen J, Garrisi GJ, Congedo-Ferrara TA, *et al.* Cryopreservation of single human spermatozoa. *Hum Reprod* 1997; **12**: 994–1001.

43. European Union. 2004 Directive 2004/23/ EC of the European Parliament and of the Council of 31 March 2004 on setting standards of quality and safety for the donation, procurement, testing, processing, preservation, storage, and distribution of human tissues and cells. *Official Journal of the European Union* 2004; L 102/48.

44. Mortimer D. A critical assessment of the impact of the European Union Tissues and Cells Directive (2004) on laboratory practices in assisted conception. *Reprod Biomed Online* 2005; **11**: 162–76.

45. The ESRHE Task Force on Ethics and Law. Taskforce 7: Ethical considerations for the cryopreservation of gametes and reproductive tissues for self use. *Hum Reprod* 2004; **19**: 460–2.

46. Horne G, Atkinson AD, Pease EH, *et al.* Live birth with sperm cryopreserved for 21 years prior to cancer treatment: case report. *Hum Reprod* 2004; **19**: 1448–9.

47. American Society for Reproductive Medicine (ASRM). Guidelines for gamete and embryo donation. *Fertil Steril* 2006; **86** Suppl 1: 38–50.

48. British Andrology Society (BAS). *Guidelines for the Screening of Semen Donors for Donors Insemination.* London: British Andrology Society 1999.

49. Gamete donation guidelines. The Corsendonk consensus document for the European Union. *Hum Reprod* 1998; **13** Suppl 2: 7–12.

50. Health Canada Directive. *Technical Requirements for Therapeutic Donor Insemination.* July 2000 (Ottawa, Canada). Available at: www.hc-sc.gc. ca/dhp-mps/alt_formats/hpfb-dgpsa/ pdf/prodpharma/semen-sperme_ directive-eng.pdf (viewed 23/07/2008).

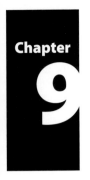

Preparation of surgically retrieved spermatozoa

Background

For many men with azoospermia, of both excretory and secretory types, spermatozoa can be recovered directly from the male reproductive tract (i.e. the epididymis or testis), and the retrieved spermatozoa used in an ICSI procedure. Because this is a laboratory handbook, clinical procedures for surgically recovering spermatozoa from the male reproductive tract have not been covered; interested readers are referred to a recent review article [1].

With obstructive azoospermia, or in the absence of vas deferens, the first approach is percutaneous sperm aspiration (PESA) or micro-epididymal sperm aspiration (MESA). If no spermatozoa can be recovered from the epididymis, then testicular sperm recovery can be attempted.

In secretory (or non-obstructive) azoospermia the cause is at the level of the seminiferous epithelium, with extremely low levels of spermatogenesis. Testicular biopsy can provide tissue in which some foci of spermatogenic activity can be found and a few spermatozoa recovered by testicular sperm aspiration (TESA) or testicular sperm extraction (TESE) [2]. These procedures are usually performed under local anesthetic.

Several studies have compared the outcome of various methods for retrieving spermatozoa for non-obstructive azoospermia, but with inconclusive results (reviewed in [1]). Furthermore, a recent Cochrane review concluded that there is insufficient evidence to recommend any specific technique for sperm retrieval from the testis or epididymis [3]. However, prior screening of azoospermic men for microdeletions in the azoospermia factor (AZF) region of the Y-chromosome can be clinically useful in excluding some men with extremely poor prognosis. This testing should be a part of the man's clinical work-up prior to attempting surgical retrieval of spermatozoa [4].

Preparation of epididymal spermatozoa

Principle

Fluid is aspirated from the epididymis through a fine needle (PESA), or obtained by making a small cut into the epididymis (MESA). The spermatozoa are ideally isolated from the epididymal fluid by density gradient centrifugation (DGC), although in extreme cases, when there are very few spermatozoa simple centrifugal washing has to be used in spite of the risk of ROS-induced damage to the spermatozoa, especially their DNA.

Specimen

- Aspirated epididymal fluid

Equipment (see also Appendix 2)

- Microscope configured for andrology with phase contrast optics (10×, 20× and 40× objectives)
- Centrifuge
- Tally counter
- Air-displacement pipette, 500-μl volume
- Rubber bulb to control Pasteur pipettes

Disposable materials

- Centrifuge tubes
- Glass Pasteur pipettes (sterile)
- Microscope slides
- Coverslips, 22 × 22 mm, #1½ or #2 thickness
- Pipette tips

Reagents

Sperm Buffer: Any HEPES- or MOPS-buffered ART culture medium known to support human spermatozoa that is supplemented with at least 5 mg/ml (ideally 10 mg/ml) of HSA. The medium must be at 37°C prior to use.

Calibration

The incubator used to warm the media must be set at 37°C and its operation verified using an independent temperature measuring device.

Quality control

No special QC procedures are required for this technique.

Procedure

1. Upon receiving a specimen of aspirated fluid, empty the syringe into a sterile Falcon tube, pumping the plunger several times to expel all the fluid.

2. Prepare a wet preparation using 10 μl of the diluted aspirate on a clean slide with a 22 × 22 mm coverslip. Examine under the microscope at 200× magnification.

3. Check for the presence of spermatozoa, and assess their approximate concentration (e.g. as "high/average/low") and motility (e.g. <1%, 1%, 5%, 20%, etc.); 5–10 motile spermatozoa per 20× objective field constitutes an average quality specimen.

4. Report the findings immediately to the surgeon and record the % motility on the Falcon tube from which the sample was taken. Also note on the tube anything that might affect the freezing process, e.g. a lot of blood or low sperm concentration, compared to the other samples.

5. Once the sample has been evaluated, store it in a 37°C air (non-CO_2) incubator.

6. Repeat steps 1 through 5 for each aspirated specimen.

Note: If cases are done in or adjacent to the surgical procedure room the urologist will likely ask when there is "enough specimen to freeze." Individual judgment is required here and, while not going too far, estimates should be on the cautious side.

7. Combine all aspirates which contain motile spermatozoa into one tube using 5.75″ sterile Pasteur pipettes and measure the total volume for cryopreservation.

8. Determine the concentration and motility of the total sample using a Makler chamber; evaluate the amount of debris at the same time.

9. If the concentration of the sample is so low as to likely provide insufficient motile spermatozoa per straw post-thaw to perform ICSI, the sample can be concentrated by centrifuging at 500 g for 10 min and resuspending the pellet in Sperm Buffer. Re-assess the sperm concentration of the concentrated specimen using a Makler chamber.

10. If possible, perform a semen analysis on the final specimen.

11. a. If the specimen has to be held for some time before performing ICSI this should be done at ambient temperature rather than 37°C to protect the spermatozoa from ROS-induced damage.

    b. Ideally, specimens should always be cryopreserved for later use, i.e. the procedure should have been performed before the ART treatment cycle. Even if the procedure is performed on the day of oocyte retrieval, always try to cryopreserve some of the specimen for use in a subsequent ICSI cycle.

Calculations and results

Ensure that all laboratory forms and reports are completed.

Notes

1. Samples showing extremely poor sperm motility (even as low as 0%) can be treated with pentoxifylline to try and stimulate sperm motility immediately prior to use. Spermatozoa to be used for ICSI are treated post-thaw, but any likely effect should be established by an earlier trial if there is sufficient material. Spermatozoa must be washed free of any pentoxifylline before being used to inseminate oocytes [5,6].

Preparation of testicular spermatozoa

Principle

Seminiferous tubule tissue is aspirated from the testis into a needle (TESA), or excised as one or more open testis biopsies (TESE). The spermatozoa must be recovered from the seminiferous tubules and washed using techniques that will not cause harm to them, in particular to their DNA. This is achieved by simple mincing of the tissue. Enzymatic digestion and/or physical homogenization (e.g. using a micro-tissue grinder) seriously compromise the quality of the spermatozoa and can result in substantial levels of ROS-induced damage to the sperm DNA. Also the sample often ends up as a gelatinous mass that is hard to handle.

Incubation of the retrieved testicular spermatozoa can lead to the acquisition of sperm motility. While this can sometimes be seen after just 3–4 h, many workers culture specimens overnight and even for up to three days.

Specimen

Testicular tissue samples, containing seminiferous tubules. Specimens should be placed in a HEPES- or MOPS-buffered medium as quickly as possible. This will allow the specimen to be kept under an air atmosphere without compromising the pH of the medium. Specimens must be kept within a temperature range of 20–38°C.

Equipment (see also Appendix 2)

- Microscope configured for andrology with phase contrast optics (10×, 20× and 40× objectives)
- Air incubator
- CO_2 incubator
- Centrifuge
- Tally counter
- Air-displacement pipette, 500-μl volume
- Sterile fine dissecting scissors
- Rubber bulb to control Pasteur pipettes

Disposable materials

- Scalpels with disposable blades
- Sterile fine (e.g. 25G) hypodermic needles, use 1-ml syringes as handles
- Culture dishes, e.g. Falcon #1007
- Centrifuge tubes
- Glass Pasteur pipettes (sterile)
- Microscope slides
- Coverslips, 22 × 22 mm, #1½ or #2 thickness

Reagents

Sperm Buffer: Any HEPES- or MOPS-buffered ART culture medium known to support human spermatozoa that is supplemented with at least 5 mg/ml (ideally 10 mg/ml) of HSA.

Sperm Medium: Any bicarbonate-buffered ART culture medium known to support human spermatozoa that is supplemented with 10 mg/ml of HSA.

All culture media must be at 37°C prior to use.

Calibration

1. Incubators must be set at 37°C and their operation verified using an independent temperature measuring device.
2. The CO_2 incubator must be set at the appropriate pCO_2 for the proper equilibration of the Sperm Medium and the %CO_2 verified by an independent CO_2 analyzer.

Quality control

No special QC procedures are required for this technique.

Procedure

Processing the tissue (see Note 2 for acknowledgement of the source of this protocol):

1. Place the testicular biopsy tissue in a small Falcon Petri dish in a small volume of Sperm Buffer. Tease the tissue apart into very small pieces using small dissecting scissors, fine scalpel blades and small-gauge hypodermic needles. (Do not try disrupting the tissue by aspirating it in and out of the needles.)
   Hint: Bend an additional small-gauge needle in the middle at 90° and use this to press on the small pieces in the dish in order to extrude material from the tubules by compression.

2. Examine the cell suspension using an inverted (ICSI) microscope by phase contrast or Hoffman optics. Only if there are large numbers of spermatozoa showing significant motility should you proceed directly to step 5.

3. Add some more Sperm Medium and place the dish at 37°C in a CO_2 incubator overnight. This will increase the motility and result in more motile spermatozoa per straw later.

4. a. Following overnight incubation, rinse the contents out of the dish and transfer them into a Falcon #2095 conical centrifuge tube.

   b. Centrifuge at 200–300 g for 10 min.

   c. Remove the supernatant and resuspend the pellet with Sperm Buffer to 1.0–2.0 ml according to its size.

   d. Make a standard wet preparation (10 µl under a 22 × 22 mm coverslip) and assess the specimen for motile spermatozoa under phase contrast optics.
   If there are sufficient motile spermatozoa, go to step 5.

   If there are no motile spermatozoa, advise the patients and the urologist. Proceed to step 5.

   Note: All further washing and preparation of the spermatozoa will be done after thawing (see step 11), not before cryopreservation.

5. a. Transfer the specimen into a small Falcon dish, and return it to culture at 37°C in the CO_2 incubator overnight.

   b. The following morning repeat step 4, unless the specimen has already been cultured for 72 h, in which case proceed to step 6.

   c. At step 4d, if there are sufficient motile spermatozoa, go to step 7; if not, then the specimen can be incubated for a third night (maximum) – repeat this step (5) once more.

6. If there are still no motile spermatozoa after 72 h in culture advise the patients and the urologist.

Freezing the spermatozoa

7. Process the specimen for cryopreservation (see Chapter 8). If there is a high concentration of motile spermatozoa, extend the specimen using Sperm Buffer before adding the

cryoprotectant medium so as to be able to freeze more straws. Ensure that the man has signed a sperm cryopreservation consent form.

8. Perform a test-thaw. See Note 3.

9. Complete the laboratory report form and transcribe the relevant information onto the necessary clinical report form(s). Make sure the nurse or clinician managing the woman's stimulation cycle is advised of the results as soon as possible.

Thawing the spermatozoa for use in ICSI

10. Thaw one or more straws of the specimen as necessary (see Chapter 8).
The dilution step should use at least a 5× volume of Sperm Buffer, and ideally a 10× volume.
Make a standard wet preparation (10 µl under a 22 × 22 mm coverslip) and assess the specimen for motile spermatozoa under phase contrast optics.

11. Depending on the number of motile spermatozoa seen, either:

   a. If there are very few motile spermatozoa, wash the sample by centrifugation (500 g × 10 min) and resuspend the pellet in *ca.* 100 µl Sperm Buffer, regardless of the amount of debris present.

   b. For more typical specimens, wash the spermatozoa using a single layer (2.0–4.0 ml) of 40% gradient colloid only (i.e. do not use a 2-layer gradient) by centrifuging at 500 g × 10 min. Discard the entire supernatant and resuspend the pellet in *ca.* 100 µl Sperm Buffer, regardless of the amount of debris present.

12. Make a standard wet preparation (10 µl under a 22 × 22 mm coverslip) and assess the specimen for motile spermatozoa under phase contrast optics. Record your observations on the lab form.

13. Proceed to preparing the sperm dish for ICSI.

Calculations and results

Ensure that all laboratory forms and reports are completed.

Notes

1. Processing testicular tissue on the day of an ICSI procedure is not recommended due to the risk of not having any spermatozoa after the woman has undergone stimulation.

2. This protocol was generously provided by Carole Lawrence (Laboratory Director, Pacific Centre for Reproductive Medicine, Burnaby, BC, Canada; see www.pacificfertility.ca). Experience using this protocol over several years, including sperm cryopreservation using Nidacon's SCP cryoprotectant medium and a CryoLogic programmable freezer (i.e. not cooling in a static vapor phase), has shown that:

   a. If there are motile spermatozoa pre-freeze (even <1%) then there should always be motility post-thaw.

   b. There should be no need to resort to using any "motility-enhancing" chemicals such as pentoxifylline.

   c. Clinical pregnancy rates of >70% per oocyte retrieval can be achieved after ICSI in women <40 years of age.

3. While some workers advocate lysing the red blood cells (RBCs) present there seems to be little real need for this and it not only results in the release of large amounts of potassium from the lysed RBCs, but all the cell "ghosts" remain in the specimen. Experienced operators have little trouble picking up spermatozoa from around intact RBCs.

References

1. Donoso P, Tournaye H, Devroey P. Which is the best sperm retrieval technique for non-obstructive azoospermia? A systematic review. *Hum Reprod Update* 2007; **13**: 539–49.

2. Wald M, Makhlouf AA, Niederberger CS. Therapeutic testis biopsy for sperm retrieval. *Curr Opin Urol* 2007; **17**: 431–8.

3. van Peperstraten A, Proctor M, Johnson N, Philipson G. Techniques for surgical retrieval of sperm prior to intra-cytoplasmic sperm injection (ICSI) for azoospermia. *Cochrane Database Syst Rev* 2008; **16**: CD002807.

4. Rowe PJC, Vomhaire FH, Hargreave TB, Mahmous AMA. *WHO Manual for the Standardized Investigation, Diagnosis and Management of the Infertile Male.* Cambridge: Cambridge University Press 2000.

5. Kovačič B, Vlaisavljević V, Reljič M. Clinical use of pentoxifylline for activation of immotile testicular sperm before ICSI in patients with azoospermia. *J Androl* 2006; **27**: 45–52.

6. Tournaye H, Devroey P, Camus M, *et al.* Use of pentoxifylline in assisted reproductive technology. *Hum Reprod* 1995; **10** Suppl 1: 72–9.

Chapter 10

Quality management and accreditation

Overview of quality management

Quality concepts

Quality is the degree to which a product or service conforms to accepted standards and/or to the requirements of internal and external customers, thus quality is definitely in the eyes of the beholder. Before beginning the discussion of quality, we must consider which dimensions or perceptions of quality the customer/consumer may have. The following is a quick overview of the possibilities:

1. Administration and management focus on continuous quality improvement in an effort to improve the level of performance across the entire organization and achieve higher levels of customer satisfaction. (Culture of quality.)

2. Clinical and laboratory personnel, i.e. physicians, nurses and scientists, focus on the delivery of medical care while consistently incorporating current professional knowledge. (Clinical quality.)

3. Employers, health care purchasers, patients and families may assess the quality of their health care delivery based on personal treatment, courtesy, environment, access to care and medical outcomes, i.e. "do they get better?" (Quality of service.)

The quality of a product or service is not random, but rather can be programmed, measured, and improved: quality is part of everyday management. The approach to quality issues is not a science – hence there is not, and can never be, a single "ideal solution." It is the job of management to assess and choose from the many possible solutions or approaches which one they think will be appropriate for their particular needs. Quality can be managed. For quality management to be considered "total" (TQM), the following three components must be employed: quality control (QC), quality assurance (QA) and quality improvement (QI).

QC   is an activity designed to ensure that a specific element within the laboratory is functioning correctly by means of the monitoring of indicators [1]. QC is about making sure that each task is done correctly. QC also includes corrective measures to ensure that procedures are up to standard.

QA   is a comprehensive program designed to look at a laboratory procedure as a whole and to identify problems or errors that exist in an attempt to improve the process. QC is a component of QA. QA is the overall program that ensures that the final results reported by the testing laboratory are correct, e.g. the sperm provided by a cryobank are valid for use in artificial insemination. QA relates to the way in which work is done. QA also prevents problems [2].

QI   is a comprehensive, perpetually reiterative, monitoring process designed not only to detect and eliminate problems, but also to enhance a laboratory's performance by exploring innovation and developing flexibility and effectiveness in all processes. This process refers to the Plan-Do-Check-Act (PDCA) circle, also known as the "Deming wheel" [3]. It is a very simple concept which helps coordinate an organization's quality improvement efforts: just as a circle has no end, the PDCA cycle repeatedly executes in pursuit of continual improvement. It emphasizes and demonstrates that improvement programs must start with careful planning, must result in effective action, and must move on again to careful planning in a continuous cycle (Figure 10.1).

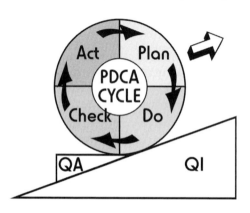

Figure 10.1 The Deming wheel ("PDCA Cycle") for continual improvement [3]. Plan: evaluate the current situation, and define a plan about how and which activities need improvement; Do: conduct a small-scale implementation of the plan; Check: monitor and evaluate the plan; adopt and adjust the plan where necessary; Act: implement the definitive plan. The process is iterative; a new cycle starts in order to continually improve the system and assure quality. QA = quality assurance; QI = quality improvement.

Hence, when a clinical laboratory such as an andrology laboratory is considering adopting TQM as an operating framework, it aims for integration consistency, an increase in efficiency and a continuous drive for improvement. With TQM, the challenge shifts from a simple question such as "was the test done correctly?" to "was the right test carried out on the right specimen and was the right result and right interpretation delivered to the right patient at the right time and all done with the lowest cost possible?"

A quality management system (QMS)

A QMS is the entire system developed by an organization that involves the establishment of a quality policy and quality objectives, and the processes to achieve those goals. In order for a QMS to be effective, the objectives must be measurable, reflect the laboratory's overall goals, and be clearly defined. It must also be practical, reviewed regularly, measured for effectiveness, and be accessible to all employees. A QMS consists of documented policies and procedures for the establishment and effective implementation of the system itself, as well as records to provide evidence that the system is in compliance. The documents include: quality manual (philosophy of the laboratory); procedures (principles and strategy); test methods (standard operating procedures or SOPs); and records (results, evidence, proof). There are software packages that facilitate the implementation of a QMS.

Process analysis

A series of continuous actions or tasks, or a method by which something is done, is termed a process. The group of techniques used to understand all factors involved in a process is called process mapping, with examples being flowcharts, top-down process maps, swim-lane analysis, and the IDEF0 modeling method [4].

Standard operating procedure (SOP)

An SOP is a document which describes the regularly recurring operations relevant to the performance and quality of an investigation. The purpose of an SOP is to carry out the operations correctly and always in the same manner. An SOP should be available at the place where the work is done, and is a compulsory instruction. If deviations from this instruction are allowed, the conditions for these should be documented, including who can give permission for this and what exactly the complete procedure will be. The original SOP should be kept in a secure place while working copies should be authenticated with stamps and/or signatures of authorized persons [4].

Process control to monitor the performance of a process over time

The two techniques most often used are control charts and rolling averages [5]. Monitoring requires the definition and use of indicators. An indicator is a measurable aspect of a process (e.g. care provided) for which there is evidence that it represents quality on the grounds of scientific research, or consensus among experts. From the viewpoint of measurement, there are three types of indicators: (a) structural; (b) technical (including pre-analysis, post-analysis and analytical) and clinical process; and (c) outcome indicators (see Table 10.1). Some indicators are more suitable for internal quality improvement (clinical indicators) and others are especially appropriate for external appraisal (outcome indicators).

Accreditation

Within quality assurance, accreditation is an effective tool for implementing internationally recognized quality systems in medical service and health care. Accreditation of management systems is internationally accepted for conformity assessment. Accreditation is defined as a collegial process based on self- and peer-assessment whereby an authoritative body (usually a non-government organization) gives formal recognition that an organization is in voluntary compliance with one or more standards set by the authoritative body. Accreditation "standards" are published documents that contain technical specifications or criteria to be used consistently as rules, guidelines, or definitions of characteristics to ensure that materials, products, processes and services are fit for their purpose.

Note: "Accreditation standards" must not be confused with "performance standards" or "minimum standards" (also called "quality specifications" or "performance specifications") since these define the minimum technical requirements for a process to be performed or undertaken, and do not usually consider anything beyond basic quality control.

Nevertheless, certain semantic confusions exist between the terms "accreditation" and "certification" and "registration." The International Organization for Standardization (ISO) Council Committee on Conformity Assessment has attempted to resolve the semantics problem by standardizing the following definitions:

1. Accreditation: A procedure by which an authoritative body gives formal recognition that a body or person is competent to carry out specific tasks. A planning for typical steps in the accreditation process can be seen in Figure 10.2.

Table 10.1 Examples of quality indicators in the andrology laboratory.

Type of indicator	Semen analysis	Sperm cryopreservation
RESOURCE	Number of semen analyses per microscope	Consumption of liquid nitrogen per cryopreservation procedure
	Number of semen analyses per technician	
	Smoother workflow	Number of samples stored per cryotank
	Reagent and culture medium wastage	Number of broken transport containers per month
PROCESS		
Technical		
Pre-analytical	Request illegible or unintelligible	Error in donor identification
	Inadequate or inappropriate transportation conditions	Incomplete semen sample
	Patient waiting time for an appointment	Donor or patient waiting times
	Patient waiting time at the lab	
	Specimen requested but not collected	
Analytical	Imprecision below analytical quality specification	Cryosurvival rate
		Verification of cooling rate
	Incubator temperature is within control limits (control chart)	Testing of a new medium when freezing a known donor
	Sperm preparation recovery rate	
	Proficiency test performance	
Post-analytical	Average time to communicate test results to patients	Average time to communicate cryopreservation results to patients
	Prepared sperm specimen delivered outside the specified time	Cryosurvival rate below benchmark
	Test not performed	
	Test performed that was not requested	
Clinical	In case of abnormal semen analysis result, perform at least one extra semen analysis	Patient has not had appropriate serological testing
	In case of normozoospermia, semen analysis not repeated	Patient specimen accepted for cryopreservation without a written order
OUTCOME	Pregnancy rate following AIH	Fertilization rate when used for IVF
		Pregnancy rate following IUI

2. Certification: A procedure by which a third-party gives written assurance (certificate of conformity) that a product, process or service conforms to specified requirements.

3. Registration: A procedure by which a body indicates relevant characteristics of a product, process or service, or particulars of a body or person, in an appropriate publicly available list.

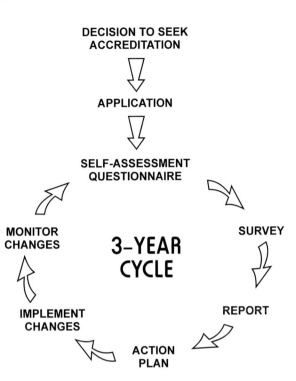

DECISION TO SEEK ACCREDITATION

APPLICATION

SELF-ASSESSMENT QUESTIONNAIRE

MONITOR CHANGES

3-YEAR CYCLE

SURVEY

IMPLEMENT CHANGES

REPORT

ACTION PLAN

Figure 10.2 Steps in the accreditation process. Reproduced from ref. 4 with permission.

Note: Internationally, certification has become the dominant term. But common terminology in the United States is not always in harmony with this international guidance, nor with European practice. The European approach is to label both quality system registrars and product certifiers as certification bodies. There is very little, if any, use of the term "registration" in Europe.

In general terms, "accreditation" is a formal recognition that a body is competent to carry out specific tasks, while "certification" is a formal evaluation by a third-party that a product conforms to a standard, and "registration" commonly refers to certification of quality systems. Hence laboratory accreditation is defined as a formal recognition that a laboratory is competent to carry out specific tests, or specific types of tests (i.e. ISO 15189:2007); and quality system registration or certification is a formal attestation that a supplier's quality system is in conformance with an appropriate quality system model (i.e. ISO 9001:2008).

Worldwide accreditation infrastructure

The standards of accreditation most often followed were established by the International and Regional Standards and Conformance Bodies. The international organization responsible for the "Documentary Standards Development" is the International Organization for Standardization (ISO) and the body specifically designated for laboratories is the International Laboratory Accreditation Cooperation (ILAC). At a regional level accrediting bodies have been established (e.g. the European Cooperation for Accreditation, or ECA, and the InterAmerican Accreditation Cooperation, or IAAC). In each country accreditation is performed by qualified government agencies, or private sector professionals or trade organizations operating in accordance with appropriate international requirements such as ISO/IEC 17011. A listing of international accreditation bodies that are signatories to the "ILAC mutual recognition arrangements" may be found on the ILAC website, www.ilac.org. (Figure 10.3).

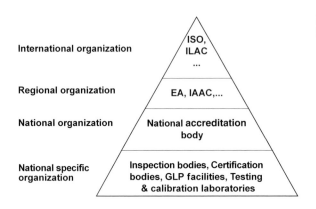

International organization

Regional organization

National organization

National specific organization

Figure 10.3 Worldwide accreditation infrastructure.

Most of the national accreditation bodies [6,7] follow an international guideline developed by the International Organization for Standardization (ISO) for testing laboratories in general (ISO/IEC 17025:2005, entitled "General Requirements for the Competence of Testing and Calibration Laboratories") and one in particular for medical laboratories (ISO 15189:2007, entitled "Medical Laboratories – Particular Requirements for Quality and Competence") [8,9,10]. Some countries prefer a "local" guideline such as CCLK (Coördinatie Commissie ter bevordering van de Kwaliteitsbeheersing op het gebied van Laboratoriumonderzoek in de Gezondheidszorg) in the Netherlands, or CPA (Clinical Pathology Accreditation) in the UK. Other models of accreditation are the European Foundation for Quality Management (EFQM) and the US Clinical Laboratory Improvement Amendments (CLIA).

Clinical quality

Another aspect of quality is clinical quality, the degree to which health care systems, services and supplies for individuals and populations increase the likelihood for positive health outcomes. The tools used in clinical quality management are:

1. Evidence-based clinical practice guidelines: These are documents containing systematically developed recommendations, algorithms and other information to assist healthcare decision-making for specific clinical circumstances. The Appraisal of Guidelines Research and Evaluation (AGREE) Instruments provide a framework for assessing the quality of clinical practice guidelines (see http://www.agreetrust.org).

2. Clinical quality indicators: These should measure quality in a valid and reliable manner with little inter- and intra-observer variability so that they are suitable for comparison between professionals, practices and institutions. Indicators are selected from research data with consideration for optimal patient care (preferably an evidence-based guideline), supplemented by expert opinion. In the selection procedure, feasibility, such as their measurability and improvability, is important alongside validity and reliability [11,12]. Nevertheless, problems can appear at the time of interpreting the results [8].

3. Health technology assessment (HTA) may be defined as a form of research which systematically analyzes: health, social, economical, ethical and legal consequences derived from the use of technology that is produced in both the short- and long-term; such analyses include both the desired effects as well as undesired ones. The International Network of Agencies for Health Technology Assessment (INAHTA) is grouped to national agencies of health technology assessment (http://www.inahta.org).

Training

Standardization of semen analysis requires clear, detailed and robust methods. However, these alone are not enough. There must also be an effective training system for staff, and this must be followed-up by ongoing QC and QA. Reading even the most detailed manual or handbook can never replace proper, basic technical training; practical hands-on training is essential. Many technicians, through no fault of their own, are performing semen analysis using inappropriate methods, with inadequate training [9]. Importantly, this can easily be addressed using proven training methods [10]. We encourage all those involved in andrology laboratory work to determine/assess if their current systems comply with current best practice.

Training of new personnel to perform techniques in an andrology laboratory constitutes the cornerstone of the quality assurance. The "learning curve" is the effort required to acquire a new skill over a specific period of time. The type of curve (steep or gradual) depends on the inherent technical difficulty as well as the heterogeneity of the caseload. Thus, sperm preparation is technically easy, but one might need to individualize the techniques employed for each step to ensure optimum results; hence, the learning curve will be a gradual progression. Meanwhile, sperm cryopreservation is technically complicated, but generally the same protocol is employed for all semen samples. A standardized training system is essential to avoid future problems. Training progress has to be closely followed, documented, and be approved by the laboratory director. Therefore, it is important to establish training criteria and performance thresholds that should be met in order to attain the experience necessary to perform procedures independently. Equally, it is desirable that appropriate quality control measures be implemented in order to ensure that such performance thresholds, once achieved, are maintained. Different levels of ability have been described for the andrology laboratory: (a) basic understanding established; (b) able to work under supervision; (c) allowed to work without supervision; and (d) able to train other people [13].

Step-by-step (slow but steady)

The first requirement should be that the trainee is fully conversant with the setting-up and operation of the andrology laboratory equipment. This may seem like an obvious statement, but an eagerness to perform semen analysis sometimes enables trainees to convince themselves, and others, that they know how to use the equipment properly when in fact they do not. Once the trainee has become familiar with the equipment and material, and after observing an experienced staff member perform the technique, the trainee can practice with "left-over" semen not required for analysis. Familiarity with the material and reagents allows the trainee to progress to using them concurrently so that they can manipulate the semen in a way that mimics a "real" scenario. Only once these techniques have been perfected should the trainee proceed to attempt to prepare or cryopreserve a "real" semen sample, under supervision.

Criteria for competence

1. For cryopreservation, an expected survival rate for donor semen of $\geq 25\%$ (ideally, $>30\%$).
2. For sperm preparation by direct swim-up from semen (DSUS), a recovery rate $\pm 10\%$ of the progressively motile spermatozoa with a $\geq 20\%$ increase in progressive motility.
3. For sperm preparation by DGC, $>95\%$ progressive motility in the final preparations from normal semen samples [13].
4. For semen analysis, competence should be based on an expectation of meeting generally accepted analytical quality specifications [14].

Once a trainee has demonstrated an ability to achieve this goal, they can be considered ready to progress to dealing with half of the semen samples in a given case, under supervision. When a trainee has demonstrated an ability to achieve the goal on three consecutive occasions, they can progress to handling an entire case independently, under supervision. A trainee will be allowed to work independently after 10 cases of sperm cryopreservation or perhaps 50 cases of ejaculated semen preparation with optimum results. Only after completing training, and after gaining experience from a certain number of cases, can someone instruct beginners. Annual reports on the percentage of recovery rate or cryosurvival rate provide a good form of quality assurance. Naturally, pregnancies resulting from sperm preparation or cryopreservation provide further quality assurance, but they are also subject to variables other than andrology laboratory techniques.

In addition to the processes already described, for proper training in semen analysis it is advisable that trainees attend a technique standardization course. The effectiveness of these courses to diminish the variability between observers has been demonstrated with the completion of a single course [10], or of refresher courses [15]. After an introductory course future training is mandatory until the individual is fully trained [16]. This can only be done with serious commitment. To support continued training "at home" control material from an EQA scheme can be used, or a specific program for continuous training can be employed [17]. When proper training has been completed, IQC should be implemented as a tool to decrease both inter- and intra-technician variability, and to ensure that semen analysis technical skills are maintained at a high standard.

Comparing the results of an expert and a trainee

Discrete variables

Comparing a discrete variable with two categories requires use of the Kappa statistic. With more categories, use the weighted Kappa [18].

Continuous variables

Continuous variables can be compared using paired t-tests or Wilcoxon matched pairs tests, interclass correlation coefficients, or Bland and Altman charts (Figure 10.4; see also the section on "Selecting methods" later in this chapter) using the mean of the differences between observers and ± 2 SD (standard deviation) control limits, or using the combined inherent coefficient of variation (CV) of each observer as a control limit [19].

A training scheme based on goal-orientated targets using libraries of reference materials has also been described [20].

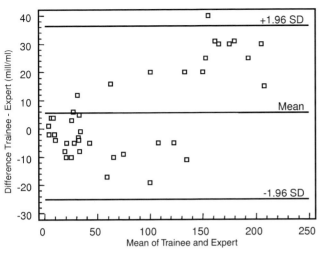

Figure 10.4 A Bland and Altman chart (see ref. 37) revealing a trainee's tendency to count more spermatozoa when analyzing semen samples with higher sperm concentration.

Training for sperm morphology assessments

Process

For sperm morphology evaluation training the trainee is first given a lecture on the biology of spermiogenesis and the theoretical aspects of sperm morphology evaluation [21], followed by the practical application of this information taught in a one-on-one situation using a double-headed microscope or video imaging system attached to a microscope. In these sessions the basic normal and abnormal morphological forms are seen and described under the microscope. The trainee is then allowed to evaluate routine morphology samples without the knowledge of the results of the original assessments. The results of the trainee are then compared to the routine laboratory results and then taken back to the one-on-one situation to discuss the trainee's results along with possible reasons for discrepancies e.g. misinterpretation of sperm size where, especially in the case of large-headed spermatozoa, mis-classification as normal can be common. In this situation the trainee should be encouraged to use a built-in eyepiece micrometer to first routinely measure the size of spermatozoa until the image of a morphologically normal, and especially normal-sized spermatozoa, is imprinted on her/his mind.

The general tendency will be that the trainee will first over-estimate the percentage of morphologically normal spermatozoa and then, after the first few training sessions, become over-critical and under-estimate the percentage of morphologically normal spermatozoa. With proper guidance the trainee will move closer to the target value so that, after about three weeks of daily training sessions, they will be able to produce acceptable results.

Extreme care must continue to be taken as there will always be a general tendency to be over-critical, and thus to under-estimate the percentage of morphologically normal spermatozoa, especially when working in isolation in a small laboratory. For this reason it is important to take part in a refresher course within a year after the initial training, as well as to participate in an EQC program. The availability of reference slides representative of the three diagnostic morphological classes [22] i.e., normal (≥14% normal forms), good prognosis pattern (5–14% normal) and the poor prognosis pattern (≤4% normal), will be highly beneficial.

Evaluation

Because of the uniqueness of sperm morphology results, a system equivalent to the z-score measurement has been developed [23], using a so-called SD-score, where the results of a trainee can be monitored on a quarterly basis and expressed as marginal, good or excellent (excellent is where the [quarterly] readings are always within –0.2 to +0.2 SD-score levels). The SD-score is calculated according to the following formula:

$$SD = \frac{\text{Trainee score} - \text{Reference laboratory score}}{\text{SD of reference laboratory}}$$

Where: $SD = \sqrt{p(100 - p)}$
  p = morphology score (%normal) for the smear evaluated by the personnel from the reference laboratory.

This system is especially useful for small laboratories which receive slides on a regular (quarterly) basis for EQC purposes. The results can be plotted on a graph and trends, scoring too strict or too lenient, can be observed.

Quality control

Control is the action of measuring, examining, testing and calibrating one or several characteristics of a product or of a service, and the comparison with the specified requirements in order to establish their conformity. Control is used for different aspects of quality in the laboratory andrology: (a) Control of an analytical process: pre-analytical, analytical and post-analytical (e.g. semen analysis); (b) Control of any step necessary to guarantee the quality of sperm preparation or cryopreservation: freezer and tank temperatures, pipette calibration, liquid nitrogen level in tanks, etc.; (c) Control of the relations with the patients, clinicians, donors or clinics (e.g. complaints); and (d) Control of the quality level of the services (outcome or clinical result) associated with the andrology laboratory (e.g. pregnancy rate).

It remains inevitable that errors will be made. Therefore, the control system should have checks to detect them. In this text we will concentrate on the quality control of analysis techniques.

Internal QC

The internal QC (IQC) involves in-house procedures for continuous monitoring of operations and systematic day-to-day checking of the produced data to decide whether these are reliable enough to be released. Two types of material can be used: control material or patient samples. An internal quality control scheme requires several steps:

Control material

- Selection of material: (a) similarity to "real" patient specimens; (b) availability in large enough quantities to allow evaluation over a long period of time; (c) similarity in concentration from aliquot to aliquot (precision); and (d) stability over a period of use. Frozen sperm samples do not meet all these conditions for semen analysis [24,25,26]. The quality control materials recommended are: for sperm concentration pools of formalin (1%) semen suspension; for sperm motility videotape or DVD recording; for sperm morphology unstained and stained smears; and for sperm vitality eosin Y/nigrosin smears; for biochemical analysis of semen, frozen or lyophilized (freeze dried) seminal fluid; and positive frozen serum or seminal fluid for antisperm antibodies [24,26,27]. No certified reference material exists at the moment for semen quality control. However, "sufficient" homogeneity and stability can be established for in-house control material [28,29].

- Selection of levels (decision points): Test material should be available in important medical decision-making levels: low (lower than reference limit), medium (near reference limit), and high (above reference limit).

- Definition of the quality requirement: The maximum allowed analytical error can be defined by various strategies [30,31]. Ideally, quality specifications should be derived from the clinical needs. However, it not possible to simply measure how much, for example, the pregnancy rate decreases with an increased variability in sperm motility analysis. Other strategies include components of biological variation, analysis of clinicians' opinions, guidelines by national or international experts, regulations or by external quality assessment schemes (EQASs) [14,24,32,33]. These quality specifications can vary according to the quality requirement (toxicological or epidemiological studies) [31].

- Variation of a method: To assess the variability (imprecision) of a method, the control material is assessed repeatedly over a period of time (e.g. at least 20 days). Independent control checks during this period should verify that the method is under control for the entire assessment time. The mean and standard deviation (SD) of the assessed control values are used to calculate the within-observer analytical CV. If the obtained value is less than the specified requirements, the performance of the method is acceptable. The values obtained should also be plotted into a classic control chart (also called Shewhart chart or Levy–Jennings chart). Note that this assessment only reflects the variability of the method, not the accuracy, which can only be evaluated with external quality assessment [34,35].

- Stability of method: Aliquots of the same control material (e.g. fixed sperm suspension) are analyzed on consecutive days and the obtained values are plotted in a Shewhart control chart [36]. As long as the control values recorded on the Shewhart chart vary randomly around the control mean with no more than 5% of the points falling outside the ±2 SD control limits, the method is in control. Points falling outside the ±2 SD control limits are taken to be warning signals, while a single point falling outside the ±3 SD control limits signals rejection of the associated assay and immediate action is required to investigate and rectify any problem that could have caused the error. Note that a stable method is not the same as a clinically useful method, but an unstable method cannot produce clinically useful results.

Patient samples

When patient samples are used, repeated measurements need to be carried out in order to establish the same basic parameters as is the case for control material (see above).

Inter-observer quality control

All methodology described previously, including control charts, can be used to assess systematic differences between technicians. Another technique is the classic Bland

and Altman chart, using the mean of the differences between observers and ±2 SD control limits, or using the combined inherent CV of each observer as the control limit [19,37].

Quality control in other areas of the andrology laboratory

In addition to the technique control chart, the accumulative histogram or rolling average has been used to control the quality in other areas of the andrology laboratory [38]. These techniques can be used to control any quality indicator (see "Overview and accreditation" section). A procedure to control the quality of all frozen semen coming out of a sperm bank should exist (see "Cryopreservation method") [39].

Coefficient of variation (CV)

Using the CV gives no indication about what the coefficient relates to, e.g. within-observer or total random error, or the level of the parameter to which the CV applies. Furthermore, a CV of 8 does not mean a 95% error range or ±8, but ±16. The interpretation of the CV is also confused because semen analysis exhibits a non-constant error variance that is proportional to the parameter level: sperm concentration is directly related, while percentages (motility, vitality and normal forms) are inversely related [16,40]. Use the CV if you must, but use it carefully, and appropriately [41].

Selecting methods

That assessments of sperm concentration, motility, and morphology are frequently subject to wide variations due to technical error is well-established and has been known for many years [16,42,43,44,45]. This is despite the availability of methods whereby intra- and inter-operator variability can be reduced, e.g. [20,36,46,47,48,49,50,51]. Yet the basic requirements for achieving accuracy, precision, and reproducibility are simple: (a) use robust methods that reduce technical error as much as possible; and (b) train staff carefully in the correct performance of the methods. This was the philosophy behind the basic semen analysis courses run by the ESHRE Special Interest Group in Andrology, courses that have provided eloquent evidence of the validity of this approach [10], which employed the goal-orientated training approach first promoted by Mortimer [20]. As a fundamental philosophical principle, expending effort on establishing standardization is logical and practical and must be preferred to expending effort on demonstrating/confirming that staff have not been properly trained and/or methods have not been correctly standardized against established definitions (e.g. [52]).

Consequently, we are left with the inescapable conclusion that the only reason sperm assessments are not performed more reliably in many diagnostic laboratories and IVF centers can only be that those responsible for the medical and scientific direction of those laboratories just do not care. As a result, the often-expressed opinion that sperm counts, etc. do not have any value becomes a self-fulfilling prophesy – how could observations with error components of up to 50% be taken seriously or used intelligently? Yet the basic standards for all medical laboratories are well-established, and clearly expounded in ISO 15189:2007 [4].

Basic requirements of a robust method

Establishing the criteria to be used for specifying a technical procedure, or for selecting one from several available (and, similarly, for choosing a particular piece of equipment) can be simplified if it is considered within the context of it being a process [53]. This approach allows the following generic questions to be used as basic principles for establishing the method's specifications and evaluating candidate methods' suitability.

What does it need to do?

Basically, what do you want to measure? If necessary define the criterion, or its sub-classifications, quantitatively. For example, the following definitions for human sperm motility classification have been established (accepted by international consensus?) since the early-/mid-1990s [20,48]:

class *a*	=	rapid progressive motility	definition:	≥ 25 µm/s progression velocity at 37°C
class b	=	slow progressive motility	definition:	5–25 µm/s progression at 37°C
class *c*	=	non-progressive motility	definition:	flagellar activity, but <5 µm/s "space gain" at 37°C
class *d*	=	immotile	definition:	no flagellar activity

How well must it do it?

What precision is necessary for the purpose of the measurement? For example, knowing the proportion of progressively motile spermatozoa to a greater precision than an integer percentage would confer no additional benefit, but would greatly increase the effort required. Also remember that results can only be presented to a degree of precision appropriate to the statistical validity of the measurement. In this regard we must consider all factors that can affect the method's accuracy and precision, including being able to establish – and respect – its "uncertainty of measurement" (see below).

What are the options?

Review the available methods, but exclude those for which no robust or validated methodology or protocols are available. Is the method being used by other respected diagnostic andrology labs? Are there established performance indicators for the method?

How well does a method do it?

Review all possible sources of error and bias within the method. Does the method control them to practical levels commensurate with achieving the necessary uncertainty of measurement? Can the method be improved so that it controls these problems better, or should a better method be designed?

How well can it be controlled? Can we make it better?

What reference materials and calibrators are available (remember that calibration ≠ quality control)? Is QC for the method practical in the routine setting (remember that QC must be continual)? Is there an EQAP for the method (remember that participating in an EQAP cannot replace QC, and that, for it to be useful, an EQAP must also include both QA and QI capabilities)?

Is it practical?

Evaluate each method's feasibility in terms of the equipment, reagents and time that will be required, as well as the method's complexity and any need for specialized training. Basically, undertake comparative cost/benefit analyses.

Will help be available?

What training courses are available? Will specialized training be required from the originator of a particular technical procedure (e.g. the SCSA™)? For specialized equipment, will support be needed/available from the manufacturer or distributor?

Uncertainty of measurement

Every measurement has an error associated with it and, without a quantitative statement of the error, a measurement lacks worth, even credibility. The parameter that quantifies the boundaries of the error of a measurement is the "uncertainty of measurement" [54,55]. An uncertainty statement must have an associated confidence level, most usually a 95% confidence level, i.e. effectively 2× the combined uncertainty. In practical terms, for diagnostic semen analysis purposes, an uncertainty of ±10% is adequate and readily achievable in practical terms (the methods described in this handbook, if properly implemented, will achieve this).

Sources of uncertainty

As per the ISO Guide [54]:

1. Incomplete definition of the measurand.
2. Incomplete realization of the definition of the measurand.
3. Non-representative sampling.
4. Inadequate knowledge of the effects of environmental conditions on the measurand (or imperfect measurement of those conditions).
5. Personal bias in reading analog instruments – or making subjective assessments!
6. Finite instrument resolution or discrimination threshold.
7. Inexact values of measurement standards and reference materials.
8. Inexact values of constants and other parameters obtained from external sources.
9. Approximations and assumptions incorporated in the measurement method and procedure.
10. Variations in repeated observations of the measurand under apparently identical conditions ("repeatability").

Determining/controlling the uncertainty for a method

This process is very similar to undertaking a failure modes and effects analysis or "FMEA" [4]:

1. Construct a model of the measurement system (process mapping).
2. List all the factors that can contribute errors to the final result (this requires a good understanding of the measurement principles, the equipment and environment) and then categorize each one as either random or systematic.

3. Ensure that each source of error has been controlled, as far as is practical, within the method.
4. Either compute their combined uncertainty [55] or derive it by comparing results with known reference values.

Comparing methods
Discrete variables

Discrete variables such as modal progression ratings or subjective rankings of debris or round cells should never be averaged. Instead frequency distributions should be compared or proportion above/below a particular threshold. When comparing two series of assessments (e.g. novice and expert), individual pairs of values should not differ by more than one rank, and be identical in, say, >90% of cases. For example, in a group of 30 paired assessments, no more than two ratings can be different, and then by no more than ±1 rank each.

Continuous variables

Continuous variables such as sperm concentration and the percentages of sperm motility, vitality and morphological normality can be analyzed using paired t-tests or, better, the method described by Bland and Altman [37], e.g. using MedCalc software (Mariakerke, Belgium, see www.medcalc.be). This latter method considers the average discrepancy between two sets of values (calculated as the mean of a series of individual difference values) compared to the average of the individual paired measurements. For training situations, the difference values should be calculated as "trainee – expert" so that an over-estimate by the trainee yields a positive difference and the expert value is used instead of the average (since there is no evidence that the trainee is able to generate reliable values, e.g. Figure 10.4 [20]). For subsequent analyses, e.g. for post-training proficiency testing or QC, the original method of plotting the difference against technician-average values should be employed. Arcsin transformation of percentage values should not be necessary, but because the range of sperm concentration values is extremely wide, each difference value is expressed as a percentage of either the expert's value for training situations, or of the average value for other purposes.

The aim is to achieve consistency between the methods (or competence of a trainee against an expert). Consequently, the goal is to achieve a zero mean difference and a 95% range of differences that is within a pre-determined level of acceptability, e.g. ±5%. The 95% range of discrepancy is calculated by multiplying the SD by the value of the "t" statistic for that number of observations and the appropriate level of significance. For example, for a 5% significance level with n = 20, t = 2.086; for n = 30, t = 2.042 (the SD is not multiplied by 2.0 until n = 60).

Making your lab better
For each technical procedure, employ the quality cycle ("Plan, Do, Check, Act" or "PDCA" cycle) [4].

A. Review your methods
1. Take your current method apart (process mapping).
2. Assess component steps and procedures (process analysis).
3. Identify all possible sources of error/bias.
4. Are they all being "trapped," avoided or at least minimized?

5. Is there anything else that can be done?
6. Compare your method with others.
7. Should (can) you change anything?

B. Uncertainty of measurement
1. Can you determine what it is?
2. Do you report results appropriately?
3. Do the report recipients understand the implications?

C. Review your quality control procedures
1. Do they relate to reality? (Calibration ≠ QC)
2. Do they actually increase reproducibility: between observers?; over time?

D. External quality assurance
1. Is it more than proficiency testing?
2. Does the feedback help you apply corrective action?
3. Does it include ongoing quality improvement?

EQA schemes

External quality assurance (EQA)

Participation in an EQA program allows an evaluation of the analytical performance of a laboratory by comparison with the results of other laboratories. In addition, these schemes can be a useful source of reference samples which can be put to good use internally by participating laboratories. The main objective in using an EQA program in laboratory andrology is to compare the results with other laboratories, thereby achieving a measurement as to how correct the results are (accuracy). There are different types of EQA, some giving approval only to laboratories achieving results within certain limits (proficiency testing), others mainly providing a measure for the participating laboratories as one tool in their own work for improved quality (educational schemes), and other schemes mainly giving the opportunity for participating laboratories to compare the results (peer comparison).

Analytical performance evaluation

The usual procedure is that sub-samples of a large sample are distributed to participating laboratories at regular intervals. Furthermore, sub-samples of certain large samples can be sent repeatedly without the participants knowing this [56]. When sub-samples have been analyzed by participating laboratories for one or more attributes the results are sent to the scheme organizer. Here the data are processed and reports of each round are returned to the participants. After a number of distributions, a more extensive report can be made since more data allow more and better statistical conclusions. Participating laboratories are supposed to analyze their results and, when significant or systematic deviations are noticed, they are supposed to take corrective action in the laboratory.

The design of each proficiency testing (PT) differs according to goals chosen, and schemes for the same seminal parameter can, under the management of different organizers, produce varying information on laboratory performance [57]. These variations depend, in particular, on the difference in methods used for the selection of control materials, statistical procedures (identification of assigned value), and the assessment of laboratory performance.

The use of human frozen semen in EQA poses several difficulties, and is therefore not recommended.

It is very important that a "target" value is assigned for each sample and each assessment type. There are two ways to obtain such values:

1. Value from expert laboratories: Average (and variation) of result from at least three expert laboratories. This method is used by the ESHRE EQA.

2. Average value from all participating laboratories: The mean or median (and variation by standard deviation, or central 50 percentiles, respectively) calculated from the results from all participating laboratories. When the "target" value is calculated on the basis of all results, it will be influenced by the results from the majority of the laboratories, irrespective of if they use the correct methods or not.

External QC/QA schemes

A number of external quality control and quality assurance schemes now exist around the world (see Table 10.2). However, the QA functionality of some schemes is higher than others and laboratories should investigate whether a particular scheme meets their needs before enrolling (and take out a trial subscription).

Table 10.2 Examples of external quality control/quality assurance (EQC/QA) schemes.

Country	Scheme name & website	Contact person
International	FertAid (Internet-based) www.fertaid.com	Dr. James Stanger office@fertaid.com
Europe	ESHRE Special Interest Group in Andrology www.eshre.com	Dr. Lars Björndahl Lars.Bjorndahl@ki.se
UK	UKNEQAS www.ukneqas.org.uk	Mrs. K Cumming andrology@ukneqas.org.uk
Spain	Programa Español de Control de Calidad Externo de Análisis de Semen (Banco de semen CEIFER) www.ceifer.com/indexCalidad.htm	Dr. Jose Antonio Castilla info@ceifer.com
Netherlands	Stichting Kwaliteitsbewaking Medische Laboratoriumdiagnostiek www.skml.nl	Dr. Frans van der Horst horstf@rdgg.nl or office@skml.nl
Germany	The German External Quality Control Program for Semen Analysis (QuaDeGA)	Barbara Hellenkemper (MTA) barbara.hellenkemper@ukmuenster.de
Denmark	DEKS www.deks.dk	Inger Plum inger.plum@deks.dk
Finland	Labquality www.labquality.fi	Minna Loikkanen Tel. +358 9 8566 8237
Belgium	National External Quality Assessment Scheme www.iph.fgov.be/ClinBiol/bckb33/activities/external_quality/_nl/sperma.htm	Jean-Claude Libeer Institute of Public Health jean-claude.libeer@iph.fgov.be
USA	Fertility Solutions www.fertilitysolutions.com	Dr. Susan Rothman srothmann@fertilitysolutions.com
Mexico	Programa Mexicano de Control de Calidad Externo de Análisis de Semen www.ceifer.com/html/es/mexico.htm	Dr. Gerardo Cerezo semenanalysis@yahoo.com.mx

Regulatory aspects

Overview

Increasingly, there are clear regulatory guidelines for semen analysis, sperm preparation for assisted conception treatment, and for sperm banking. It is essential that laboratory personnel are aware of both the national and international regulatory/legislative environment they operate within. While each country has (or is likely to have) its own particular system, e.g. CLIA in the USA, NATA in Australia, CPA and HFEA in the UK (see below), there are also international systems of regulation. For example, the EU Tissues and Cells Directive (2004/23/EC), which came into operation in 2007, sets standards of quality and safety for the donation, procurement, testing, processing, preservation, storage and distribution of human tissue and cells. While this directive does not cover basic semen assessment, any processing of the specimen (e.g. sperm preparation for IUI) is subject to the regulations under the directive. As such, any laboratory performing IUI within the European Union (EU) (and in the European Economic Area [EEA], which includes Iceland, Liechtenstein, and Norway) will need to be licensed under this directive. IVF clinics and cryobanks storing either patient or donor spermatozoa also require a license.

ISO standards

The ISO Standard 15189:2007 is the recently revised version of the earlier standard ISO 15189:2003 that was based on the more general ISO 17025 that specifies requirements for quality and competence in testing laboratories [4,53]. ISO 15189:2007 is more specific for medical laboratories and assists them in developing their quality management systems and processes for assessing their competence. The overall aim of the standards is to define a management system for quality assurance, including working systems for internal and external audits of all aspects of the laboratory and its administration. ISO 15189 also helps accreditation bodies in confirming or recognizing the competence of medical laboratories.

Regulatory environments

The requirement for accreditation or licensing of laboratories varies widely between countries and some examples are given below. Good Laboratory Practice (GLP) refers to a system of management controls for laboratories to ensure the consistency and reliability of results; various regulatory and non-government bodies have GLP guidelines, rules or regulations. There are great similarities in the expectations of all these schemes, notably in their focus on quality management principles. Consequently, the principles espoused in ISO 15189 can be considered as fundamental for good andrology laboratory management.

European Union (and EEA)

The EU Tissues and Cells Directive (2004/23/EC) is a wide-ranging and comprehensive document covering all handling of human cells and tissues for therapeutic use in humans. In addition to the parent directive there are two technical directives (Directives 2006/17/EC and 2006/86/EC) which detail the implementation of the primary directive. Together, these directives cover a wide range of topics, from administrative organization and quality management to traceability of sample origin and all components, materials, and equipment that come into contact with the tissues and cells during their procurement, processing, storage and distribution. The implementation of these directives has been debated in many different forums [58,59] and ESHRE has presented a position paper on the directives [60].

The EU member states were supposed to have implemented the directives via national legislation by 1 July 2008. A few countries (e.g. the UK) have been very progressive in implementing the directive, and the UK's Human Fertilisation and Embryology Authority (HFEA, www.hfea.gov.uk) has performed a detailed review, provided a comprehensive document on "Standards for Assisted Conception" and provided a series of updates for licensed ART centers. The national authorities responsible for the accreditation of tissue establishments covering gametes and zygotes in accordance with the EU directives are given support for their audit work by the EU organization EUSTITE (www.eustite.org).

Australia

The National Association of Testing Authorities (NATA) accredits all testing facilities including medical laboratories. NATA has assessed all laboratories according to ISO 17025 since January 2000, and medical laboratories according to ISO 15189 since 2004. Any laboratory performing diagnostic testing (e.g. andrology or endocrine) must be NATA accredited to operate. Although IVF labs are not required to have NATA accreditation, an increasing number are seeking it, recognizing that their "sperm tests" are, in fact, diagnostic tests and must therefore be performed in accordance with proper standards for such tests.

USA

The Clinical Laboratory Improvement Amendments (CLIA) of 1988 established three levels of laboratory testing: "waived," moderate complexity, and high complexity, with tests being classified according to the risk of harm to patients, the likelihood of erroneous results and the simplicity of testing. Almost any test that involves microscopic assessment is rated as high complexity, and only laboratories that meet the regulatory requirements of CLIA 88 can perform moderate or high complexity tests. These laboratories must undergo registration and periodic on-site inspections, and meet a range of other requirements, including: (a) having a QA program; (b) specific personnel standards; (c) participation in an approved proficiency testing program; and (d) ensuring that the testing equipment and assays are reliable, including having specified QC measures [61]. A number of organizations have received federal authorization to implement the inspection, licensing, and accreditation of andrology laboratories, including the Joint Commission on Accreditation of Healthcare Organizations (JCAHO), the College of American Pathologists (CAP), the Commission on Laboratory Accreditation (COLA), the American Association of Tissue Banks (AATB), and various state regulatory agencies.

References

1. Tomlinson MJ, Barrat CL. Internal and external quality control in the andrology laboratory. In: Keel BA, May JV, De Jonge CJ, eds. *Handbook of the Assisted Reproduction Laboratory*. Boca Raton: CRC Press 2000: 269–77.

2. Centola GM. Quality control, quality assurance, and management of the cryopreservation laboratory. In: Keel BA, May JV, De Jonge CJ, eds. *Handbook of the Assisted Reproduction Laboratory*. Boca Raton: CRC Press 2000: 303–25.

3. Deming, WE. *Out of the Crisis*. Cambridge, MA: MIT Press 1986.

4. Mortimer D, Mortimer ST. *Quality and Risk Management in the IVF Laboratory*.

Cambridge: Cambridge University Press 2005.

5. McCulloh DH. Quality control and quality assurance. *Obstet Gynecol Clin N Am* 1998; **9**: 285–309.

6. Huysman W, Horvath AR, Burnett D, *et al.* Accreditation of medical laboratories in the European Union. *Clin Chem Lab Med* 2007; **45**: 268–75.

7. Burnett D. *A Practical Guide to Accreditation in Laboratory Medicine*. London: ABC Venture Publications 2002.

8. Castilla JA, Hernandez J, Cabello Y, *et al.* Defining poor and optimum performance in an IVF programme. *Hum Reprod* 2008; **23**: 85–90.

9. Riddell D, Pacey A, Whittington K. Lack of compliance by UK andrology laboratories with World Health Organization recommendations for sperm morphology assessment. *Hum Reprod* 2005; **12**: 3441–5.

10. Björndahl L, Barratt CLR, Fraser LR, *et al.* ESHRE basic semen analysis courses 1995–1999: immediate beneficial effects of standardized training. *Hum Reprod* 2002; **17**: 1299–305.

11. Mourad SM, Hermens RP, Nelen WL, *et al.* Guideline-based development of quality indicators for subfertility care. *Hum Reprod* 2007; **22**: 2665–72.

12. Wollersheim H, Hermens R, Hulscher M, *et al.* Clinical indicators: development and applications. *Neth J Med* 2007; **65**: 15–22.

13. Keck C, Fischer R, Baukloh V, *et al.* Staff management in the in vitro fertilization laboratory. *Fertil Steril* 2005; **84**: 1786–8.

14. Aguilar J, Alvarez C, Morancho-Zaragoza J, *et al.* Quality specifications for seminal parameters based on clinicians' opinions. *Scand J Clin Lab Invest* 2008; **68**: 68–76.

15. Toft G, Rignell-Hydbom A, Tyrkiel E, *et al.* Quality control workshops in standardization of sperm concentration and motility assessment in multicentre studies. *Int J Androl* 2005; **28**: 144–9.

16. Auger J, Eustache F, Ducot B, *et al.* Intra- and inter-individuality variability in human sperm concentration, motility and vitality assessment during a workshop involving ten laboratories. *Hum Reprod* 2000; **15**: 2360–8.

17. Björndahl L, Tomlinson M, Barratt CLR. Raising standards in semen analysis:

Professional and personal responsibility. *J Androl* 2004; **25**: 862–3.

18. Viera AJ, Garrett JM. Understanding interobserver agreement: The kappa statistic. *Fam Med* 2005; **37**: 360–3.

19. Petersen PH, Stöckl D, Blaabjerg O, *et al.* Graphical interpretation of analytical data from comparison of a field method with reference method by use of difference plots. *Clin Chem* 1997; **43**: 2039–46.

20. Mortimer D. Technician training and quality control aspects. In: *Practical Laboratory Andrology*. Oxford: Oxford University Press 1994: 337–347.

21. Menkveld R, Stander FSH, Kotze TJvW, Kruger TF, Van Zyl JA. The evaluation of morphological characteristics of human spermatozoa according to stricter criteria. *Hum Reprod* 1990; **5**: 586–92.

22. Kruger TF, Acosta AA, Simmons KF, Swanson RJ, Matta JF, Oehninger S. Predictive value of abnormal sperm morphology in in vitro fertilization. *Fertil Steril* 1988; **49**: 112–7.

23. Franken DR, Menkveld R, Kruger TF, Sekadde-Kigondu C, Lombard C. Monitoring technologist reading skills in a sperm morphology quality control program. *Fertil Steril* 2003; **79**: 1637–43.

24. Alvarez C, Castilla JA, Martinez L, *et al.* Biological variation of seminal parameters in healthy subjects. *Hum Reprod* 2003; **18**: 2082–8.

25. Johnson JE, Blackhurt DW, Boone WR. Can Westgard Quality Control Rules determine the suitability of frozen sperm pellets as a control material for computer assisted semen analyzers? *J Assist Reprod Genet* 2003; **20**: 38–45.

26. Clements S, Cooke ID, Barratt CL. Implementing comprehensive quality control in the andrology laboratory. *Hum Reprod* 1995; **10**: 2096–106.

27. Lu JC, Xu HR, Chen F, *et al.* Standardization and quality control for the determination of alpha-glucosidase in seminal plasma. *Arch Androl* 2006; **52**: 447–53.

28. Fearn T, Thompson M. A new test for 'sufficient homogeneity'. *Analyst* 2001; **126**: 1414–7.

29. ISO. ISO 13528. *Statistical Methods for Use in Proficiency Testing by Interlaboratory Comparisons*. Geneva, Switzerland:

International Standardization Organization 2005.

30. Fraser CG, Harris EK. Generation and application of data on biological variation in clinical chemistry. *Crit Rev Clin Lab Sci* 1989; **27**: 409–37.

31. Fraser CG, Kallner A, Kenny D, Petersen PH. Introduction: strategies to set global quality specifications in laboratory medicine. *Scand J Clin Lab Invest* 1999; **59**: 477–8.

32. Ricos C, Alvarez V, Cava F, *et al.* Current databases on biological variation: pros, cons and progress. *Scand J Clin Lab Invest* 1999; **59**: 491–500.

33. Castilla JA, Morancho-Zaragoza J, Aguilar J, *et al.* Quality specifications for seminal parameters based on the state of the art. *Hum Reprod* 2005; **20**: 2573–8

34. Westgard JO. Use and interpretation of common statistical tests in method comparison studies. *Clin Chem* 2008; **54**: 612.

35. Cooper TG, Atkinson AD, Nieschlag E. Experience with external quality control in spermatology. *Hum Reprod* 1999; **14**: 765–9.

36. World Health Organization. *WHO Laboratory Manual for the Examination of Human Semen and Sperm-Cervical Mucus Interaction.* 4th edn. Cambridge, UK: Cambridge University Press 1999.

37. Bland JM, Altman DG. Statistical methods for assessing agreement between two methods of clinical measurement. *Lancet* 1986; **i**: 307–10.

38. McCulloh DH. *Quality Control and Quality Assurance. Record Keeping and Impact on ART Performance and Clinical Outcome.* In: May JV, Diamond MP, De Cherney AH, eds. Infertility and Reproductive Medicine: Clinics of North America 1998: 285–309.

39. Castilla JA, Sanchez-Leon M, Garrido A, *et al.* Procedure control and acceptance sampling plans for donor sperm banks: a theoretical study. *Cell Tissue Bank* 2007; **8**(4): 257–65.

40. Alvarez C, Castilla JA, Ramirez JP, *et al.* External quality control program for semen analysis: Spanish experience. *J Assist Reprod Genet* 2005; **22**: 379–87.

41. Strike PW. *Statistical Methods in Laboratory Medicine.* Oxford: Butterworth Heinemann 1991.

42. Jequier AM, Ukombe EB. Errors inherent in the performance of a routine semen analysis. *Br J Urol* 1983; **55**: 434–6.

43. Neuwinger J, Behre HM, Nieschlag E. External quality control in the andrology laboratory: an experimental multicenter trail. *Fertil Steril* 1990; **54**: 308–14.

44. Matson PL. External quality assessment for semen analysis and sperm antibody detection: results of a pilot scheme. *Hum Reprod* 1995; **10**: 620–5.

45. Keel BA, Quinn P, Schmidt CF Jr., *et al.* Results of the American Association of Bioanalysts national proficiency testing program in andrology. *Hum Reprod* 2000; **15**: 680–6.

46. Eliasson R. Standards for investigation of human semen. *Andrologie* 1971; **3**: 49–64.

47. Eliasson R. Analysis of semen. In: Burger H, de Kretser D, eds. *The Testis.* New York: Raven Press 1981: 381–99.

48. Mortimer, D. Laboratory standards in routine clinical andrology. *Reprod Med Rev* 1994; **3**: 97–111.

49. Belsey MA, Eliasson R, Gallegos AJ, et al. *Laboratory Manual for the Examination of Human Semen and Semen-Cervical Mucus Interaction.* Singapore: Press Concern 1980.

50. World Health Organization. *WHO Laboratory Manual for the Examination of Human Semen and Semen-Cervical Mucus Interaction.* 2nd edn. Cambridge: Cambridge University Press 1987.

51. World Health Organization. *WHO Laboratory Manual for the Examination of Human Semen and Sperm-Cervical Mucus Interaction.* 3rd edn. Cambridge: Cambridge University Press 1992.

52. Yeung CH, Cooper TG, Nieschlag E. A technique for standardization and quality control of subjective sperm motility assessments in semen analysis. *Fertil Steril* 1997; **67**: 1156–8.

53. International Standard ISO 15189. *Medical laboratories – Particular Requirements for Quality and Competence.* Geneva: International Organization for Standardization 2007.

54. ISO. *Guide to the Expression of Uncertainty in Measurement.* Geneva: International Organization for Standardization 1993.

55. Cook RR. *Assessment of Uncertainties in Measurement for Calibration and Testing*

Laboratories. Sydney: National Association of Testing Authorities 1999.

56. Matson PL. External quality assessment for semen analysis and sperm antibody detection: Results of a pilot scheme. *Hum Reprod* 1995; **10**: 620–5.

57. Cooper TG, Björndahl L, Vreeburg J, *et al.* Semen analysis and external quality control schemes for semen analysis need global standardization. *Int J Androl* 2002; **25**: 306–11.

58. Mortimer D. A critical assessment of the impact of the European Union Tissues and Cells Directive (2004) on laboratory practices in assisted conception. *Reprod Biomed Online* 2005; **11**: 162–76.

59. Hartshorne GM. Challenges of the EU 'tissues and cells' directive. *Reprod Biomed Online* 2005; **11**: 404–7.

60. European Society of Human Reproduction and Embryology. ESHRE position paper on the EU Tissues and Cells Directive EC/2204/23, November 2007. http://www.eshre.com/emc.asp?pageId=685 (viewed 01/08/2008).

61. Carrell DT, Cartmill D. A brief review of current and proposed federal government regulation of assisted reproduction laboratories in the United States. *J Androl* 2006; **23**: 611–7.

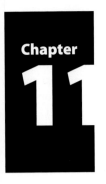

Risk management

Overview

Risk management is a rapidly growing area of concern in modern medicine, with primary areas of focus being on reducing medical errors and enhancing patient and staff safety. Risk management was originally an engineering discipline dealing with the possibility that some future event might cause harm or "loss," leading to a generic description of "risk" as being any uncertainty about a future event that might threaten an organization's ability to accomplish its mission. Risk management, therefore, includes strategies and techniques for recognizing and confronting any such threat – ideally before it happens – and provides a disciplined environment for proactive decision-making for the purpose of assessing on a continuous basis what can go wrong, determining which risks need to be dealt with, and implementing strategies to deal with these risks [1,2,3,4].

1. "Proactive risk management" is concerned with "What can go wrong?" and "What will we do to prevent the harm from occurring?"

2. "Retrospective risk management" is concerned with "If something happens, how will we resolve it, put things right (and pay for it) and prevent it from recurring?"

In an effective risk management program, risks are continuously identified, analyzed and minimized, mitigated or eliminated, and problems are prevented before they occur. In layman's terms, there is a cultural shift from "fire-fighting" and "crisis management" to proactive decision-making and planning. Conversely, failing to pursue risk management means that catastrophic problems will occur without warning, and that there will likely be no ability to respond rapidly to such "surprises" – making recovery very difficult and/or costly, requiring resources having to be expended to correct problems that could have been avoided.

Risk management tools

There are two main tools used in risk management: a proactive tool called "failure modes and effects analysis" or FMEA, and a reactive tool called "root cause analysis" or RCA [1,5]. While FMEAs work towards the prevention of risk, RCAs are used to deal with actual adverse events and with troubleshooting. Both tools depend on systems and process analysis, whereby every step or component process in a system is identified (process mapping): each process must be reduced to its fundamental steps, with no lower-level derivative processes, so that the factors acting on every component process can be identified and analyzed.

Detailed descriptions of FMEA and RCA methodology are available elsewhere [1,5], but to be effective both require an enlightened, positive management philosophy and staff committed to quality and risk management. Obviously an RCA can only be effective if it is accepted throughout the organization that its goal is to aid improvement, and not to assign blame (in keeping with the principles of continuous improvement intrinsic to a "total quality management" or TQM philosophy). Moreover, it must be understood that most errors result from faulty systems rather than human error: poorly designed processes put people in situations where errors are more likely to occur [1,6,7,8].

Risk management and regulation

Laboratory accreditation and certification schemes (e.g. ISO 15189:2007 [9,10]) integrate risk management and quality management (especially quality assurance and quality improvement) into an overall operational system. However, laboratory licensing perforce relates to regulations, and typically focuses much more on a perceived need to control risk, most often within the broad-reaching context of "public safety." A good example of this, and an illustration of risk analysis and communication, can be seen in the extent to which extreme precautionary measures have been deemed necessary to avoid the theoretical transmission of variant Creutzfeldt–Jakob disease (vCJD) via sperm donors [11].

What can make an andrology lab "high risk?"

As in all areas of laboratory medicine, continual training and proficiency testing are imperative. But these tactics alone will neither ensure quality nor prevent potentially catastrophic errors. The following list covers the most likely areas where risk factors can be found in an andrology laboratory.

Inadequate physical resources

Laboratories that are forced to operate with the minimum physical facility or equipment resources will be at greater risk; there must be sufficient capacity in all critical equipment to deal with the busiest of times. All laboratory equipment must be included in a preventative maintenance program, and all "mission critical" equipment must be monitored on a continual basis, e.g. cryostorage tanks, incubators, CO_2 supply, liquid nitrogen supply. In addition, an out-of-hours alarm system that can call or page a list of contact persons capable of resolving the issue is essential. Real-time monitoring systems are also being installed in more andrology laboratories, especially those with cryobanks. Continuity of electrical power supply to critical equipment must be ensured (e.g. by an in-house generator), while items sensitive to power fluctuations need to be protected by an "uninterruptible power supply" (UPS).

Inappropriate methods, kits, reagents, devices or products

Use of inappropriate methods, e.g. ones with poor accuracy and/or precision, or which cannot provide results with the required uncertainty of measurement, will prevent a laboratory from providing proper service, and can lead to misdiagnosis. All kits and reagents must be "suitable for purpose," have been stored correctly and not have expired. Similarly, all devices or products used in therapeutic procedures (e.g. sperm preparation for IUI or sperm cryopreservation) must have been approved for medical use by the appropriate regulatory authorities, e.g. the Food and Drug Administration in the USA, CE-marking in Europe, etc., wherever possible; non-approved products, or veterinary products must not be used.

Inadequate human resources

Staffing levels must also reflect the maximum caseload [1,9,10], with some slack in the system so that staff are not constantly working at maximum capacity [1,12] and are able to be alert and not distracted by tiredness – and hence be able to perform all aspects of their jobs accurately and reliably, with the lowest possible risk of making mistakes. Any circumstances that contribute to over-tiredness or exhaustion represent serious risk factors. Even with effective training programs, a high staff turnover increases the number of people who are less sure of the laboratory's systems, standard operating procedures (SOPs) and usual practices. Laboratories with a higher proportion of relatively inexperienced staff are less equipped to recognize and deal with operational problems as they arise. Comprehensive, formal programs are essential for training all laboratory staff in new techniques and procedures, and for the orientation, and re-training as necessary, of staff coming from other laboratories. Finally, there is the issue of staff not accepting professional responsibility, e.g. when a member of a team does not take enough care to ensure that (s)he has performed – and completed – all assigned tasks. This can be either intentional or unintentional, but in all cases is unprofessional.

Inadequate systems

Laboratory standard operating procedures (SOPs) must include sufficient technical/procedural detail for anyone with basic competence to perform the procedure exactly as intended. Methodological variations are thereby excluded, and the incursion of factors that can adversely affect the process prevented. Proper specification of an SOP requires understanding not just how the process in question is regulated by biology, chemistry and physics (and hence engineering), but also how it might be impacted by extrinsic factors, the lab environment, or ergonomics. Incomplete or poorly written SOPs create opportunities for laboratory staff to make mistakes, and all staff must follow the laboratory's SOPs exactly. Any changes to documented SOPs must be authorized by the Laboratory Director: the introduction of variations, short-cuts or perceived "improvements" without authorization must be prevented. Every time that a specimen is labeled, or moved from one container to another, identity checks must be followed strictly and verified either by a competent witness or some validated process or technological solution [1,13]. Likewise, great care must be taken when completing all documentation to ensure that all records are complete and accurate. Repeated incidents of carelessness or lack of attention to detail (i.e. risk) must be followed-up and remedied; the use of a comprehensive, documented system of notifications and/or task lists to ensure that the laboratory staff know exactly what has to be done each day, will greatly decrease the risk of critical tasks being forgotten. Unless a comprehensive system of Incident Reports ("nonconformity reports" in ISO 9001:2008 parlance) for all adverse events is in place, enforced, and employed constructively, many mistakes will never be recognized or remedied [10]. In this context, an "adverse event" can be defined as any event that potentially or actually affects staff safety, patient safety or the provision of testing or treatment according to the patient's care plan or the expected outcome of their treatment [1].

Specimen provenance

Specimen provenance refers to establishing the origin of a specimen. This encompasses the following main areas:

Identification of the patient who produced a specimen

It is important to clearly identify the patient correctly. This might sound obvious, but it is necessary to be certain of the identity of the patient who provides a specimen. In cases where the patient does not speak the local language there could be particular difficulties. Identification using name, address and date of birth are commonly used. But in some circumstances, particularly if ART treatment is used, more robust methods of identification might be required, such as presenting a driver's license, passport, or other "government-issued" identification. In these cases laboratory personnel can be confident who produced the sample.

In all cases the patient should sign a laboratory form saying that they produced the sample, regardless of whether the specimen was collected on-site or off-site. Especially important is dealing with situations where the woman delivers to the laboratory a specimen produced at home. Here, the deliverer must be identified, and provide a statement of provenance as to the origin of the specimen, e.g. "I, Mrs. Angelina Smith, have today delivered to the Fertility Laboratory a semen specimen collected at home by my partner, Mr. Brad Smith." From a risk management perspective, even if the semen specimen were to have been produced by Mrs. Smith's "friend," she has stated that it was from Mr. Smith, so the laboratory would not be "at risk" for specimen misidentification, the fraud having been committed intentionally by Mrs. Smith.

Processing of a specimen and reporting of the results

We have stated in this handbook that two unique identifiers must be assigned to each specimen to assist in its correct identification as it is processed through the laboratory. During this process the individual identifiers are routinely checked when performing specific procedures, e.g. sperm morphology assessments. Additionally, when the final results are collated and the report forms prepared, a final check related to the specimen provenance should be made to verify that the result being prepared does relate to the particular man named on the report.

Witnessing

It has already been noted that every time a specimen is labeled, or moved from one container to another, identity checks must be followed strictly and verified either by a competent witness or some validated process or technological solution [1,13]. But whether "double witnessing" – which is merely one tool that can be used to address the problem – can eliminate all risk has been questioned [1,13]. It is the responsibility of each laboratory to undertake a formal risk assessment of their specimen provenance and identification processes to ensure that the risk of specimen misidentification or confusion is reduced to as low a level as possible (recognizing that risk elimination is rarely possible when a process depends on the people actually performing the process).

Cryobanking

The prevalence of adverse events related to staff and sample safety is unknown in a sperm bank, although a recent survey suggests that they are frequent [14]. Moreover, there is an obsession with analyzing the unknown or minuscule risk of cross-contamination between straws, instead of paying attention to other more common risks, such as staff safety or premature warming of specimens during handling (e.g. during audit) [14,15,16].

General measures

Restricted access to the cryobank itself should clearly stipulate that only authorized personnel will be granted entry; patients and donors must not be allowed entry into either the andrology laboratory or the cryobank. There should be a written security procedure and contingency plan for different risks, and registers to record personnel statements that they have read and understood these policies.

Staff safety

General training in the use of liquid nitrogen and in the use of pressurized nitrogen vessels is a key element in the prevention of risk in the cryobank. Personal protective equipment and suitable equipment for the job must be available. Oxygen monitoring systems must be installed (sensors must currently be replaced annually) and linked to an alarm or some other form of external warning system. There should be adequate low-level ventilation (forced air change) and the inside of the cryobank should be visible from outside the room (e.g. a glass door panel).

Liquid nitrogen transport

Avoid unnecessary liquid nitrogen transport. Provide easy access for the liquid nitrogen delivery vehicle. Stores should be located on the ground floor. Supply vessels should be checked regularly. There must be a written procedure for the safe handling of liquid nitrogen and a register to record personnel statements that they have read and understood the procedure. Nobody should accompany a vessel being transported in an elevator [17].

Mistaken identity

Witnessing has been proposed to verify all processes involving transfer of gametes, and is mandatory in some countries, e.g. the UK. However, the cost-effectiveness of this measure has not been evaluated. Straws must be identified individually. Automatic labeling systems for straws, or self-adhesive labels, should be used. Labels must be able to withstand immersion in liquid nitrogen. There must be a written procedure for dealing with straws with labels that are illegible or missing, and records of samples that are lost.

Dual storage

The storage of samples in geographically separate storage facilities or in the same bank but in different containers, and their potential security advantages, should be analyzed in a risk management process. If adequate risk management and security measures are in place then duplicate storage is not essential for a sperm bank [1].

Transmission of infection

While there is a risk of cross-contamination during storage in the same cryotank, this risk can be minimized significantly by using various strategies such as those described in Chapter 8 "Sperm cryopreservation." Briefly:

1. High security straws must be used as the packaging system following Good Laboratory Practice: the outside of the straw must not be allowed to come into contact with either the semen or the sides of the container (e.g. fill using a filling nozzle); disinfect the outside of each straw using hypochlorite solution, followed by rinsing with sterile water and drying

after sealing – and again before opening; and after thawing use a sterile (disposable?) device to cut the straw.

2. Use different types of containers according to the serological status of the patient.
3. Keep donor and patient spermatozoa in different vessels.
4. Use emergency tanks when necessary.

If these measures are followed, vapor phase or supercold containers, previous sample processing, quarantine containers for sperm donors, and high quality air in the sperm bank are not necessary [18,19].

Premature warming of cells
Freezing
A contingency plan for malfunction of the controlled-rate freezer during sperm cryopreservation (e.g. have a spare controlled-rate freezer) should be in place.

Monitoring system: For secure and effective long-term storage of spermatozoa it is recommended that a triple-layer alarm system for the storage tanks be employed. Any temperature increase of more than 10% above −196°C must trigger a series of progressive alarms.

- Local alarm (audible and visual) in the room where the containers are located and in a nearby room.

- Distant alarm (audible and visual). If, in a set period of time, the local alarm has not been attended to, an alarm will be activated in a distant room in the same building or complex which is manned by maintenance or security staff 24 hours per day. This alarm will not be effective unless clear and concise written instructions are left indicating which protocol should be followed.

- In the absence of either local or distant alarms being effective, or if there is no maintenance staff station, a dial-out system should be installed that will contact a series of pre-programmed telephone numbers. It is recommended that a contingency plan be developed and clearly displayed close to the repository, in particular, detailing the location of other tanks of similar dimensions and characteristics into which the samples may be transferred in the event of a breakdown or when the tank is being cleaned.

Packaging system
The packaging system should be related to the type of container. If straws are used then liquid nitrogen tanks are recommended. Straws have a higher warming rate than cryovials, and the risk of warming when handling specimens outside the cryogenic storage tank for brief periods is higher. Consequently, straws should remain submerged in liquid nitrogen to reduce the risk of premature warming, which is not possible in the vapor phase or supercold tanks.

Supply of liquid nitrogen
Failures can be due to dewar vacuum failure, automated auto-fill system failure, refrigerator over-fills, or failure of the supply company to deliver. Possible solutions include having

emergency tanks, establishing a reciprocal cover arrangement with a nearby center, or maintaining substantial spare capacity [14,15].

Interpretation and diagnosis

Interpretation of results from semen analysis involves more challenges than most other modern laboratory services. Besides the common analytical variability discussed in Chapter 10 there is also considerable variability between men and between semen samples from one man, variability that does not necessarily imply pathology or reduction of fertility potential. It has not been possible to establish any distinct limits ("cut-offs") between results from fertile and subfertile men – the overlap between populations is considerable, giving a large range of borderline results [20]. Therefore, the risk for an incorrect diagnosis is far from negligible if decisions for further investigations or treatment options are based only on a single semen characteristic. Better support for such decisions is of course achieved if several characteristics are evaluated together [21].

Furthermore, it is essential for clinicians to be aware of the level of uncertainty for each value reported by the andrology laboratory, so as to be able to determine if, for instance, the difference between two samples from one patient is more likely to depend on random variation or rather is due to physiological or pathological changes in the male reproductive organs. It is therefore important for the laboratory to provide not only guidelines in the form of reference ranges, but also guidance on the analytical variability ("error" or "uncertainty of measurement") related to each semen characteristic, and what it means when a reported result is close to a decision limit.

A correct diagnosis cannot usually be made based only on laboratory results. The clinical diagnosis, on which decisions for further investigations or treatment choices will be made, should be based on patient history, physical examination and laboratory investigations like semen analysis, as well as on other tests such as hormone analyses.

The risks with incorrect interpretation and diagnosis comprise medical, economic and ethical issues. Among the worst complications would be the possibility of an infertility investigation with sub-optimal results from semen analysis not being followed through with an appropriate clinical investigation, where an underlying severe, or even fatal if not treated, somatic disease would have been discovered in time for proper medical treatment [22]. Less serious from a medical point of view, but with severe ethical implications, are more chronic disorders with secondary negative influence on semen parameters, where failure of discovery due to lack of proper clinical investigation will result in delayed diagnosis and unnecessarily long suffering. Over-emphasizing "male factor" infertility in general will cause an exaggerated use of intracytoplasmic sperm injection (ICSI) that will usually mean increased costs for the patient or any other party paying for treatment. On the other hand, poor diagnostic work-up can also mean that a patient with reduced chances for success with ordinary IVF procedures has an increased risk of being given a sub-optimal treatment, also causing economic losses as well as raising ethical issues [23,24].

In the communication between the laboratory and the clinicians using its service, it is important that the laboratory does not over-interpret the laboratory findings by making assumptions about clinical diagnoses. However, remarks about possible underlying problems that could cause or contribute to discovering abnormalities *should* be communicated to the clinician responsible for consideration together with other information that is usually not available to the laboratory.

References

1. Mortimer D, Mortimer ST. *Quality and Risk Management in the IVF Laboratory.* Cambridge: Cambridge University Press 2005.

2. Kennedy CR. Risk management in assisted reproduction. *Clin Risk* 2004; **10**: 169–75.

3. Kennedy CR, Mortimer D. Risk management in IVF. *Best Pract Res Clin Obstet Gynaecol* 2007; **21**: 691–712.

4. Mortimer D. Setting up risk management systems in IVF laboratories. *Clin Risk* 2004; **10**: 128–37.

5. Hutchison D. *Total Quality Management in the Clinical Laboratory.* Milwaukee: ASQC Quality Press 1994.

6. Reason JT. Foreword. In: Bogner MS, ed. *Human Error in Medicine.* Hillsdale: Lawrence Erlbaum Associates Inc. 1994.

7. Bogner MS, ed. *Human Error in Medicine.* Hillsdale: Lawrence Erlbaum Associates Inc. 1994.

8. Leape LL. A systems analysis approach to medical error. *J Eval Clin Pract* 1997; **3**: 213–22.

9. International Standard ISO 15189. *Medical Laboratories – Particular Requirements for Quality and Competence.* Geneva: International Organization for Standardization 2007.

10. Burnett D. *A Practical Guide to Accreditation in Laboratory Medicine.* London: ACB Venture Publications 2002.

11. Mortimer D, Barratt CLR. Is there a real risk of transmitting variant Creutzfeldt–Jakob Disease (vCJD) by donor sperm insemination? *Reprod Biomed Online* 2006; **13**: 778–90.

12. DeMarco T Slack. *Getting Past Burnout, Busywork, and the Myth of Total Efficiency.* New York: Broadway Books 2001.

13. Brison DR, Hooper M, Critchlow JD, et al. Reducing risk in the IVF laboratory: implementation of a double-witnessing system. *Clin Risk* 2004; **10**: 176–80.

14. Tomlinson M, Morroll D. Risks associated with cryopreservation: a survey of assisted conception units in the UK and Ireland. *Hum Fertil* 2008; **11**: 33–42.

15. Tomlinson M. Managing risk associated with cryopreservation. *Hum Reprod* 2005; **20**: 1751–6.

16. Clarke G. Sperm cryopreservation: is there a significant risk of cross-contamination? *Hum Reprod* 1999; **14**: 2941–3.

17. Air Liquide – DMC. *Cryogenic Material: Safety in Cryogenics.* Bussy-Saint-Georges: Air Liquide – DMC 2008. www.dmc. airliquide.com/en/precautions/precaution. htm (viewed 05/12/2008).

18. Mortimer D. A critical assessment of the impact of the European Union Tissues and Cells Directive (2004) on laboratory practices in assisted conception. *Reprod Biomed Online* 2005; **11**: 162–76.

19. Mortimer D. Current and future concepts and practices in human sperm cryobanking. *Reprod Biomed Online* 2004; **9**: 134–51.

20. Nallella KP, Sharma RK, Aziz N, Agarwal A. Significance of sperm characteristics in the evaluation of male infertility. *Fertil Steril* 2006; **85**: 629–34.

21. Jedrzejczak P, Taszarek-Hauke G, Hauke J, Pawelczyk L, Duleba AJ. Prediction of spontaneous conception based on semen parameters. *Int J Androl* 2008; **31**: 499–507.

22. Jequier AM. The importance of diagnosis in the clinical management of infertility in the male. *Reprod Biomed Online* 2006; **13**: 331–5.

23. Mortimer, D. Structured management as a basis for cost-effective infertility care. In: Gagnon C, ed. *The Male Gamete: From Basic Knowledge to Clinical Applications.* Vienna, IL: Cache River Press 1999: 363–370.

24. Mortimer, D. The future of male infertility and ART. *Hum Reprod* 2000; **16** Suppl 5: 98–110.

12 Reproductive toxicology

Introduction

Several compounds (environmental, therapeutical and occupational) have been shown to act as male reproductive toxicants [1,2]. Assessment of human male reproductive toxicity represents a great challenge compared to studies with animal models. Data from laboratory animal studies may not be of relevance to human health risk assessment, due to differences between species regarding dose–response relationship, metabolism of the compound and mechanism of action, as well as the high doses of toxicants often used in experimental models.

Reproductive toxicology studies in humans are mostly population-based, or use a case-control design. Several retrospective studies have indicated a decline in semen quality, and there is a growing concern for male reproductive health worldwide. This has motivated several multicenter studies including comparison of semen parameters at different centers. Standardization of methods and external quality control are essential for meaningful comparison of data collected at different centers.

Semen analysis studies

Standardization of methods

Standardization of semen analysis to improve the reliability of the results is not only important for infertility investigation, but also when assessing male reproductive toxicity, on both the individual and population levels. Standardized protocols, training of the technicians and internal quality control are essential. For multicenter studies, examination of which type of equipment (e.g. counting chambers) or methods (e.g. assessment of motility) give the best results should be evaluated as part of the external quality control [3]. Measurement of semen volume should be done by the same method, preferentially by weighing [4], and the same type of counting chamber should be used when assessing the sperm concentration [5,6]. It should be noted that in capillary-loaded chambers the sample is not uniformly distributed, introducing a significant error that varies according to semen viscosity [7,8].

For individual assessment of reproductive toxicology, or when there are few participants in a study, two samples should be collected for each observation point. In population toxicology studies, however, only one sample from each individual can be sufficient [9]. Regardless, an appropriate power analysis should be undertaken to quantify the number of individuals necessary to detect differences if they exist. When evaluating changes in sperm concentration, in a population or between populations, abstinence time is an important consideration. Although a specific time is recommended, there will be variations which can influence the results. This must be included in the model when performing the statistical analyses. Furthermore, the study populations should be comparable regarding age, ethnicity, and medical history. In exposure studies, the interval between the sampling should be carefully considered. For detecting toxicologic effects on spermatogenesis the "follow-up" sample should be collected after at least one completed spermatogenic cycle (approximately 10–12 weeks).

Training of technicians

Studies have revealed large variation between laboratories, even when the same standardized protocols are used [10,11,12], and meaningful comparisons depend on strict quality control [3]. In a pilot study, inter- and intra-technician coefficients of variation should be calculated for each technique. Furthermore, the mean percent difference from a chosen standard value should be calculated. Actions to correct errors should be performed when necessary [3]. If possible, technicians from each center should come together and perform the various assessments side-by-side in order to minimize differences in method performance. Detailed discussion of robust semen analysis methods can be found in Chapter 3.

Sperm chromatin integrity tests

Chemical toxicants can induce DNA damage affecting fertility and pregnancy outcome. The harmful effect on the spermatozoa will not necessarily be detected by a standard semen analysis, therefore reproductive toxicology testing should include measurements of sperm DNA damage. Several DNA fragmentation tests have been developed during the last 20 years, and information obtained from these tests can be overlapping, but also supplementary. Especially for human semen, it is recommended that several tests are performed in order to measure different types of chromosome damage. However, there are challenges related to standardization of the techniques, and some of them are also expensive to perform. The methods listed below involve detection of fluorescence labeling by flow cytometry or microscopy (for detailed discussion of the methods, see [13,14]; see also Chapter 5).

Sperm chromatin structure assay (SCSA)

By this method the amount of single-stranded DNA is measured after denaturation of the sperm DNA [15], and spermatozoa are classified as abnormal when the amount of single-stranded DNA exceeds a certain limit. Flow cytometry of acridine orange-stained spermatozoa measures the relative amount of single-stranded DNA (red) compared to double-stranded (green), and the percentage of abnormal spermatozoa in the sample can be calculated. Reproducibility requires that the analysis is performed under identical conditions, and centralized equipment and performance of testing can reduce the variability of the method.

Enzymatic tests for DNA damage (TUNEL and NT)

In the terminal deoxynucleotidyl transferase (TUNEL) and in situ-nick translation (ISNT) assays, single-stranded or double-stranded DNA breaks are detected by the addition of fluorescently labeled nucleotides which bind to the DNA at the breaks [13]. The cells are scored by either fluorescence microscopy or flow cytometry.

Single cell electrophoresis (Comet) assay

This method is based on the electrophoresis of single cells and identification of a "tail" of damaged DNA detected using a fluorescent dye. The length of DNA migration and the percentage of DNA in the tail reflect the amount of single-stranded and double-stranded DNA breaks [13].

Sperm chromatin dispersion test (SCD)

The SCD test also involves electrophoresis and identification of DNA damage by fluorescence microscopy. It is based on the principle that fragmented DNA fails to produce a halo of dispersed DNA loops that can be observed in spermatozoa with non-fragmented DNA following acid denaturation and removal of nuclear proteins [16].

References

1. Phillips KP, Tanphaichitr N. Human exposure to endocrine disrupters and semen quality. *J Toxicol Environ Health B Crit Rev* 2008; **11**: 188–220.

2. Kumar S. Occupational exposure associated with reproductive dysfunction. *J Occup Health* 2004; **46**: 19.

3. Brazil C, Shanna SH, Tollner CR, *et al.* Study for Future Families Research Group. Quality control of laboratory methods for semen evaluation in a multicenter research study. *J Androl* 2004; **25**: 645–56.

4. Cooper TG, Brazil C, Swan SH, Overstreet JW. Ejaculate volume is seriously underestimated when semen is pipetted or decanted into cylinders from the collection vessel. *J Androl* 2007; **28**: 1–4.

5. Brazil C, Swan SH, Drobnis EZ, *et al.* Study for Future Families Research Group. Standardized methods for semen evaluation in a multicenter research study. *J Androl* 2004; **25**: 635–44.

6. Haugen TB. In search of an accurate and rapid method for sperm counting. *Scand J Clin Lab Invest* 2007; **67**: 436–8.

7. Tomlinson M, Turner J, Powell G, Sakkas D. One-step disposable chambers for sperm concentration and motility assessment: how do they compare with the World Health Organization's recommended methods? *Hum Reprod* 2001; **16**: 121–4.

8. Douglas-Hamilton DH, Smith NG, Kuster CE, *et al.* Capillary-loaded particle fluid dynamics: effect on estimation of sperm concentration. *J Androl* 2005; **26**: 115–22.

9. Stokes-Riner A, Thurston SW, Brazil C, *et al.* One semen sample or 2? Insights from a study of fertile men. *J Androl* 2007; **28**: 38–43.

10. Jørgensen N, Auger J, Giwercman A, *et al.* Semen analysis performed by different laboratory teams: an intervariation study. *Int J Androl* 1997; **20**: 201–8.

11. Auger J, Eustache F, Ducot B, *et al.* Intra- and inter-individual variability in human sperm concentration, motility and vitality assessment during a workshop involving ten laboratories. *Hum Reprod* 2000; **15**: 2360–8.

12. Björndahl L, Barratt CL, Fraser LR, *et al.* ESHRE basic semen analysis courses 1995–1999: immediate beneficial effects of standardized training. *Hum Reprod* 2002; **17**: 1299–305.

13. Perreault SD, Aitken RJ, Baker HW, *et al.* Integrating new tests of sperm genetic integrity into semen analysis: breakout group discussion. *Adv Exp Med Biol* 2003; **518**: 253–68.

14. Chohan KR, Griffin JT, Lafromboise M, *et al.* Comparison of chromatin assays for DNA fragmentation evaluation in human sperm. *J Androl* 2006; **27**: 53–9.

15. Evenson DP, Wixon R. Environmental toxicants cause sperm DNA fragmentation as detected by the Sperm Chromatin Structure Assay (SCSA®). *Toxicol Appl Pharmacol* 2005; **207**: 532–7.

16. Fernández JL, Muriel L, Rivero MT, *et al.* The sperm chromatin dispersion test: a simple method for the determination of sperm DNA fragmentation. *J Androl* 2003; **24**: 59–66.

Appendix 1: Reference values

Introduction

While most readers might expect a simple table of values in this Appendix, to do so would only promulgate many current misconceptions and misunderstandings about such "normal ranges" or "reference values." Since the goal of this handbook has been to improve the standardization and quality of semen assessments and other andrology lab procedures, improving the understanding and clinical application of the results from semen analysis and other sperm assessments must be a corollary. However, there are a number of major issues that must be borne in mind when developing, or using, reference values:

1. There is a big difference between a "normal range" and a "reference value" in laboratory medicine, and this has been discussed at length elsewhere [1]. However, in brief, using reference values is an important step toward establishing a scientific basis for clinical interpretation of laboratory results, and eliminates the confusion arising from three very different meanings of the word "normal" relating to the Gaussian statistical distribution, "normal" vs. "abnormal" in the epidemiological sense, and the clinical sense, where normal equates to healthy or non-pathological. Understanding, and applying, these concepts is of great importance to andrology because there is no specific disease "infertility"; subfertility is a problem of a *couple* where either – or neither – partner might be "normal" (i.e. unaffected by relevant disease). Moreover, fertility is age-related and also affected by many environmental factors. Consequently, a normal population cannot be either readily defined or studied, but "reference values" can be defined that relate more to the likelihood that a given characteristic is a contributory factor in determining an endpoint of interest.

2. There are fundamental differences in the endpoints of interest, for which semen analyses and other sperm assessments are made. Clearly there is a great difference between attempting to diagnose the etiology of a couple's infertility and attempting to provide a prognosis for any given outcome. But there are also great differences between outcomes such as spontaneous pregnancy without treatment (which must also be considered in regard to the time required to achieve such pregnancies, perhaps integrated as an expression of the fecundity rate) and the likelihood of a successful outcome of a particular treatment modality (which, again, needs to include a consideration of time). There are, of course, also substantial differences between treatments, which bypass different levels of the normal process of conception *in vivo* – and hence compensate for different underlying abnormalities in the man's (and/or woman's) physiology, e.g. timed intercourse, cervical insemination, IUI, IVF or ICSI.

3. A reference value derived for a particular purpose or in a particular way, e.g. based on the risk of poor or no fertilization at IVF ("in-vitro subfertility"), cannot be used to diagnose in-vivo subfertility (i.e. whether a couple will achieve a pregnancy without treatment, or with some systemic therapy) – or vice versa. Moreover, the high intra- and inter-individual variability of semen characteristics can result in a man providing a semen sample that shows one or more characteristics that are very unusual for him, but the

values are well within the reference value(s) for the population [2,3]. As a result, semen analysis reference values are unsuitable for following longitudinal monitoring and detecting whether change has occurred in an individual.

4. Any reference value will be dependent upon the technical method by which it was determined, and this also includes the presumption of proper training and adequate internal and external quality control. If a value is derived according to a specific protocol then it cannot be used with the same confidence – or perhaps even the same relevance – when derived by another technique. An obvious example of this is the now generally accepted change to using "strict criteria" for evaluating human sperm morphology [4,5,6,7], necessitating entirely different reference values to those used for assessments made using other sperm morphology classification schemes (e.g. [8,9]). Further examples of this problem are given in the following section of this Appendix.

5. Semen analysis characteristics are also affected, to varying degrees, by the duration of prior ejaculatory abstinence (and also ejaculatory frequency), as well as post-ejaculatory specimen holding conditions and pre-analysis delay (e.g. [10]).

6. When considering endpoints of interest, there will be further confounding factors related to the clinical management of the couple (e.g. the use of ovarian stimulation, handling of follicular aspirates during oocyte retrieval, and handling of embryos during embryo transfer). Similarly, we must recognize that aspects of laboratory quality will affect the likelihood of achieving success: not just the sperm handling and processing technique, but also the handling of oocytes and embryos during IVF and ICSI, and the general physico-chemical quality of the culture environment for achieving fertilization *in vitro* and for supporting embryo development through to transfer.

7. Reference values should be based on data obtained from well-defined populations, and derived using statistical techniques. Consequently, they are subject to a certain degree of uncertainty, and not therefore necessarily as robust when applied to individual cases. They are *not* "cut-offs" and there are no absolute values that allow the definition of binary states, e.g. "normal" vs. "abnormal" or "fertile" vs. "subfertile"; while this has been known for many years, far too many workers still seem to believe in such false interpretations. Even what might seem an "absolute" cut-off of azoospermia cannot necessarily be used in the modern day to define a man as "sterile": many men who presented with azoospermia have become fathers following surgical sperm retrieval from their testes and ICSI.

8. Issues of ethnicity and geography should also be taken into account. Several studies have revealed ethnic differences concerning the so-called testicular dysgenesis syndrome (a.k.a. the "falling sperm counts" theory). Furthermore, geographical differences in various semen parameters have also been reported between countries or regions that are comparable with respect to ethnicity (e.g. the Nordic countries). But since there are as yet no indications of differences in fertility between these regions/countries, it might be wrong to use common reference ranges. Finally, genetic variations between different ethnic groups could also be of relevance to at least some of the semen parameters.

Almost all expert publications on semen analysis have recommended that each laboratory should derive its own reference values (e.g. [11,12,13]) – yet this has very rarely ever occurred. But even using a population of men who have recently become fathers to define "normal ranges" for semen analysis remains fraught with confounding factors:

1. Was the age range of the female partners controlled? This is a significant factor affecting a couple's fecundity.

2. How many cycles of trying did it take for the couple to achieve a pregnancy?

3. Were either or both partners affected by external factors, e.g. tobacco smoking, recreational drug use, environmental or workplace reproductive toxins?

4. Is the man actually the biological father? Without paternity testing this cannot be assumed – and there is a generally accepted non-trivial prevalence of non-paternity in many western societies at least.

5. Was any treatment employed but not admitted to? With the growth in "reproductive tourism" in recent years, especially with the increasing scarcity of gamete donors in many countries, more and more couples go overseas for treatment and then conceal that fact from at least the regulatory authorities, if not family and friends as well.

Probably the most insightful approach for simple guidelines for interpreting semen analysis results was that promoted by Eliasson in the late 1970s, in which semen analysis evaluation guidelines were provided using *three* categories: normal, doubtful and pathological or not normal, derived from frequency distribution studies on populations of men whose wives were pregnant in the first trimester and men with a barren union [8,9]. Equivalent values can also be derived from the analysis of the clinical fertility of men attending a fertility clinic after a 20-year follow-up period [14]. This three-category approach was adopted and promoted by Mortimer [15,16] but not by the WHO [11,12,13]. As a final comment in this regard, it must be biologically obvious that no single semen characteristic can be expected to confirm a man's diagnosis of subfertility, nor adequately classify a couple's fertility potential. Indeed, Guzick et al. concluded that while threshold values for sperm concentration, motility, and morphology can be used to classify men as subfertile, of indeterminate fertility, or fertile (see Figure A1.1), none of the measures were diagnostic of infertility [17]. Table A1.1 provides an example of this approach, derived by consensus and updated for the use of "strict criteria" sperm morphology assessments. It is well-known that, on a population basis, the quantitative aspects (i.e. sperm concentration and total sperm count) and qualitative aspects of sperm production (i.e. sperm morphology, motility and vitality) are positively inter-correlated [18].

From the above discussion it is evident that a simple table of reference values, no matter how well defined the source population, how rigorous the lab methodology and staff training and QC, or how much statistical analysis or manipulation the data were subjected to, cannot be expected to provide answers for more than one endpoint of interest. Consequently, in the following paragraphs, the applicability of the various reference values, and guidelines for their interpretation, will be provided when available.

Semen characteristic	Fertility status	
	Subfertile - - - Indeterminate fertility - - - Fertile	
Sperm concentration (10⁶/ml)	13.5	48.0
% motile spermatozoa	32	63
% morphologically normal	9	12

Source: Guzick et al. NEJM 2001; 345: 1388-93.

Figure A1.1 Figure illustrating the threshold values defined by Guzick et al. (2001).

Table A1.1 General (consensus-based) guidelines for the evaluation of human semen, in relation to a general classification of in-vivo fertility potential only (may be considered comparable to a diagnosis of subfertility). Values are provided relative to the usual precision of reporting, and assume that semen analysis is carried out as per the technical methods, training, and QC standards described in this handbook only (given this, all values should be considered to have an uncertainty of measurement of 10%).

Characteristic	Units	Normal	Borderline	Pathological	Notes
Volume	ml	2.0–6.0	1.5–1.9	<1.5	a
Sperm concentration	10^6/ml	20–250	10–20	<10	a,b
Total sperm count	10^6/ejaculate	≥80	20–79	<20	a,b
Motility	% motile	≥60	40–59	<40	c,d
	% progressive	≥50	35–49	<35	c,d
	% rapid	≥25			c,d,e
	progression grade	3 or 4	2	1 or 0	c,d,f
Morphology	% typical forms	≥14	4–13	<4	g
	TZI	≤1.60	1.61–1.80	>1.80	g,h
Vitality	% live (vital)	≥60	40–59	<40	i
Leukocytes	10^6/ml			>1.0	j
Antisperm antibodies	% binding	<50	50–79	≥80	k

a) Evaluated after 2–4 days of abstinence.
b) For specimens with 2.0–6.0-ml volume.
c) Evaluated at 30 min post-ejaculation.
d) Evaluated at 37°C.
e) Cut-off for rapid is 25 µm/s "space gain"; only a normal threshold value is available.
f) Based on a scale of 0–4: 0 = no progression; 1 = poor; 2 = medium; 3 = good; 4 = very good/excellent.
g) Evaluated using Tygerberg "strict criteria."
h) Evaluated as per refs [12,16] from Papanicolaou-stained smears.
i) Evaluated by eosin dye exclusion at 30 min post-ejaculation.
j) Evaluated by cytochemical staining for peroxidase; only a pathological threshold value is available.
k) Evaluated using the Immunobead or MAR test methods for IgG and/or IgA.

Semen analysis values

Note: For all semen characteristics it is assumed that robust technical methods, careful operator training, and both internal QC and external QC/QA, as described in this handbook, have been implemented.

Ejaculate volume

Prerequisites

A known period of prior ejaculatory abstinence; reference range assumes 2–4 days.

In-vivo significance

Only if the volume is very low is there a risk of the acidic vaginal milieu adversely affecting the spermatozoa. A high volume (>6.0 ml) can also be regarded as an abnormal value, due to likely loss of semen from the vagina. However, no specific risks amenable to routine diagnostic or therapeutic application have been quantified and validated.

In-vitro significance

No specific relevance.

Sperm concentration

Prerequisites

Assumes 3 ± 1 days prior ejaculatory abstinence, and a complete collection.

Cautionary note

On a population basis, sperm quality (i.e. motility and progression, vitality and morphology) are positively correlated with sperm concentration; but higher sperm "quality" (i.e. functional potential) can mitigate the impact of a simple decrease in sperm concentration.

In-vivo significance

In general, fecundity is decreased with values below 20×10^6 spermatozoa per ml, but only below 5×10^6 per ml will the man's fecundity likely be substantially reduced [14,19]. However, no specific risks amenable to routine diagnostic or therapeutic application have been quantified and validated.

Notes:
1. Only valid where the entire ejaculate has been collected for analysis (the first fraction contains most of the spermatozoa).
2. In cases of hypothalamic hypogonadism undergoing hormonal initiation of spermatogenesis these reference values are invalid, conception can occur with as few as 0.5×10^6 spermatozoa per ml.
3. One out of 2000 vasectomized men have been reported to father children in spite of a laboratory finding of no spermatozoa, i.e. azoospermia [20].

In-vitro significance

No generally applicable thresholds beyond whether sufficient spermatozoa can be obtained post-processing for a potential treatment modality.

Total sperm count

Prerequisites

Only valid for complete ejaculates with normal volumes (i.e. 2.0–6.0 ml) collected after 3 ± 1 days prior ejaculatory abstinence.

Cautionary note

On a population basis, sperm quality (i.e. motility and progression, vitality and morphology) are positively correlated with the total sperm count; lesser impairment of sperm quality will reduce the impact of lower total sperm count.

In-vivo significance

Decreasing fecundity with values below 80×10^6 per ejaculate, and fecundity will likely be substantially reduced below 20×10^6 per ejaculate. However, no specific risks amenable to routine diagnostic or therapeutic application have been quantified and validated.

Notes:
1. Only valid where the entire ejaculate has been collected for analysis (the first fraction contains most of the spermatozoa).
2. In cases of hypothalamic hypogonadism undergoing hormonal initiation of spermatogenesis these reference values are invalid, conception can occur with as few as 0.5×10^6 spermatozoa per ml.
3. One out of 2000 vasectomized men have been reported to father children in spite of a laboratory finding of no spermatozoa, i.e. azoospermia [20].
4. The total sperm count can also be useful when deciding on an ART treatment regimen, since it indicates the total number of potentially functional spermatozoa that might be available.

In-vitro significance

No generally applicable thresholds beyond whether sufficient spermatozoa can be obtained post-processing for a potential treatment modality.

Sperm motility

Since sperm function requires progressive motility, simple assessments of the proportion of motile spermatozoa regardless of progression should be expected to have less biological, and hence, clinical relevance. For this reason they are not recommended for routine clinical use within the context of either diagnosis or prognostic management.

Sperm progressive motility

Prerequisites

Must be evaluated soon after completion of semen liquefaction, and assessments must be made at 37°C for physiological relevance.

Cautionary note

On a population basis, progressive motility is positively correlated with other aspects of sperm quality (i.e. concentration, vitality and morphology). Isolated reductions of sperm motility might have less impact upon fertility or fecundity than when seen in conjunction with other evidence of decreased sperm quality. Simple "bulk" assessment of progression grade (see Table A1.1) has limited value compared to the determination of the proportions of spermatozoa showing grades of progression.

In-vivo significance

At least 50% of the spermatozoa are expected to show progressive motility (WHO grades $a + b$); decreasing values below this will be associated with an increasing likelihood of sperm dysfunction, and hence reduced fecundity. However, no specific risks amenable to routine diagnostic or therapeutic application have been quantified and validated.

In-vitro significance

Poor progressive motility, seen as a reduced proportion of progressively motile spermatozoa and/or reduced quality of progression (i.e. sperm velocity and other kinematic characteristics), is likely to be associated with other impairments of sperm function and hence there will be increased risks of poor or no fertilization at IVF – and hence a likely greater benefit of using ICSI. However, no specific risks amenable to routine diagnostic or therapeutic application have been quantified and validated.

Sperm rapid progressive motility

Prerequisites

Must be evaluated soon after completion of semen liquefaction, and assessments must be made at 37°C using an objective definition for "rapid" (i.e. space gain of ≥25 μm/s) for optimum physiological relevance.

Cautionary note

On a population basis, progressive motility is positively correlated with other aspects of sperm quality (i.e. concentration, vitality and morphology), and is essential for effective penetration into and migration through the cervical mucus *in vivo*. An isolated reduction in the proportion of rapid progressive spermatozoa might have less impact upon fertility or fecundity than when seen in conjunction with other evidence of decreased sperm quality.

In-vivo significance

A reduced proportion of rapid progressive spermatozoa will decrease the potential of an ejaculate being able to achieve effective colonization of the cervical mucus and establish the sperm reservoir within the female reproductive tract [21,22,23]. However, no specific risks amenable to routine diagnostic or therapeutic application have been quantified and validated.

In-vitro significance

Poor penetration of cervical mucus (assessed either *in vivo* or *in vitro*), which is often due to impaired sperm motility, has been associated with an increased risk of impaired fertilization at IVF [24,25]. However, no specific risks amenable to routine diagnostic or therapeutic application have been quantified and validated.

Sperm progression grading

Since this is a population-averaged subjective assessment its routine use is no longer considered appropriate in a specialized andrology laboratory. However, various clinicians believe that it is useful to them, and some laboratories will need to continue providing these evaluations to the maximum practicable level of objectivity and standardization.

Sperm vitality

Prerequisites

Must be evaluated soon after completion of semen liquefaction. Typically only assessed when there are <40–50% motile spermatozoa.

Cautionary note

On a population basis, vitality is positively correlated with other aspects of sperm quality (i.e. concentration, motility and progression and morphology); hence isolated reductions of sperm motility might have less impact upon fertility or fecundity than when seen in conjunction with other evidence of decreased sperm quality. Sperm vitality typically exceeds the proportion of motile spermatozoa by at least a small margin, representing those spermatozoa that are "live" but not motile.

In-vivo significance

Sperm vitality assessments can clarify cases of "necrozoospermia" (e.g. due to the presence of spermotoxic antibodies), and help differentiate such cases from ones of immotile cilia syndrome (where motility is essentially zero but many spermatozoa are live). However, no specific risks amenable to routine diagnostic or therapeutic application have been quantified and validated, and the routine assessment of sperm vitality on all semen samples is not recommended.

In-vitro significance

No specific relevance beyond that for in-vivo endpoints.

Sperm morphology: typical forms

Prerequisites

Should be evaluated soon after completion of semen liquefaction. Properly prepared and appropriately stained smears are essential, as are proper training using the defined Tygerberg strict criteria and both IQC and EQC/EQA (see Chapters 3 and 10 of this handbook for further information).

Cautionary note

While sperm morphology is positively correlated with other aspects of sperm quality (i.e. concentration, motility and progression, and vitality) on a population basis, isolated reductions of sperm morphology can impact fertility or fecundity even when seen in conjunction with evidence of apparently normal sperm quality. Of further importance is the situation where there is an apparent disagreement between "normal" morphology and the teratozoospermia index (TZI: see below), and therefore it is strongly recommended that these results should always be interpreted in conjunction with an assessment of the TZI.

In-vivo significance

A proportion of morphologically typical or ideal spermatozoa of at least 14% indicates that sperm morphology is less likely to be a contributory factor to a couple's subfertility, or an adverse factor influencing prognosis.

In-vitro significance

A proportion of morphologically typical or ideal spermatozoa of at least 14% indicates that sperm morphology is less likely to be a contributory factor to poor or no fertilization at IVF; with values between 13% and 4% there is an increasing risk of poor or no fertilization at IVF, and ICSI might be a cautious approach; and with <4% many experts recommend the use of ICSI. However, these interpretations should be made in conjunction with the sperm morphology patterns present (small heads, large heads, etc.), and with an assessment of the TZI, since many abnormal spermatozoa show multiple anomalies, reflecting a greater disturbance of spermiogenesis and/or abnormalities arising during maturation and storage in the epididymis.

Sperm morphology: teratozoospermia index (TZI)

Prerequisites

Properly prepared and appropriately stained (Papanicolaou) smears are essential.

Cautionary note

The TZI provides an additional dimension of information on the production of competent spermatozoa via the process of spermiogenesis [7,26,27]. An elevated TZI indicates an increased risk of abnormal spermiogenesis, and the concomitant existence of sperm dysfunction, even though spermatozoa appear superficially normal at the level of observation used in the sperm morphology evaluation.

In-vivo significance

A TZI of >1.80 indicates that sperm morphology is more likely to be a contributory factor to a couple's subfertility or a man's fertility potential; with values ≤1.60 there is considered to be no increased risk over what can be identified from the proportion of ideal forms.

In-vitro significance

A TZI of >1.80 indicates that sperm morphology is likely to be a contributory factor to poor or no fertilization at IVF and that ICSI should be employed. With values of 1.60–1.80 there is an increased risk of poor or no fertilization at IVF and ICSI might be a cautious approach. With a TZI <1.60 there is considered to be no increased risk over what can be identified from the proportion of ideal forms.

Computer-aided sperm analysis (CASA)

The conclusions and recommendations of the consensus workshop organized by the ESHRE Special Interest Group in Andrology, San Miniato 1997, must be fully considered in any clinical (or research) application of computer-aided sperm analysis (CASA) of human spermatozoa [28]. Further discussion of these issues can be found in Appendix 4 of this handbook. Key points to be noted are:

1. Determination of sperm concentration in semen using CASA is subject to a wide range of error factors, and values must be considered suspect unless a special staining technique, validated against determinations made using the methods described in this handbook, has been used.

2. Determination of the percentages of motile and progressively motile spermatozoa in semen using CASA is subject to a wide range of error factors, and values must be considered suspect unless the technique has been validated against determinations made using the methods described in this handbook.

3. Population-averaged kinematic values are of limited value. Median and range or centile values will be statistically more meaningful than mean values, but multiparametric kinematic definitions (allowing the classification of individual spermatozoa into specific sub-populations that are correlated with relevant functional endpoints, e.g. "good mucus penetrating" spermatozoa) will have greater biological, and hence clinical, relevance.

4. Differences between CASA instruments, in both hardware and software, can preclude using reference values derived using one type of instrument to interpret values obtained using a different type of instrument.

5. There are no population-based studies using the current generation of CASA systems, to define either:

   a. the limits of normal semen quality in fertile men;

   b. the relationships between CASA variables and the time to pregnancy; or

   c. the relationships between CASA variables (especially hyperactivation) and IVF outcome.

Antisperm antibodies

In general, controversy continues regarding the prevalence and clinical significance of antisperm antibodies (ASABs) in the diagnosis of subfertility and its treatment; their evaluation remains an integral part of the basic semen analysis according to WHO, and guidelines for the use of this information in managing the subfertile couple have been established by the WHO (see below) [13,27,29,30].

Circulating ASABs, especially when they coat the majority of spermatozoa, are directed against the sperm head, and are of both IgG and IgA isotypes simultaneously (IgA alone has a worse prognosis than IgG alone), are a definite risk factor for impaired sperm transport *in vivo* and fertilization. Serum ASABs should also be considered a contraindication for both IUI and GIFT, and obviously preclude using affected serum as a supplement for IVF culture medium. ASABs identified in cervical mucus, either by abnormal sperm–mucus interaction tests or by their detection in solubilized cervical mucus, often cause a failure of sperm transport – although this can be amenable to treatment by IUI.

- Tail-tip IBT/MAR only   Not clinically relevant
- <50% IBT/MAR head/midpiece/tail   Not clinically important
- 50–80% IBT/MAR midpiece/tail   Try IUI, or perhaps go straight to IVF
- 50–80% IBT/MAR head   IVF (increase motile sperm numbers to compensate)
- >80% IBT/MAR midpiece/tail   Try IVF, or perhaps go straight to ICSI
- >80% IBT/MAR head   ICSI

The detection of IgM ASABs is definitely pathological, and can indicate either recent trauma to the male tract or perhaps testicular cancer. Any man in whom such ASABs are detected should be referred to a clinical andrologist for a thorough investigation.

In biological terms it must be remembered that ASABs can have three different biological effects: sperm agglutination, cytotoxicity, or just coating the spermatozoa. While the presence of agglutinating antibodies is usually apparent from examination of a wet preparation during semen analysis, and cytotoxic ASABs will result in severely diminished, or even zero sperm vitality, there is no indication of sperm-coating antibodies within a semen analysis. However, sperm-coating antibodies will reduce, or even block, sperm penetration of cervical mucus, and can be readily identified using in-vitro tests of sperm–mucus interaction, especially "shaking" as seen in the SCMC test (see Chapter 6 of this handbook).

Seminal plasma biochemistry

Zinc
Prerequisites
A completely collected semen sample.

Cautionary note
For clinical interpretation it is essential that the complete ejaculate was collected; low semen volume, few motile spermatozoa and low zinc can be caused by incomplete sample collection. If an incomplete sample is provided for analysis, provide information to the patient about the importance of reporting any missed part of the ejaculate before allowing collection of a repeat sample.

In-vivo significance
Low zinc content can be due to reduced secretory function of the prostate, either because of an ongoing prostatitis or as a concomitant of chronic or iterated inflammatory disease of the prostate. A low contribution of prostatic secretion in the sperm-rich ejaculate fractions reduces sperm motility, survival and chromatin stability.

In-vitro significance
A normal zinc content indicates that prostatic fluid was contributed to the ejaculate.

Fructose
Prerequisites
A completely collected semen sample.

Cautionary note
The main source of fructose in semen is from the seminal vesicles. The seminal vesicular fluid typically constitutes the last 2/3 of the ejaculate volume, explaining why incomplete collection of the later fractions of the ejaculate can give false too low values. Because live spermatozoa kept in seminal plasma for an extended period of time will metabolize fructose, seminal plasma for fructose determination should be centrifuged free from spermatozoa within 60 minutes after ejaculation.

In-vivo significance
Absence of spermatozoa and low fructose levels indicate possible agenesis of the Wolffian duct system, including the vasa deferentia and seminal vesicles.

In-vitro significance
A normal fructose content indicates that seminal vesicular fluid was contributed to the ejaculate.

α-Glucosidase

Prerequisites

A completely collected semen sample.

Cautionary note

Glucosidase is considered mainly a secretory product of the epididymal epithelium, although significant contributions also come from the prostate.

In-vivo significance

Low glucosidase activity in semen primarily indicates a low contribution of epididymal secretion to the ejaculate. This can be due to a partial blockage (in which case spermatozoa can also be lacking in the ejaculate) or due to reduced function of the epididymal epithelium (where sperm function, especially motility, and the reduction of cytoplasmic residues, could be impaired).

In-vitro significance

A normal α-glucosidase content indicates that epididymal fluid was contributed to the ejaculate.

Sperm function tests

Reactive oxygen species measurement

There are no defined reference values available. However, using the assay method described in this handbook, values of $>0.2 \times 10^6$ cpm per 20 million spermatozoa can be considered abnormal (see Chapter 5 of this handbook).

In-vivo sperm–mucus interaction testing – the post-coital test (PCT)

Prerequisites

Appropriate timing of the procedure during the immediate pre-ovulatory period.

Cautionary note

A cervical mucus Insler Score of <10, and/or pH <7.0 can cause a poor PCT. Reading a PCT after a long post-coital delay can show increased numbers of non-progressive spermatozoa (as distinct from shaking spermatozoa), downgrading the test result.

In-vivo significance

A satisfactory result can be reported when there are either >2500 progressively motile spermatozoa per mm^3 in the cervical mucus, or >1000 rapid progressive spermatozoa per mm^3.

A result of <500 spermatozoa per mm^3, especially when associated with slow progressive or non-progressive motility, indicates decreased sperm penetration ability of the mucus, and/or abnormality of the cervical mucus.

Note: Interpretation of the clinical significance of a PCT must be the responsibility of the physician requesting the test. A negative PCT is not always a true negative clinical finding.

In-vitro significance

None established from population-based evidence.

In-vitro sperm–mucus interaction tests (SMITs)
Prerequisites

Appropriate timing of the mucus collection during the immediate pre-ovulatory period and the collection of a complete semen sample after 3 ± 1 days prior ejaculatory abstinence.

Cautionary note

A cervical mucus Insler score of <10, and/or pH <7.0 can affect sperm–cervical mucus interaction and lead to a poor test result.

In-vivo significance

See Chapter 6 of this handbook for the specific interpretation criteria for the Kurzrok–Miller slide test, the Kremer capillary tube sperm penetration test, and the sperm–cervical mucus contact (SCMC) test, as well as the value of crossed-hostility format testing.

> Note: Interpretation of the clinical significance of any test of sperm–cervical mucus interaction must be the responsibility of the physician requesting the test.

In-vitro significance

None established from population-based evidence.

Tests of sperm fertilizing ability

There are no evidence-based, population-derived reference values for any in-vitro test of human sperm fertilizing ability. See the report from the consensus workshop organized by the ESHRE Special Interest Group in Andrology, Hamburg 1995, and Chapter 5 in this handbook for further information [31].

Sperm DNA tests

Sperm chromatin structure assay (SCSA®)

The SCSA provides a measure of the stainability of double- and single-stranded DNA in the sperm chromatin by acridine orange following acidic pH-induced denaturation *in vitro*, which has been interpreted as a measure of the susceptibility of the sperm chromatin to fragmentation, the "DNA fragmentation index" (DFI), as well as an indication of the proportion of spermatozoa that show nuclear immaturity, the "high DNA stainable" (HDS) fraction. It is the only test of sperm DNA/chromatin for which validated clinical interpretation criteria exist, and these are based on many thousands of tests and hundreds of clinical treatment cycles (although the complete nature of the accessibility and stainability of the sperm DNA has not been fully clarified). While there is some controversy in the field regarding the use and interpretation of the SCSA, rational understanding by some workers seems to be confounded by unreasonable expectations (e.g. that the SCSA can predict fertility – no single sperm test can do this, see above), by inappropriate use of the test (e.g. that it is a first-line screening test for all infertile couples), by the uncertainty derived

273

from a number of factors that directly impinge on the predictive value of DNA fragmentation tests [32], including confusing different endpoints, iatrogenic induction of DNA damage due to inappropriate semen processing for ART, the DNA repair ability of the oocyte or whether the type of sperm DNA damage is repairable or not [33], not taking proper account of the female partner's fertility status, and uncritical consideration of some clinical trials.

Because published DFI and HDS results were defined using the SCSA's highly specific testing protocol and objective analysis of the raw flow cytometer data (SCSAsoft®, SCSA Diagnostics Inc.), the results from modified or "improved" assays can only be considered equivalent to DFI or HDS if a directly equivalent test protocol and data analysis algorithms were employed. Unless these basic scientific criteria are met then the established and validated clinical interpretation criteria for the SCSA cannot be used with such assays, and independent results and clinical interpretation criteria must be established.

In-vivo significance

While results of >30% DFI do not preclude a natural full-term successful pregnancy, they are associated with a significant reduction in the prevalence of term pregnancies (up to a 7.5-fold difference), and increase in the time required to achieve a pregnancy, and an approximate doubling of miscarriages (due to damaged paternal genes). Also, if there are >15% HDS spermatozoa, a couple should expect a longer time to natural pregnancy.

When IUI treatment is considered, a DFI >25% has been associated with a substantial reduction in fecundity and fertility (at least an 8-fold difference) and the couple should be recommended to consider IVF or ICSI.

In-vitro significance

The relationship between DFI and HDS values and fertilization *in vitro*, and with subsequent embryonic development, remains unclear, although there does seem to be some association between elevated DFI and impaired sperm function. With >15% HDS spermatozoa there is a risk of a reduced fertilization rate with IVF, although ICSI might overcome this factor.

Other tests of sperm DNA or chromatin

No specific risks or interpretation criteria amenable to routine diagnostic or therapeutic application have been quantified and validated for any test of sperm DNA fragmentation or chromatin structure or stability other than the SCSA. Tests awaiting the development of such criteria include the TUNEL and Comet assays, as well as various tests for sperm chromatin condensation or dispersion (e.g. the "Halo Test"). As noted above, such assays do not give results that are the same as the SCSA's DFI result, and attempts to apply or adapt the threshold DFI values for use with any of these other tests are scientifically unjustifiable. Large-scale prospective clinical trials will be required to develop, and then validate, interpretation criteria for each of these tests separately.

References

1. Solberg HE. Establishment and use of reference values. In: Burtis C, Ashwood ER, Tietz NW, eds. *Tietz Textbook of Clinical Chemistry*. 3rd edn. Philadelphia: WB Saunders Co. 1999: 336–56.

2. Heuchel V, Schwartz D, Czyglik F. Between and within subject correlations and variances for certain semen characteristics in fertile men. *Andrologia* 1983; **15**: 171–6.

3. Álvarez C, Castilla JA, Martínez L, Ramírez JP, Vergara F, Gaforio JJ. Biological variation in seminal parameters in healthy subjects. *Hum Reprod* 2003; 18: 2082–8.

4. Menkveld R. The influence of environment factors on spermatogenesis and semen parameters. PhD. dissertation (Afrikaans), Faculty of Medicine, University of Stellenbosch, South Africa, August 1987.

5. Menkveld R, Stander FSH, Kotze TJvW, et al. The evaluation of morphological characteristics of human spermatozoa according to stricter criteria. *Hum Reprod* 1990; 5: 586–92.

6. van Zyl JA, Kotze TJvW, Menkveld R. Predictive value of spermatozoa morphology in natural fertilization. In: Acosta AA, Swanson RJ, Ackerman, SB, Kruger TF, van Zyl JA, Menkveld R, eds. *Human Spermatozoa in Assisted Reproduction.* Baltimore: Williams & Wilkins 1990: 319–24.

7. Mortimer D, Menkveld R. Sperm morphology assessment – historical perspectives and current opinions. *J Androl* 2001; 22: 192–205.

8. Eliasson R. Semen analysis and laboratory workup. In: Cockett ATK, Urry RL, eds. *Male Infertility. Workup, Treatment and Research.* New York: Grune & Stratton 1977: 169–88.

9. Eliasson R. Analysis of semen. In: Burger H, de Kretser D, eds. *The Testis.* New York: Raven Press 1981: 381–99.

10. Mortimer D, Templeton AA, Lenton EA, Coleman RA. The influence of abstinence and ejaculation-to-analysis delay upon semen analysis parameters of suspected infertile men. *Arch Androl* 1982; 8: 251–6.

11. World Health Organization. *WHO Laboratory Manual for the Examination of Human Semen and Semen-Cervical Mucus Interaction.* 2nd edn. Cambridge: Cambridge University Press 1987.

12. World Health Organization. *WHO Laboratory Manual for the Examination of Human Semen and Sperm-Cervical Mucus Interaction.* 3rd edn. Cambridge: Cambridge University Press 1992.

13. World Health Organization. *WHO Laboratory Manual for the Examination of Human Semen and Sperm-Cervical Mucus Interaction.* 4th edn. Cambridge: Cambridge University Press 1999.

14. Bostofte E, Serup J, Rebbe H. Interrelationships among the characteristics of human semen, and a new system for classification of male infertility. *Fertil Steril* 1984; 41: 95–102.

15. Mortimer D. The male factor in infertility. Part I: Semen analysis. *Curr Prob Obstet Gynecol Infertil* 1985; VIII(7): 87pp.

16. Mortimer D. *Practical Laboratory Andrology.* New York: Oxford University Press 1994.

17. Guzick DS, Overstreet JW, Factor-Litvak P, et al. Sperm morphology, motility, and concentration in fertile and infertile men. *NEJM* 2001; 345: 1388–93.

18. Mortimer D, Templeton A A, Lenton EA, Coleman RA. Semen analysis parameters and their interrelationships in suspected infertile men. *Arch Androl* 1982; 8: 165–71.

19. Jouannet P, Ducot B, Feneux D, Spira A. Male factors and the likelihood of pregnancy in infertile couples. I. Study of sperm characteristics. *Int J Androl* 1988; 11: 379–94.

20. Smith JC, Cranston D, O'Brien T, Guillebaud J, Hindmarsh J, Turner AG. Fatherhood without apparent spermatozoa after vasectomy. *Lancet* 1994; 344: 30.

21. Mortimer D, Pandya IJ, Sawers RS. Relationship between human sperm motility characteristics and sperm penetration into human cervical mucus in vitro. *J Reprod Fertil* 1986; 78: 93–102.

22. Aitken RJ, Warner PE, Reid C. Factors influencing the success of sperm-cervical mucus interaction in patients exhibiting unexplained infertility. *J Androl* 1986; 7: 3–10.

23. Mortimer ST. A critical review of the physiological importance and analysis of sperm movement in mammals. *Hum Reprod Update* 1997; 3: 403–39.

24. Barratt CLR, Osborn JC, Harrison PE, et al. The hypo-osmotic swelling test and the sperm mucus penetration test in determining fertilization of the human oocyte. *Hum Reprod* 1989; 4: 430–4.

25. Berberoglugil P, Englert Y, Van den Bergh M, Rodesch C, Bertrand E, Biramane J. Abnormal sperm-mucus penetration test predicts low in vitro fertilization ability of apparently normal semen. *Fertil Steril* 1993; 59: 1228–32.

26. Mortimer D. Sperm form and function: Beauty is in the eye of the beholder. In: Van der Horst G, Franken D, Bornman R, de Jager T, Dyer S, et al., eds. *Proceedings of the 9th International Symposium on Spermatology.* Bologna: Monduzzi Editore SpA. 2002: 257–62.

27. Rowe PJ, Comhaire FH, Hargreave TB, Mahmoud AMA, *et al. WHO Manual for the Standardized Investigation, Diagnosis and Management of the Infertile Male.* Cambridge: Cambridge University Press 2000.

28. ESHRE Andrology Special Interest Group. Guidelines on the application of CASA technology in the analysis of spermatozoa. *Hum Reprod* 1998; **13**: 142–5.

29. Hjort T. Antisperm antibodies. Antisperm antibodies and infertility: an unsolvable question? *Hum Reprod* 1999; **14**: 2423–6.

30. Chamley LW, Clarke GN. Antisperm antibodies and conception. *Semin Immunopathol* 2007; **29**: 169–84.

31. ESHRE Andrology Special Interest Group. Consensus workshop on advanced diagnostic andrology techniques. *Hum Reprod* 1996; **11**: 1463–79.

32. Evenson DP, Wixon R. Data analysis of two in vivo fertility studies using Sperm Chromatin Structure Assay – derived DNA fragmentation index vs. pregnancy outcome. *Fertil Steril* 2008; **90**: 1229–31.

33. Alvarez JG. The predictive value of sperm chromatin structure assay. *Hum Reprod* 2005; **20**: 2365–7.

Appendix 2: Equipment required for a basic andrology laboratory

The following equipment is required in order for an andrology laboratory to be capable of performing the basic procedures described in this handbook. Sufficient equipment must be available for the number of staff working in the laboratory and for the laboratory to function efficiently at maximum caseload. Backup equipment should also be available in order for the laboratory's services not to be compromised by equipment failure. Recommendations reflect one or more of the authors' preferences, but do not indicate that other manufacturers or models are not suitable (unless specifically stated).

The equipment has been listed in three general categories:

- Basic andrology laboratory
- Cryobanking equipment
- Equipment for specialized assays: e.g. CASA system, flow cytometer, fluorescence microscope, luminometer

See Appendix 3 for manufacturers' contact details.

Basic andrology laboratory

This section covers the equipment required by any andrology laboratory wishing to employ the methods described in this handbook and operate to proper levels of technical quality and quality control.

Equipment – microscope

A **microscope** with good quality phase contrast optics is fundamental to a serious andrology laboratory. General features of a microscope configured for andrology (see Figure A2.1) include:

- 10×, 20×, 40× objectives, all PL (positive low) phase contrast;
- 100× oil immersion objective (*not* phase contrast);
- wide-field eyepieces, minimum 10× (12.5× are recommended for sperm morphology assessments);
- extra eyepiece with built-in *grid reticle*;
- phase telescope (for proper alignment of the phase rings);
- intermediate magnification capability (vital for sperm motility assessments using video);
- trinocular head with camera oculars, as necessary, and *camera's adapter(s)*, e.g. C-mount for video camera;
- green (45G533: IF550), daylight and diffuser filters; and

- *heated stage*, ideally built into the microscope's own stage, not one that sits on top of the stage, as these stages will adversely affect proper illumination and phase contrast optics (e.g. the Minitüb system with HT-200 controller which also has a warm plate on top of the controller).

Notes:

1. Sufficient microscopes should be available for efficient working at maximum caseload.

2. A dedicated sperm morphology workstation microscope would not require either phase contrast optics or a heated stage.

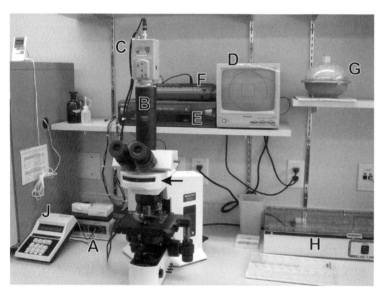

Figure A2.1 Illustration of a typical andrology workstation built around an Olympus BX51 microscope (fitted with intermediate magnification changer module; **arrow**) and attached video display and recording equipment for sperm motility assessments, training and quality control. **A** = Minitüb HT-200 heated stage controller unit; **B** = camera adapter with additional camera ocular; **C** = monochrome video camera; **D** = 9″ monochrome video monitor with acetate overlay showing 25-micron-equivalent ruled grid; **E** = VHS videocassette recorder; **F** = video titler device; **G** = Nalgene desiccator used as humid chamber for settling hemocytometers; **H** = large warming place with hinged clear acrylic cover; and **J** = electronic multichannel counter.

A videomicrography system is extremely useful for sperm motility assessments (see Figure A2.1). Ideally a monochrome system, but these are "surveillance"-type CCTV units and sometimes harder to source and may be more expensive than "low-end" color systems. A *digital video camera* (with C-mount, no lens) and *small monitor* are required as a minimum. The monitor should not be too large since it will be viewed close-up (a screen size of about 9″ or 23 cm is ideal); ideally, the total magnification on the video screen should be such that 70–90 mm on the screen represents 100 µm in the sample. To facilitate estimating sperm velocity an acetate sheet with a central circular field and a grid with squares corresponding to 25 × 25 µm under the microscope can be attached to the video monitor screen. Video recording is best performed using a *combination hard-drive/DVD recorder* so recordings can be saved to the hard drive and only burnt to disk when necessary or convenient (VHS videocassette recorders have been largely superseded by these devices); alternatively, the camera can be linked to a suitably equipped computer to record video clips. Ideally, a *video character generator or titler* should be connected between the camera and video recorder to allow identifying text to be added to the recordings.

> Note: Although video recording would not be necessary on a dedicated sperm morphology workstation microscope, still-image capture or photography capability is highly recommended.

General equipment

Other general requirement equipment items are listed alphabetically, below.

Balances

Top-load balance (maximum 100 g, readout to 0.1 g) for weighing semen specimens and their containers.

Analytical balance (maximum 100 g, readout to 0.1 mg) for weighing reagents.

Centrifuge with swing-out rotor and sealed buckets

Ideally this centrifuge should be programmable for ease of use. Adapters should be available for each type of tube to be centrifuged in the laboratory, including the Falcon 15-ml conical tubes for density gradients and the 50-ml Falcon "Blue Max" tubes for retrograde ejaculation urine specimens. There are many possible models from a wide variety of manufacturers, but the Eppendorf model 5804 performs extremely well and is very quiet with minimal vibration (very important if it has to be located on the same bench as the microscope). There should be sufficient centrifuges for efficient working at maximum caseload.

Counting chambers

Hemocytometers should be the Improved Neubauer pattern and in sufficient quantity for efficient operation of the laboratory. Remember to buy spare cover glasses.

Makler chambers for assessing washed sperm preparations. Again more than one should be available so that the chamber can be warmed back up to 37°C after washing before re-use (total number required will depend on maximum caseload). It is advisable to have at least one spare cover glass.

Dry bath or warming block

With drilled metal blocks for the particular type(s) of tubes to be used.

Freezer

For storing reagents and specimens frozen at –25 to –30°C. Can be a combined refrigerator–freezer having separate compartments.

Fume hood or fume adsorber

For working with fixatives, stains and solvents, in accordance with local safety and fire regulations.

Heated stirrer (combination hot plate and magnetic stirrer)

For making some reagent solutions and stains.

Hotplate

Capable of at least 55°C for running the fructose spot test.

Humid chamber

For allowing hemocytometers to "settle," e.g. a 15-cm diameter Nalgene desiccator (cat. no. 5315–0150) containing gauze swabs wetted using sterile water. One per workstation is recommended.

Incubators

Air incubator where semen samples can be left at 37°C to liquefy after delivery to the laboratory. A gravity convection-type model is adequate. If an orbital mixer can be placed inside the incubator then the specimens will mix as they liquefy, facilitating their analysis.

CO_2 incubator for sperm function tests. Most bicarbonate-based culture media that support sperm capacitation require 5.8–6.0% CO_2-in-air when used close to sea level (i.e. pCO_2 of 44 mmHg). If a CO_2 incubator is not available then tubes can be gassed with pre-mixed gas (containing the same amount of CO_2), capped tightly and mixed by inversion to equilibrate with the gas, and then placed in a 37°C incubator with an air atmosphere.

Miscellaneous minor items

Calculator for calculating test results (one per workstation).

Forceps of various types and sizes for handling slides and coverslips during fixing/staining/ mounting, small centrifuge tubes, processing surgical sperm retrieval tissue, and also for handling straws and cryovials when frozen (see Figure A2.2).

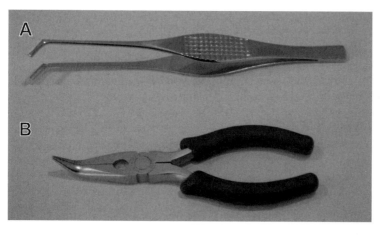

Figure A2.2 A: Straw-handling forceps (Rocket Medical, Watford, UK; cat.no. R30.722 for 0.5-ml straws, and R30.721 for 0.25-ml straws). B: Bent-nose radio pliers, ideal for attaching and removing cryovials to/ from canes while in cryogenic storage.

Glassware

Bottles for storing stains and other reagents.

Coplin jars for fixation and staining of slides.

Filter funnels for filtering the hemocytometry diluent and stains.

Measuring cylinders (ideally with stoppers) for preparing fixatives and staining solutions. Staining dishes and racks for sperm morphology staining (e.g. the preferred Papanicolaou method).

Iris scissors (stainless steel) for cutting cervical mucus specimens. Several pairs should be available so they can be washed thoroughly and decontaminated after use.

Marker pens for labeling tubes and slides, also special *cryogenic marker pens* for writing on straws.

Pencils for writing on frosted-end microscope slides; *not* to be used for completing laboratory forms or any other permanent record.

Pens for completing laboratory forms and other paperwork; must be indelible (i.e. not water-based gel pens).

Rubber bulbs for using glass Pasteur pipettes. For volumetric work, use either a 3-ml syringe with a short tubing connector or a suitable macro-pipetter device.

Safety glasses to protect operators whenever there is a risk of aerosol contamination (as distinct from protection while using liquid nitrogen).

Scissors, general purpose. Not to be used for opening straws as there is a high risk of cross-contamination; even with in-house "sterilization" (a process that would, of course, require regular validation).

Spatulas of various types and sizes (as per operator preference) for weighing chemicals to prepare diagnostic reagents and stains.

Spotting plates, porcelain for the fructose spot test; can also be used for mixing semen with eosin-nigrosin stain.

Stage micrometer for calibration of microscope fields and magnification.

Pipetters

Air-displacement pipetters for dispensing reagents and loading hemocytometers; several models to cover the range from 5–10 µl to 1000 µl, preferably fitted with tip ejectors (e.g. Gilson Pipetman P20, P200 and P1000 units).

Positive-displacement pipetter for taking accurate samples of semen. The Gilson M100 unit (1–100 µl) is recommended as it avoids cross-contamination between samples and its tips are available pre-assembled (unlike those for the M50 model).

Macro-pipetter to allow volumetric use of glass Pasteur pipettes, for example when preparing density gradients, e.g. the VWR Pipettor (VWR cat. no. 53499–605). Alternatively, use a 3-ml syringe with a short tubing connector.

Pipette controller for using volumetric pipettes. Ideally a motorized unit or else Pi-Pump manual units (the models with an integral release valve are not recommended due to their tendency to leak).

Note: A set of pipetters is recommended for each workstation.

Refrigerator

For storing culture media and other reagents at *ca.* +4°C. Can be a combined refrigerator–freezer with separate compartments.

Solvent storage cabinet

For safe storage of all flammable solvents and reagents in the laboratory, as per local safety and fire regulations.

Safety cabinets

Class II biosafety cabinet for working with potentially infectious semen samples, as per local regulations.

Vertical laminar flow cabinet as a "clean" workstation for handling density gradient preparations and processing spermatozoa for freezing (as per local regulations), and filter-sterilizing diagnostic reagents.

> Note: Sufficient cabinets should be available for efficient, safe working at maximum caseload.

Slide warmer

To keep slides, coverslips, Makler chambers, pipette tips, etc., warm. Should be a large model, ideally with hinged cover. One per workstation is recommended.

Tally counters

Single-channel hand tally counters for counting in hemocytometers.

Multi-channel counters, mechanical or electronic, for performing differential counts of sperm motility, vitality and morphology.

> Note: There should be one of each type of counter at each workstation.

Thermometers

For calibrating and checking (operational qualification) all temperature-controlled equipment, including daily use electronic thermocouple-type devices as well as a calibrated *reference thermometer* for in-house calibration/verification of the daily use thermometers.

> Note: Electronic thermometers are strongly recommended; spirit-filled thermometers are acceptable but easily broken. Thermometers containing mercury should not be used due to occupational safety concerns.

Vortex mixer

For mixing diluted hemocytometry specimens, *Accu-Beads*®, *Immunobeads*®, etc. One per workstation is recommended. Warning: Do *not* vortex live spermatozoa!

Waterbath

For heat-inactivating sera and seminal plasma samples for antisperm antibody testing. Also for thawing cryopreserved semen and spermatozoa.

Cryobanking equipment

Controlled-rate freezer

For cryopreserving semen and washed sperm preparations. Ideally it should have built-in programs that allow the specimens to be cooled to at least $-160°C$ before transferring them into storage. Numerous instruments are available from several manufacturers, e.g. *Freeze Control® CL8800* (CryoLogic, Victoria, Australia), *CTE 2104* (MTG Medical Technology, Altdorf, Germany), *Labotec Cryo Unit* (Labotec, Göttingen, Germany), *Kryo 360–1.7* and *Kryo 360–3.3* (Planer, Sunbury-on-Thames, UK), *Asymptote EF600* (Grant Instruments, Cambridgeshire, UK), and *Nicool MS21* (Air Liquide, Cryogenic Material, Marne La Vallée Cedex, France).

Cryogenic safety gear

At *each location* where cryogenic materials will be handled, as per local safety regulations. Should include **gauntlets** (not "gardening" gloves), a **full-face visor** and **apron** specifically designed for use with cryogenic materials wherever liquid nitrogen is being handled, and at least gauntlets and safety glasses (but ideally a full-face visor) at other locations where only cryogenic specimens are being handled.

Cryogenic storage dewars

Vessels for the cryogenic storage of biological specimens in liquid nitrogen. These are available from a number of manufacturers, e.g. Air Liquide, MVE, Taylor-Wharton. Where they will be moved around within the laboratory or cryobank they must be on **roller bases**. Also, it is highly recommended (and is required in an increasing number of jurisdictions) that each tank used for storing specimens be fitted with at least a low-level alarm sensor, and ideally a combined temperature and level sensor; these are available from a variety of manufacturers including many of those that manufacture the storage vessels, as well as others including Gordinier Electronics, Labotect, LEC, and MidAtlantic Diagnostics.

> Note: While some authorities recommend storage of specimens in the vapor phase, or in supercold air, this is inherently more risky due to the existence of frequent opportunities for storage temperatures to rise above the transition point of water (i.e. above $-132°C$) as other specimens are being transferred into/out of storage. Given the biocontainment that is inherent in the use of **High Security Straws** (CryoBioSystem, Paris, France), the use of storage other than immersed in liquid nitrogen is not recommended.

Dry shipper

For transport of cryopreserved samples (e.g. Air Liquide's *Voyageur*, or Taylor-Wharton's *X*).

Label printer

For secure labeling of straws, e.g. the various models manufactured by Brady that are sold by many distributors, e.g. TLS 2200 and LabXpert models.

Liquid nitrogen supply vessel(s)

These dewars are required for the supply of liquid nitrogen to the laboratory for use with the controlled-rate freezers and for refilling storage and shipper tanks (note that tanks containing patient specimens must never leave the control of laboratory or cryobank personnel, and must never be filled directly by the delivery person). The size(s) and number of supply vessels needed will depend on each laboratory's particular requirements, but the following principles must be considered:

- Liquid supply tanks must be on **roller bases** and, ideally, **tipper stands** so that liquid can be poured from the tank without having to lift the tank.
- Large volume users should consider a self-pressuring "PGS"-type supply vessel, available from major liquid nitrogen suppliers. These vessels require the use of supply hoses fitted with a phase separator.
- Some controlled-rate freezers (e.g. Planer's Kryo-10 models) require the liquid nitrogen to be supplied under pressure; this can be achieved using a **thermal transfer pump** fitted to a standard 25-liter supply dewar.

Sealing device for straws

The *SYMS* sealer must be used with the *CBS High Security Straws* (the recommended packaging system for cryobanking semen and washed sperm preparations: CryoBioSystem, Paris, France). **Automated systems** for labeling, filling and sealing straws are available from CryoBioSystem (Paris, France), e.g. the MAPI, PACE and SIDE units, although these are too large-scale for the great majority of human sperm cryobanks.

> Note: The *Ultraseal 21*™ ultrasonic sealing device from Penetrating Innovations (Verona, WI, USA) is not validated for use with CBS *High Security Straws*.

Equipment for specialized assays

CASA instrument

The Hamilton Thorne IVOS computer-aided sperm analyzer is the most common instrument worldwide and the Boolean sort criteria provided in Chapter 4 have been validated for this instrument. The unit should ideally operate at a 60 Hz image capture rate and have the "HDATA," "Edit Tracks" and "Sort" function software options installed.

Flow cytometer

As an optional means of reading TUNEL assays, e.g. Becton Dickinson FACScan (San Jose, CA, USA) equipped with a 15 mW argon-ion laser for excitation and green FITC fluorescence detection in the FL1 sensor (550 nm dichroic long-pass filter and 525 nm band-pass filter).

Fluorescence microscope

For visualization of fluorescently labeled lectins (acrosome reaction testing) or TUNEL assays. A dedicated epifluorescence microscope system is recommended and must include the appropriate filter sets for the particular fluorescent probes being used:

FITC: excitation at 494 nm (blue); emission at 520 nm (green) and barrier filter (dichroic mirror) at 510–515 nm.

TRITC: excitation at 541 nm (green); emission at 572 nm (red) and barrier filter (dichroic mirror) at 570–580 nm.

H33258: excitation at 343 nm (*u.v.*); emission at 480 nm (blue) and barrier filter (dichroic mirror) at 400 nm.

An attached or integral imaging system is also recommended.

Inverted microscope

For working with zonae pellucidae (see Chapter 5)

Luminometer

For assaying reactive oxygen species, e.g. LKB model 953 (Wallac Inc., Gaithersburg, MD, USA).

Macro-pipetter

For volumes of 1–10 ml (see Chapter 4).

Magnetic stirrer

For biochemistry assays (see Chapter 4).

Microcentrifuge

For use in the TUNEL assay (1.5-ml Eppendorf tubes).

Micromanipulator attachments

Required for the *hemizona assay* for bisecting the hemizonae, and 10× and 40× phase contrast objectives are needed. For the *competitive (intact) zona binding assay*, phase contrast optics giving total magnification of 160× or 250× are needed.

Microtiterplate reader

For biochemistry assays (see Chapter 4).

Multi-stepper pipette

For volumes in the range 50–1000 µl (see Chapter 4).

Appendix 3: Supply companies

The following table provides contact information for the companies whose products are mentioned in this handbook. Many companies have networks of distributors, details of which can be found on the manufacturer's websites.

Company	Product(S)	Location	Website
Air Liquide (Cryogenic Material Division)	Cryogenic storage equipment, MiniCool controlled-rate freezers, Nicool LM10 vapor phase controlled-rate freezer	Marne La Vallée Cedex, France	www.airliquide.com
Becton Dickinson	Falcon plasticware, FACScan flow cytometer	San Jose, CA, USA	www.bd.com
Biotronics Ltd.	DB1 controlled-rate freezer	Leominster, UK	ww.biotronics.net
Brady	Labeling systems	Milwaukee, WI, USA	ww.bradyid.com
Chart Biomed	MVE Biological Systems, cryogenic storage systems	Marietta, GA, USA	www.chartbiomed.com
Conception Technologies	Microcell fixed-depth chambers, Culture media for human spermatozoa	San Diego, CA, USA	www.conceptiontechnologies.com
Cook Medical	Sydney IVF culture media for human assisted reproduction, MINC benchtop incubator		www.cookmedical.com
Cooper Surgical	Aspirette cervical mucus aspiration device, Sage Quinn's Advantage® culture media for human assisted reproduction	Trumbull, CT, USA	www.coopersurgical.com
CryoBioSystem	Aspiglaire cervical mucus aspiration device, High Security Straws SYMS sealing device for High Security Straws	Paris, France	www.cryobiosystem-imv.com
CryoLogic	Controlled-rate freezer systems	Mulgrave, Vic, Australia	www.cryologic.com
Dako Corp	Immunodiagnostic reagents	Carpinteria, CA, USA	www.dakousa.com
Dow Corning	High vacuum silicone grease	Midland, MI, USA	www.dowcorning.com/applications/search
Embryotech Laboratories	Baby Start™ Male Fertility Test, MARQ™ Liquefaction Cups	Wilmington, MA, USA	www.embryotech.com
FertAid	Internet-based training, QC and QA schemes	Newcastle, NSW, Australia	www.fertaid.com

Company	Product(S)	Location	Website
FertiPro	LeucoScreen™ leukocyte detection kit, Sil-Select™ density gradient material culture media for human spermatozoa	Beernem, Belgium	www.fertipro.com
Fisher Scientific (ThermoFisher)	General laboratory equipment and supplies	Springfield, NJ, USA	country-specific: www.fishersci.com www.fisher.co.uk www.fishersci.ca
Genosis	Fertell male fertility test		www.fertell.com
Hamilton Thorne Biosciences	IVOS computer-aided sperm analyzer (CASA) instruments	Beverly, MA, USA	www.hamiltonthorne.com
Heraeus	Biosafety and laminar air flow cabinets, centrifuges, incubators		www/heraeus.com
INGfertility	Pre' and pre' MD lubricant for external use, Pre~Seed vaginal lubricant	Valleyford, WA, USA	www.preseed.com/ MedicalProfessionals/ People_Products.php
Irvine Scientific	Immunobead test reagents, PBS ISolate density gradient material	Santa Ana, CA, USA	www.irvinesci.com
Kendall	Monoject blunt syringe needles		www.kendallhq.com
MedCalc Software	Statistical software	Mariakerke, Belgium	www.medcalc.be
MediCult	Culture media for human assisted reproduction	Jyllinge, Denmark	www.medicult.com
Merck	Entellan mountant, colorpHast pH test strips	Darmstadt, Germany	Global network of sites: www.merck,com
MidAtlantic Diagnostics	General laboratory equipment and supplies for assisted reproduction and cryobanking	Mount Laurel, NJ, USA	www. midatlanticdiagnostics. com
Millipore	Filters and water systems	Billerica, MA, USA	www.millipore.com
Minitüb	Heated stages, PETG cryo straws; Note: products for human applications are sold through MTG	Tiefenbach, Germany	see MTG
MTG	General laboratory equipment and supplies for assisted reproduction and cryobanking	Altdorf, Germany	www.mtg-de.com
Nalge NUNC International	NUNC A/S	CryoTube range of products, Plastic culture ware	www.nalgenunc.com

Company	Product(S)	Location	Website
Nidacon International	PureSperm density gradient products, Sperm CryoProtec-II cryoprotectant medium, Sperm VitalStain	Gothenburg, Sweden	www.nidacon.com
NUNC A/S	CryoTube range of products, Plastic culture ware	Roskilde, Denmark	www.nuncbrand.com
Planer	Assure24seven laboratory equipment monitoring system, Controlled-rate freezers	Sunbury-on-Thames, UK	www.assure24seven.com www.planer.co.uk
Research Instruments	Products for human assisted reproduction laboratories, including IVF Witness and IVF Tracker systems	Falmouth, UK	www.research-instruments.com
Roche Diagnostics	Immunodiagnostic reagents and kits TUNEL assay kit	Mannheim, Germany	www.roche-applied-science.com
Rocket Medical	Disposable suture scissors, Straw-handling forceps	Watford, UK Hingham, MA, USA	www.rocketmedical.com
Santa Cruz Biotechnology, Inc.	Immunodiagnostic reagents	Santa Cruz, CA, USA	www.scbt.com
SCSA Diagnostics	SCSA assay service	Brookings, SD, USA	www.scsadiagnostics.com/
Sefi Medical	Makler chamber	Haifa, Israel	www.sefimedical.com
Sigma	Chemicals and reagents	St Louis, MO, USA	Global access website: www.sigmaaldrich.com
Taylor-Wharton	Cryogenic storage equipment	Theodore, AL, USA	www.taylorwharton.com
VitroCom	Microslide rectangular glass capillary tubes	Mountain Lakes, NJ, USA	www.vitrocom.com
Vitrolife	Culture media for human assisted reproduction	Kungsbacka, Sweden Englewood, CO, USA	www.vitrolife.com
Wako Chemicals GmbH	Zinc assay	Neuss, Germany	www.wako-chemicals.de
VWR International	General laboratory equipment and supplies	Global	Global network of websites

Appendix 4: Recommendations on the application of CASA technology in the analysis of spermatozoa

This Appendix repeats, essentially verbatim, the recommendations on the practical application of CASA technology included in the 43 guidelines put forward by the ESHRE Special Interest Group in Andrology following a consensus workshop held in San Miniato (Italy) in April 1997 [1]. Guidelines that referred to the further development of the technology have been omitted.

General recommendations for all mammalian species

- Standardization and quality control (both internal and external) are paramount fundamental requirements for CASA, just as they are for any other diagnostic andrology laboratory procedure.

- As for all measurement systems, it is the responsibility of users to ensure that an appropriate number of cells are sampled in order to achieve the statistical requirements for a proper interpretation of the obtained results with CASA, including sensitivity and specificity.

- It is mandatory that technicians are trained to understand the theory behind CASA, as well as the influence that the initial settings can have on the data produced.

- Each laboratory using CASA must have quality control (QC) procedures.

- In any manuscript or report, methods should be presented in sufficient detail to establish that accepted relevant CASA guidelines were followed. These include: image acquisition rate, track sampling time, smoothing algorithm employed, number of cells sampled, type of chamber including its depth, as well as instrument model and software version numbers, and microscope optics and magnification.

- Chamber depth must be sufficient for unconstrained sperm motion. This will vary depending on the species. Chamber depth must match optics to achieve appropriate depth of focus.

- In all CASA analyses, the user must verify that all motile spermatozoa in the field of view are being tracked.

Basic instrumentation

- When used for kinematic analysis of non-capacitated spermatozoa in seminal plasma, the magnification of the CASA instrument should be such that the majority of spermatozoa are tracked for 0.5 s before leaving the field of view. Hence, for human spermatozoa, the minimum field of view should be no less than 200 μm by 200 μm, allowing optimal tracking of spermatozoa with VSL values up to 100 μm/s.

- For human spermatozoa, an objective with maximum 10× magnification and suitable numerical aperture must be used so as to provide an adequate depth of focus.
- Reliable analysis of human sperm motility ideally requires a minimum acquisition frequency of 50 Hz.
- A minimum sampling time of 0.5 s is needed to acquire reliable kinematic values for a track (see [1] for further details).

Determination of sperm concentration

- This must not be a primary reason for acquiring a CASA instrument.
- A user wishing to use a CASA instrument to determine sperm concentration must establish that the intended measurement procedure provides accurate results compared to established, reliable techniques (e.g. WHO hemocytometry method).

  Note: This is further compounded by the specific error associated with the capillary-loading of shallow chambers, as are used by many laboratories using CASA [2,3], although it might be possible to apply a correction factor in order to achieve the correct result [4].

- The current generation of CASA instruments does not provide accurate, reproducible values for sperm concentration unless the method can differentiate sperm from other cells and debris by a specific staining method, e.g. fluorescent staining of DNA with quantitative determination of nucleus size.

Determination of the proportion of motile spermatozoa

- This should not be considered a primary reason for acquiring a CASA instrument.
- *If* used in the routine analysis of seminal spermatozoa, CASA should be used to determine the *concentration* of progressively motile spermatozoa. CASA can determine this value accurately if care is taken with specimen preparation, instrument use and appropriate user-defined criteria. Current CASA instruments should not be used for the determination of the *proportion* of motile spermatozoa, since they cannot be relied upon to distinguish between debris and dead spermatozoa while tracking live spermatozoa at the same time.

Determination of sperm movement

- For ejaculated spermatozoa:
  - Semen samples with sperm concentrations higher than those recommended by the CASA instrument manufacturer must be diluted using cell-free autologous seminal plasma.
  - All CASA analyses should be performed at body temperature (37°C for human spermatozoa).
  - A minimum chamber depth of 10 μm must be used. Depths >20 μm are unlikely to be of any benefit.
  - At least 200 motile spermatozoa should be analyzed per sample.
- Population-averaged kinematics are considered to be of limited value because values are often not normally distributed, making the mean an inappropriate estimate of the sample. Consequently:

a. median and range or centile values are statistically more meaningful than mean values; and

b. multiparametric kinematic definitions, which allow the classification of individual spermatozoa into specific sub-populations that are correlated with relevant functional endpoints (e.g. "good mucus penetrating" spermatozoa), should be made.

For critical analysis of data it is recommended that individual track values be saved in a database so that their distribution may be examined in order to select the most appropriate statistic for either describing the sample or comparing it with others (e.g. fertile versus infertile men or treated/exposed versus control/unexposed animals).

CASA analysis of hyperactivation

- Spermatozoa for hyperactivation studies should not be prepared from liquefied semen using techniques that have been demonstrated to have potentially deleterious effects on sperm function, e.g. initial centrifugation to separate spermatozoa from seminal plasma.

- An appropriately constituted culture medium should be employed, i.e. one capable of supporting capacitation in vitro. However, the medium must contain at least 25 mM HCO^{3-} and millimolar quantities of Ca^{2+} and glucose. Sufficient albumin must be incorporated to minimize the sticking-to-glass phenomenon, probably at least 10 mg/ml.

- All hyperactivation analyses must be performed at body temperature (i.e. 37°C for human spermatozoa).

- Preparations of sufficient depth so as not to constrain hyperactivated movement must be used. For human spermatozoa, a minimum chamber depth of 30 μm is essential. Although 50 μm is probably ideal, it can only be employed if the optical system used is capable of resolving this depth of focus.

- Definitions for hyperactivated motility must take into account the image acquisition frequency and should use kinematic criteria which have been validated for that CASA instrument.

Morphology assessment by CASA

- The current generation of CASA instruments is not capable of analyzing human sperm morphology in a manner adequate for routine clinical applications. In particular, the inability to include assessment of the midpiece and tail regions is considered to be a major weakness. Consequently, the use of CASA instruments for the clinical assessment of human sperm morphology is not supported at this time.

Clinical application of CASA

- In the context of male fertility diagnosis, CASA should not be used without first undertaking a proper clinical assessment of the patient (including a clinical history and physical examination).

- For the present, CASA should not be undertaken in a clinical setting without first having constructed a basic semen profile according to recognized (WHO [or ESHRE Andrology SIG]) guidelines.

- Clinicians should understand that correct sample handling prior to analysis is critical for obtaining useful information. This is true for all semen assessments, not just CASA. Hence the length of abstinence (ideally in hours) and the ejaculation-to-analysis delay must be known accurately.
- Studies are required, using the current generation of CASA systems, to define:
  a. the limits of normal semen quality in fertile men;
  b. the relationships between CASA variables and the time to pregnancy;
  c. the relationships between CASA variables (especially hyperactivation) and IVF outcome.

Applications of CASA in reproductive toxicology

- For toxicological studies on epididymal or vasa deferentia spermatozoa, accepting that samples must be diluted, the user must demonstrate that:
  a. the process of dilution does not damage the spermatozoa;
  b. the medium used supports consistently normal motility over the period of analysis;
  c. the sperm concentration has been adjusted and controlled to minimize artifacts induced by crowding.
- Magnification should be adjusted according to sperm size and velocity (e.g. 4× is appropriate for rat spermatozoa, which are considerably larger and faster than human spermatozoa) and chamber depth should allow unimpeded motion (e.g. >40 μm for rat spermatozoa).
- Users must verify that instrument settings have been optimized to detect all motile spermatozoa.
- Users must verify that the temperature at which images are captured is the body temperature for that species.
- With rodent sperm preparations, CASA can be used to determine both % motile and % progressively motile spermatozoa. User-defined thresholds for progressiveness should be justified based upon distributions of these endpoints in control samples.
- A permanent record of samples (e.g. video- or digital-recording) is recommended so that data can be verified at any time, and re-analyzed as necessary when improvements in software become available. Fields should be recorded in a predetermined order so that the user does not bias the results by selecting or rejecting fields on the basis of their appearance.
- New users should compare their sample preparation methods and velocity data with those in the literature to achieve minimum standards in line with current practice.

References

1. ESHRE Andrology Special Interest Group. Guidelines on the application of CASA technology in the analysis of spermatozoa. *Hum Reprod* 1998; **13**: 142–5.
2. Douglas-Hamilton DH, Smith NG, Kuster CE, *et al.* Particle distribution in low-volume capillary-loaded chambers. *J. Androl* 2005; **26**: 107–14.
3. Douglas-Hamilton DH, Smith NG, Kuster CE, *et al.* Capillary-loaded particle fluid dynamics: effect on estimation of sperm concentration. *J Androl* 2005; **26**: 115–22.
4. Rijnders S, Bolscher JG, McDonnell J, Vermeiden JP. Filling time of a lamellar capillary-filling semen analysis chamber is a rapid, precise, and accurate method to assess viscosity of seminal plasma. *J Androl* 2007; **28**: 461–5.

Appendix 5: Home testing

Semen analysis is the cornerstone of subfertility investigation in the male. On the basis of the semen analysis result, the couple are provided with diagnostic and prognostic information to assist in their management. However, many men find the production of a semen sample an embarrassing and stressful experience. In addition, there is often a significant waiting time for an initial appointment with the doctor, or at a specialist clinic, and then a further time delay before the results are available. Because all these factors heighten the anxiety associated with subfertility investigations, the development of an over-the-counter home sperm test has been an important goal in andrology for many years. Such a test should allow a man to obtain, at his own convenience, an assessment of his fertility potential, and also warn him of a potential problem so that he can go on to seek detailed investigations and possible treatment at the earliest opportunity.

Today there are several commercially available tests which can give a man an indication of either his sperm concentration (Baby Start™ Male Fertility Test [previously FertilMARQ™]; EmbryoTech Laboratories Inc.; www.embryotech.com), or his sperm motility or concentration of motile cell spermatozoa (Fertell®, Genosis plc.; www.fertell.com; [1]). Although each assay has been validated, it is critical to stress that such home tests should only be used as a screening test, and should not be seen as an alternative to a detailed, high quality, comprehensive semen assessment.

Reference

1. Björndahl L, Kirkman-Brown J, Hart G, *et al.* Development of a novel home sperm test. *Hum Reprod* 2006; **21**: 145–9.

Appendix 6: Example laboratory and report forms

Consistent routine is one important ingredient in order to achieve reliable results with low variation between different observers, and between different occasions. Elaborated work forms help the staff members to perform the techniques as intended, and such forms can also be used to document which investigator has been responsible for each of the different parts of the complete semen analysis. This documentation is a basic part of requirements for quality management in the andrology laboratory.

Example laboratory work form

SAMPLE WORK FORM

Patient

Name:_____ Date of Birth:_____ Unique ID*_____

*) Social Security Number, Laboratory Patient number or other unique identifier   ID controlled by: _____

Sample Date: _____ Date of previous ejaculation: _____

Collection time: _____ Complete collection: ❏ Yes   ❏ No:

If not complete: missed ❏ 1st   ❏ middle ❏ last part; approximately _____ % lost of the ejaculate

Start of investigations (time): _____   Fresh sample investigator: _____

Liquefaction: ❏ within 30 minutes, ❏ 30-60 minutes, ❏ incomplete at 60 minutes after ejaculation

Volume: _____ ml   Viscosity: ❏ normal; ❏ increased

Other macroscopic observations: _____

Investigation of the **wet preparation**:

Estimation of appropriate dilution for concentration ❏ 1:5 ❏ 1:10 ❏ 1:20 ❏ 1:50

Presence of: ❏ Aggregates   ❏ Agglutinates; dominant region of binding: _____

Motility assessment:	1st drop		2nd drop		Average	Diff. /•/* drops	Diff. < Limit?
	Counts	Percent	Counts	Percent			
rapid (a)							
slow (b)							
non progressive (c)							
Immotile (d)							
TOTAL		100		100			
Progressive (a+b)							
Motile (a+b+c)							

* /•/ = between   Investigator: _____

Determination of sperm concentration: Sperm counted in upper left large square: _____

1st chamber: Sperm counted _____ in _____ large squares

2nd chamber: Sperm counted _____

Total number counted (sum): _____ Difference between counts: _____ OK? ❏ Yes ❏ No

Divide total number by: _____ = _____ $\times 10^6$/ml;

Total sperm number:
volume × concentration = _____ $\times 10^6$ / ejaculate   Investigator: _____

SAMPLE WORK FORM

Sperm morphology assessment:

	Counts	Percentage	Comments
Normal			
Abnormal			
TOTAL		**100**	
Head defects			
Neck/midpiece			*Percentage of ALL spermatozoa assessed*
Tail defects			
cytoplasmic residue			
		> 100	

Teratozoospermia Index (TZI): _____

Immature germ cells:_____ / _____ spermatozoa = _____ / 100 spermatozoa

Investigator: _____

Sperm vitality: Number of spermatozoa assessed: _____

Number of live spermatozoa: _____ ; % live spermatozoa: _____

Investigator: _____

Round cells and white blood cells (leucocytes) - *Cells in wet preparation*

	Cells counted	N:o of microscope fields	Cells/field	Conc.
Round cells				$\times 10^6$/ml
White cells				$\times 10^6$/ml
Spermatozoa				$\times 10^6$/ml

Calculate round cell and white cell concentration:

Sperm concentration $\times$ (Cells/field / spermatozoa/field)   Investigator: _____

Inflammatory cells (peroxidase positive granulocytes)

Cells counted in counting chamber: _____

Factor to divide counted cells by: _____

Calculated concentration: _____ $\times 10^6$/ml   Investigator: _____

Antisperm Antibodies (ASAB)   Method used: _____   Investigator: _____

First reading (_____ min): Total sperm counted: _____ ; sperm with beads: _____ = _____ %

Second reading (_____ min): Total sperm counted: _____ ; sperm with beads: _____ = _____ %

299

General Hospital
Unit for Reproductive Medicine
Andrology Laboratory
Address:
Telephone: E-mail:

patient:	**Name**
	ID
partner:	(Name)
	(ID)	Print date
Ref. Dr:		Aug 22, 2008

											Ref.	Unit
Date:	May 8 '08	Jun 4 '08										
Sample No.	2008/1768	2008/1933										
BASIC ANALYSES												
Collection:	m	m									m	-
Complete:	y	y									y	-
Time to invest.:	0.30	0.35									<1.00	h.min
Volume:	3.2	3.7									1.5-6.0	ml
Rapid progr (a):	22	22									>25 or	%
Slow progr (b):	23	39									>50(a+b)	%
Non progr (c):	29	8										%
Immotile (d):	26	31									<60	%
%Live:	74	68									>40	%
Aggregates:	0	0									0-1	a.u.
Round cells:	0.7	0.1									<1	×10^6/ml
Abst. days:	5	3									2-7	day(s)
Sperm conc.:	115	42										× 10^6/ml
Sperm count:	368	155									>40	×10^6/ejac.
Inflam. cells:	0.2	0.0									<1	×10^6/ml
MORPHOLOGY ASSESSMENT												
% Typical:	4	12										%
Head	96	81										%
Neck/MP	41	30										%
Tail	27	11										%
Cytol. Residue:	2	4										%
TZI:	1.73	1.43									<1.60	-
Immature	0	0										
SEMEN BIOCHEMISTRY												
α-glucosidase:	18.0	22.3										mU/ml
α-G-amount:	57.6	82.5									>20.0	mU
Zinc conc.:	1.8	4.4									>1.2	mmol/l
Zinc amount:	5.8	16.4									>2.5	μmol
Fructose conc.:	15.7	18.9									>6.0	mmol/l
Fructose amount:	50.2	69.9									>13.0	μmol
Zinc/Fructose:	0.11	0.24									>0.10	-
ANTISPERM ANTIBODIES												
Test method:	IBT	SpM										
Sperm with beads	8	4									<40	%
localization:	NS	NS										

H = Head; MP = Midpiece; T = Tail; tt = tail tip; any combinations according to actual observations ; NS= non-specific

Date	Sample	Comment
May 8 '08	2008/1768	Liquefaction incomplete after 30 min; complete at 60 min
Jun 4 '08	2008/1933	A smaller, isolated gel streak left after 30 min liquefaction,

Printed from LB Andrologidata
© 2008 LB Andrologikonsult
www.andrologi.net

Figure A6.1 An example of a computer-generated report form where results from up to ten different semen samples from the same patient can be printed, together with basic information of reference ranges etc.

Explanatory notes for the example basic semen analysis report form

A sample report form with the possibility of showing up to 10 different semen analysis results for one patient (Figure A6.1, reproduced by permission from LB Andrologikonsult [www.andrologi.net]).

Left text column

Collection: Coded: m = masturbation; i = interrupted intercourse ("withdrawal"); c = collection condom.

Complete: Coded: y = yes; n = incomplete. It is advisable to give a text comment (bottom of page) explaining if the first, middle, or last part of the ejaculate was missed, and an approximate estimation of the loss.

Time to invest.: Time to investigation = time between ejaculation and initiation of analysis.

Rapid progr (a): Rapidly progressive spermatozoa (% of all spermatozoa): velocity 25 µm/s or more at 37°C.

Slow progr (b): Slowly progressive spermatozoa (% of all spermatozoa): velocity 5–24 µm/s at 37°C.

Non progr (c): Non-progressive spermatozoa (% of all spermatozoa): less than 5 µm/s at 37°C.

Immotile (d): Immotile sperm (% of all sperm).

Aggregates: Given in arbitrary units (a.u.): 0, 1, 2, 3 for none, some, many, most.

Abst. days: Days of sexual abstinence before collecting the sample for semen analysis.

Sperm conc.: Sperm concentration.

Sperm count: Total number of spermatozoa in the ejaculate (concentration × volume).

Inflam. cells: Concentration of inflammatory cells (peroxidase-positive cells).

% Typical: Proportion of spermatozoa with a morphology typical for spermatozoa that are able to reach the site of fertilization, and bind to the zona pellucida.

Head: Proportion of spermatozoa with head morphology that is not consistent with the definition of typical spermatozoa.

Neck/MP: Proportion of spermatozoa with neck/midpiece morphology that is not consistent with the definition of typical spermatozoa.

Tail: Proportion of spermatozoa with tail morphology that is not consistent with the definition of typical spermatozoa.

Cytopl. Residue: Proportion of spermatozoa with a cytoplasmic residue that is not consistent with the definition of typical spermatozoa.

TZI: Average number of abnormal regions in the abnormal (non-typical) spermatozoa; calculated as in the 1992 (3rd) edition of the WHO Manual.

Immature: Presence of immature germ cells in the ejaculate, expressed as number per 100 spermatozoa.

α-glucosidase: Concentration of marker for epididymal secretion.

α-G-amount: Total amount of epididymal marker in the ejaculate.

Zinc conc.: Concentration of marker for prostatic secretion.

Zinc amount: Total amount of prostatic marker in the ejaculate.

Fructose conc.: Concentration of marker for seminal vesicular secretion.

Fructose amount: Total amount of seminal vesicular marker in the ejaculate.

Zinc/Fructose: Zinc–Fructose molar ratio, indicating the relative contribution of prostatic and seminal vesicular secretions to the ejaculate.

Test method: Method used for sperm antisperm antibody assessment, e.g. ImmunoBead Test™ or SpermMar™.

Sperm with beads: Proportion of spermatozoa with antisperm antibodies attached.

Localization: Head, Midpiece, Tail, Tt (tail-tip), combinations of these, or NS (Non-Specific) – comment if there is a specific localization of the antibodies.

Columns to the right of result columns

Ref.: Reference limits and ranges. It should be noted that numbers given in this sample form are given as examples only. Each laboratory should determine its own reference ranges and limits. These ranges can be based on frequency distributions of results from fertile and subfertile men, respectively. When no clear cut-off can be determined, a consensus-based decision limit can function as reference.

Unit: Specification of unit used for values presented in each row.

Text comments

Date, Sample Number, and Comment – text comments regarding additional information obtained from the patient, or during laboratory investigation.

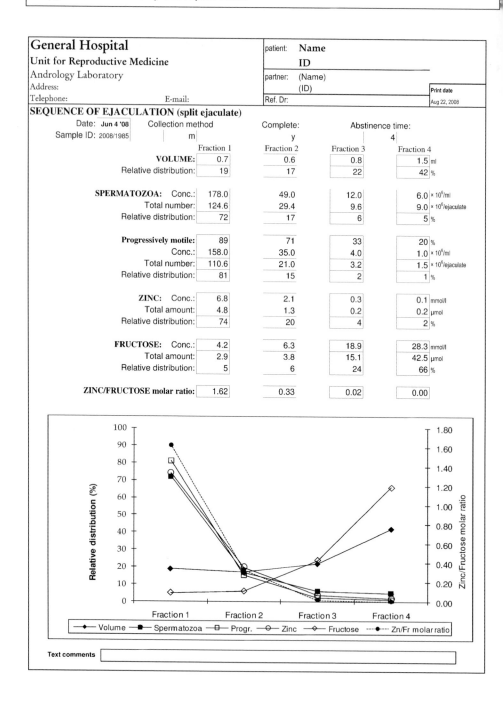

Figure A6.2 An example of a computer-generated report form, with results in numbers and graphics of a split ejaculate.

Explanatory notes for the sample sequence of ejaculation report form

A sample report form giving results from a split-ejaculate investigation (Figure A6.2, reproduced by permission from LB Andrologikonsult [www.andrologi.net]).

Collection method, completeness and abstinence time as for the basic semen analysis.

This form is based on having the patient collect the three first expelled fractions in the first three containers (Fractions 1–3), and the remainder of the ejaculate in the fourth, last container (Fraction 4).

Relative distribution of volume:	The volume in each fraction in relation to the sum of the volume of all fractions.
Progressively motile:	Proportion of spermatozoa that were progressively motile in each fraction; used to calculate concentration and total number of progressively motile spermatozoa.
Total number/amount:	Calculated from concentration and volume in each fraction.
Relative distribution:	Proportion of the measurand in each fraction of the ejaculate. 100% = sum of the four fractions.
Zinc/Fructose molar ratio:	Contribution of the prostatic marker zinc in relation to the contribution of the seminal vesicular marker fructose.
Graphic representation:	Diagram showing relative (%) distribution of volume, spermatozoa, progressively motile spermatozoa, zinc and fructose (left axis), and the zinc–fructose molar ratio (right axis).

Appendix 7: Comparison of replicate counts

Acceptable differences between replicate assessments of proportions

Table A7.1 can be used to facilitate the decision if replicate assessments of proportions (e.g. % motile spermatozoa, % typical spermatozoa, or (optional) % live spermatozoa) can be accepted. Since the recommendation is to count 200 spermatozoa in duplicate (2 × 200) values are given for this sample size. The table is *not* valid for replicate counts of 100 spermatozoa (i.e. 2 × 100). The table is calculated from a formula based on the binomial distribution required to determine asymmetrical confidence intervals for proportions (which have absolute minimum and maximum values of 0% and 100%) [1].

Table A7.1

Average %	Limit difference
0	1
1	2
02–03	3
04–06	4
07–09	5
10–13	6
14–19	7
20–27	8
28–44	9
45–55	10
56–72	9
73–80	8
81–86	7
87–90	6
91–93	5
94–96	4
97–98	3
99	2
100	1

Calculate the *average percentage* (rounded off with no decimal place) for the replicate assessments, and the *difference* between them. Look up the row corresponding to the average percentage (left column). The difference between the two assessments must be less than or equal to the limit difference given in the right column. If the difference is above the limit the assessments must be discarded and two new counts made.

Uncertainty of results due to the number of spermatozoa assessed

Table A7.2 illustrates the uncertainty of results with respect to the number of spermatozoa assessed to obtain the result. The recommended number of assessed cells in each duplicate is 200. In the table data are also given for 100 and 200 assessed spermatozoa for comparisons where less than 400 spermatozoa are available for assessment.

When a proportion is determined (as % motile or % typical spermatozoa), the total number of spermatozoa assessed will influence how certain the result is. The higher the number of spermatozoa that have been examined, the more certain the result will be. This can be expressed as the "95% confidence interval" for the obtained proportion. This interval signifies that, with a 95% probability, the true value of the proportion is within the interval.

Example

If the result is 6% typical spermatozoa after assessing 2 × 200 spermatozoa, then the true proportion is most likely in the range 4–9%. If only 100 spermatozoa had been assessed the range would be 2–13%. Thus, the uncertainty of the result is much lower when 400 spermatozoa are assessed instead of 100.

Correspondingly, a result of 50% progressively motile spermatozoa has a confidence interval of 45–55% for 400 assessed spermatozoa, but 40–60% when only 100 have been assessed.

Table A7.2

Average percentage found	Total number of spermatozoa assessed		
	400 (2 x 200)	100	200
	95% Confidence interval		
0	0–1	0–4	0–2
1	0–3	0–5	0–4
2	1–4	0–7	1–5
3	2–5	1–9	1–6
4	2–6	1–10	2–8
5	3–8	2–11	2–9
6	4–9	2–13	3–10
7	5–10	3–14	4–11
8	6–11	4–15	5–13
9	6–12	4–16	5–14
10	7–13	5–18	6–15
11	8–14	6–19	7–16
12	9–16	6–20	8–17
13	10–17	7–21	9–18
14	11–18	8–22	10–20
15	12–19	9–24	10–21
20	16–24	13–29	15–26
25	21–30	17–35	19–32
30	26–35	21–40	24–37
35	30–40	26–45	28–42
40	35–45	30–50	33–47
45	40–50	35–55	38–52
50	45–55	40–60	43–57
55	50–60	45–65	48–62
60	55–65	50–70	53–67
65	60–70	55–74	58–72
70	65–74	60–79	63–76
75	70–79	65–83	68–81
80	76–84	71–87	74–85
85	81–88	76–91	79–90
90	87–93	82–95	85–94
91	88–94	84–96	86–95
92	89–94	85–96	87–95
93	90–95	86–97	89–96
94	91–96	87–98	90–97
95	92–97	89–98	91–98
96	94–98	90–99	92–98
97	95–98	91–99	94–99
98	96–99	93–100	95–99
99	97–100	95–100	96–100
100	99–100	96–100	98–100

Acceptable difference between replicate counts

Table A7.3 can be used to facilitate deciding whether replicate assessments of sperm concentration can be accepted.

Calculate the total number of spermatozoa counted and locate the corresponding range in the left column (SUM) of the table. If the difference between the two assessments is less than or equal to the value in the right column (LIMIT) the assessments can be accepted. If the difference between the duplicates is higher than the LIMIT the assessments must be discarded and two new assessments made. The shadowed part of the table is where, according to recommendations, too few spermatozoa have been counted to achieve a result with less than 10% uncertainty (confidence interval larger than ±10% interval) [1,2].

Table A7.3

SUM	LIMIT	SUM	LIMIT
969–1000	61	376–395	38
938–968	60	357–375	37
907–937	59	338–356	36
876–906	58	319–337	35
846–875	57	301–318	34
817–845	56	284–300	33
788–816	55	267–283	32
760–787	54	251–266	31
732–759	53	235–250	30
704–731	52	219–234	29
678–703	51	206–218	28
651–677	50	190–205	27
625–650	49	176–189	26
600–624	48	163–175	25
576–599	47	150–162	24
551–575	46	138–149	23
528–550	45	126–137	22
504–527	44	115–125	21
482–503	43	105–114	20
460–481	42	94–104	19
438–459	41	85–93	18
417–437	40	76–84	17
396–416	39	67–75	16
		59–66	15
		52–58	14
		44–51	13
		38–43	12
		32–37	11
		27–31	10
		22–26	9
		17–21	8
		13–16	7
		10–12	6
		7–9	5
		5–6	4
		3–4	3
		2	2
		1	1
		0	0

Uncertainty of results in relation to the number of spermatozoa counted

Table A7.4 illustrates how the certainty, expressed as confidence intervals in relation to counted numbers, of a sperm concentration result depends on the number of spermatozoa actually counted.

If 10 spermatozoa have been counted to get the result 1×10^6/ml in, e.g. a Makler chamber, the confidence of the result is between 0.4 and 1.6×10^6/ml ($1 \times 10^6 \pm 62\%$ according to the table). Thus, the concentration may vary up to 4-fold. If, instead, 100 spermatozoa had been counted (for instance in a hemocytometer with Improved Neubauer ruling), the confidence of the result would be between 0.8 and 1.2×10^6/ml ($1 \times 10^6 \pm 20\%$). With the number of spermatozoa in this latter example (i.e. 50 per Neubauer grid area of 5×5 large squares), it would be necessary to assess 100 large squares, or the central grid, plus three peripheral 5×5 grids in each hemocytometer chamber (see Figure 3.5A), in order to reach a confidence level of $\pm 10\%$ (0.9–1.1×10^6) – or 40 Makler chamber grids.

Table A7.4

Counted	±%
1	196
5	88
10	62
20	44
30	36
40	31
50	28
60	25
70	23
80	22
90	21
100	20
150	16
200	14
250	12
300	11
400	10
500	9
600	8
700	7
1000	6

References

1. Kvist U, Björndahl L, eds. *Manual on Basic Semen Analysis. ESHRE Monographs 2*. Oxford: Oxford University Press 2002.

2. World Health Organization. *WHO Laboratory Manual for the Examination of Human Semen and Sperm-Cervical Mucus Interaction*. 4th edn. Cambridge: Cambridge University Press 1999.

Appendix 8: Safety

Safety is the responsibility of everyone working in the laboratory

Each laboratory is required to work in compliance with the local and national safety guidelines. These vary between countries with potentially each having different resources/requirements. For example in Canada there is the Workplace Hazardous Material Information Scheme (www.hc-sc.gc.ca/ewh-semt/occup-travail/whmis-simdut/index-eng.php [WHMIS]), which is a hazard communication standard. The key elements of this system are cautionary labeling of containers of WHMIS "controlled products," the provision of material safety data sheets (MSDSs) and worker education programs. There is a national standard for the classification of hazardous workplace materials and all controlled products must be properly labeled and identified using MSDSs. Additionally, workers receive education and training to ensure the safe storage, handling and use of controlled products in the workplace. In the UK the Health and Safety Executive (www.hse.gov.uk) is the national body tasked with protecting workers' health and safety by ensuring risks in the workplace are properly controlled. The HSE is responsible for enforcing health and safety at work legislation and plays a major role in producing advice on health and safety issues, and guidance on relevant legislation.

All UK laboratories using chemicals or other hazardous substances are required to perform a detailed assessment covering the following 8 points: (a) assess the risks; (b) decide what precautions are necessary; (c) prevent or adequately control exposure; (d) ensure that control measures are used and maintained; (e) monitor the exposure; (f) carry our appropriate health surveillance; (g) prepare plans and procedures to deal with accidents, incidents and emergencies; and (h) ensure employees are properly informed, trained and supervised.

These themes are common to many regulatory bodies on health and safety, and are robust guiding principles. In addition to national guidelines, there are a number of international resources that provide high quality information related to safety in the laboratory – for example the WHO Laboratory Biosafety Manual [1]. Several excellent web-based safety training programs are freely available [2].

General recommendations

These recommendations are adapted from those published by Schrader [3], the World Health Organization [4], ASRM [5] and ESHRE [6].

1. Vaccination of all laboratory personnel handling human tissues and body fluids is encouraged in accordance with the recommendations for medical personnel in general.

2. *Universal precautions.* Laboratory personnel must handle every specimen of human tissue or body fluid as if it were contaminated with an infectious organism.

3. Extraordinary precautions must be taken to avoid accidental wounds from (contaminated) sharp instruments in the laboratory. This includes any sharp edges or corners of microscope slides and coverslips. As far as possible, hypodermic needles should be eliminated from general laboratory use to minimize the risks of "finger stick" injury. Dispose of all sharp objects in a designated sharps bin.

4. Avoid contact between biological materials and open skin lesions. Disposable gloves must be worn at all times when handling fresh or frozen semen, seminal plasma, blood plasma or serum, cervical mucus, follicular fluid and urine, as well as any containers or handling devices (e.g. pipettes) that have come into contact with these materials. Gloves must be removed and discarded as contaminated waste when leaving the laboratory or handling the telephone, etc. Never reuse gloves.

5. Either surgical scrubs or a laboratory coat or gown must be worn, fastened, in the laboratory. This protective clothing must be removed on leaving the laboratory. Under no circumstances should such clothing be worn outside the laboratory or ART procedures area.

6. Suitable footwear is essential; open weave shoes and sandals do not give suitable protection.

7. A high standard of personal hygiene must be maintained at all times. Hands must be washed after removing gowns and gloves. Hands must be washed thoroughly and immediately if they become contaminated with biological material. All hand washing must be with bactericidal soap and hot water. Hand washing sinks must not be used for any other purpose, and hands must not be washed in the general laboratory sink.

8. Hands should be kept away from face, nose, eyes and mouth, as must pens, pencils and other objects used in the laboratory.

9. Long hair must be tied back.

10. If the outside of any sample container is contaminated it must be disinfected using isopropanol or ethanol.

11. Disposable laboratory supplies should be used whenever and wherever possible. After use they must be collected in special "CONTAMINATED WASTE BIOLOGICAL HAZARD" containers and properly disposed of as for other infectious material, e.g. by incineration or autoclaving.

12. All laboratory equipment that could potentially be contaminated by biological material must be disinfected or sterilized (e.g. by alcohol spray) after a spill or after work activity is completed. This includes equipment handled while wearing protective gloves, e.g. microscopes and pipetting devices.

13. Pipetting by mouth is not permitted. Mechanical pipetting devices must be used for the manipulation of all other liquids in the laboratory.

14. All procedures and manipulations of biological fluids must be performed so as to minimize the creation of droplets and aerosols. Such procedures include centrifugation or vigorous mixing (especially vortex mixing) of open containers. Only centrifuges fitted with sealed carriers should be used.

15. Laboratory work surfaces must be decontaminated with a disinfectant (see #10 and #12, above) immediately after any spill occurs, and also on completing work with biological fluids each day.

16. Eating, drinking, smoking, applying cosmetics and the wearing of strong perfume or after-shave, etc. are prohibited in the andrology laboratory. Smoking is not permitted in the laboratory. The consumption of food and drink is only permitted in the designated areas, e.g. kitchen, staffroom and office areas.

17. All working areas must be kept clean and tidy at all times.

18. Faulty equipment must be reported immediately to the Laboratory Supervisor.

19. If you come across a situation that is unsafe, do something about it yourself and report it to your senior.

Accident prevention

Supervisors' responsibilities

1. That all appropriate actions have been taken to correct any safety hazards that might exist.

2. Proper personal protective clothing and equipment is provided and used.

3. Staff are aware of, and abide by, all national, provincial, and local government safety regulations.

4. Employees receive adequate training in, and information on, safe working procedures.

5. An adequate number of workers are trained in first aid procedures.

Employees' responsibilities

1. Report all accidents and injuries to the Laboratory Supervisor.

2. All federal, provincial, and local government safety regulations are conformed to.

3. Unsafe procedures and conditions are reported immediately to the Laboratory Supervisor.

4. Be aware of hazards in the day-to-day work and that appropriate measures to eliminate any risk of accident are taken.

5. Wear appropriate personal protective clothing and equipment as required and ensure that it is maintained in good condition.

Protective clothing and equipment

While performing his/her normal duties a laboratory worker may be exposed to a variety of hazards. While all steps must be taken to control these hazards at their source(s), personal protective equipment and/or clothing must be used (see discussion of responsibilities, above).

Eye protection

Eye protection must be worn at any time there is a danger of flying particles, aerosols, irritating substances, liquids, or harmful radiation endangering the eyes.

Contact lenses are not a substitute for proper eye protection, and spectacles with plain glass lenses also pose a potential hazard. All workers wearing spectacles who are regularly exposed to this type of hazard should be encouraged to request safety lenses when having prescriptions for new spectacles filled.

Hand protection

Appropriate gloves must be worn when handling materials or equipment that could be injurious to the skin such as sharp objects, chemicals, biological or extremely hot or cold materials.

Respiratory protection

Although special equipment such as self-contained breathing apparatus or respirators are not required in an andrology/ART laboratory, suitable surgical face masks should be worn whenever there is a possibility of exposure to aerosols of biological material.

All handling of flammable or noxious substances such as solvents or fixatives should be performed in a fume hood.

Protective clothing

The general principles governing this issue are that clothing worn in the laboratories or clinical procedure areas must be protected from contamination, and any clothing worn in those areas must not be worn outside them where it might contaminate others.

Fire safety

While it is the responsibility of the institution to ensure that appropriate fire detection and suppression systems, as required by relevant building and fire safety codes, are installed and serviced – including the provision of portable fire extinguishers – laboratory staff also have specific responsibilities.

General fire safety rules

The following list is not exhaustive:

1. Never use naked flames when flammable vapors are present. Smoking is forbidden in all laboratories at all times.

2. Never block fire exit doors, fire/smoke control doors, or access to fire fighting equipment.

3. Do not store large quantities of flammable solvents in the laboratory. Highly flammable liquids (flash point below 40°C, e.g. ether) must not be stored in ordinary glass containers in quantities of more than 4.5 liters. Larger volumes, if essential, must be stored in approved safety containers.

4. Never store equipment or materials in hallways or under stairwells.

5. Use metal or other approved waste solvent containers. Plastic waste solvent containers are only suitable for small-scale use (e.g. under-bench locations).

6. Be aware of potential fire or explosion hazards of *any* chemical or material you use.

Dealing with spills

General rules

1. The primary concern in any spillage incident is the care and safety of all exposed persons, especially those at risk from infection.

2. *Always wear gloves and gowns.* Also, wear a face mask and eye protection if appropriate for the particular spill.

3. In the laboratory, to protect gametes and embryos from the toxic, and possibly terato-genic, effects of disinfectants, the only disinfectants that can be used are isopropanol

(isopropyl alcohol or "IPA") and ethanol. Ideally oxidative sanitizers should be used to avoid releasing volatile organic compounds (VOCs) into the air.

4. Always read the appropriate safety data sheets for a material before using it and understand risks, e.g. COSHH assessments.

Specific procedures for dealing with spills of biological material and other hazardous substances are described in the following sections.

Biological materials: use and disposal

Modern infection control regulations require that all human tissue samples be considered potentially pathogenic (the principle of *universal precautions*). Therefore, all ART laboratories (including embryology laboratories, andrology laboratories, semen banks, etc.) must have adequate safety programs to protect their staff against accidental contamination. This also dictates that laboratory workers recognize the potential dangers of their profession and take every precaution to ensure their own safety. The employers are obligated to provide any necessary safety clothing and equipment to protect their staff from infections or exposure to hazardous materials, and to ensure that all staff know what is required. Failure to follow declared safety procedures may in some circumstances be a disciplinary matter.

The notoriety of HIV has resulted in many individuals being preoccupied with the possibility of AIDS transmission by handling semen or blood. While this is certainly a significant concern, it must not be allowed to overshadow the wide range of other pathogens commonly found in specimens handled by laboratories. AIDS is substantially less infectious through this route than hepatitis, which is the most frequently occurring infection of laboratory workers. Hepatitis B virus (HBV) has been detected in semen, urine and saliva as well as blood, and infection can occur from contamination of even a small area of exposed skin if an open lesion such as a scratch or graze is present. Hepatitis C also has similar routes of infection.

In addition, the organisms causing many traditional sexually transmissible diseases (STDs) are found in semen. Cases of accidental *Gonorrhoea*, *Chlamydia*, *Mycoplasma* and *Streptococcus* infection of laboratory personnel have been documented. Cytomegalovirus (CMV), *Ureaplasma* and human papillomavirus (HPV) have also been isolated in semen. However, while no documented laboratory-associated infections have been reported for these other pathogens, the possibility of their transmission by exposure to mucous membranes (e.g. ingestion or inhalation of aerosolized material) or accidental inoculation (e.g. finger stick or contamination of an open wound) does exist.

Specific information on dealing with the most commonly encountered biological materials, semen and follicular fluid, follow. There is also a section on other biologically derived materials used in the ART laboratory.

Semen

Collection and specimen reception

1. Whenever possible, semen specimens should be collected on the premises into the sterile specimen jars provided. The scientist must have the patient verify that his name as printed on the sticky label provided is correct.

2. The patient should be instructed to wash his hands before and after collecting the specimen.

3. The patient must hand his specimen to one of the laboratory staff and fill in the required paperwork.

4. Place the specimen in the specimen reception incubator. If the specimen is received on behalf of another section (e.g. by andrology for embryology) then notify a member of staff from the other area that the specimen has been received.

5. The scientist handing the specimen must wear gloves from before first contact with the specimen container.

Handling and processing

This is performed according to the "General recommendations" listed above. Specifically:

1. Ideally all semen specimens should be handled inside a Class II biosafety cabinet. If working in a horizontal laminar air-flow cabinet the fan should be switched off when working with open specimens to avoid the risk of operator contamination.

2. Minimize contamination of the surrounding work area. Do not handle fixtures and fittings that might be touched by others not wearing gloves (e.g. water taps), equipment (e.g. pipettes, microscopes, counters), implements (e.g. pens, calculators), the telephone or paperwork with contaminated gloves.

3. Gloves must be removed or a paper tissue used when, for example, turning on a tap.

Disposal

1. Contaminated specimen containers, tubes and volumetric pipettes are discarded in designated contaminated waste bins. Do not over-fill these bins. The lid must be able to be put on the bin without the need for squashing down or breaking long items.

2. Used Pasteur pipettes, pipette tips, slides, and coverslips are discarded in designated contaminated sharps boxes. Do not over-fill these boxes.

Spills

1. Wear gloves.

2. Surround and cover the spillage with paper tissues or towels. Wipe up the spill using paper tissues or towels.

3. Sterilize the area of the spill using isopropyl alcohol or ethanol; wipe up excess disinfectant using clean paper tissues or towels.

4. Dispose of all paper tissues or towels in a designated contaminated waste bin.

Other biologicals

There are a number of other biologically derived materials that might be used in andrology laboratories. They arrive either in pure form or as solutions, e.g. in culture medium. Such materials include the following:

Blood products: Serum albumin (HSA)
Enzymes: Hyaluronidase, chymotrypsin, trypsin
Others: Egg yolk, heparin, hyaluronic acid

Since these biological products are obtained as pure, aseptic or sterile preparations they may, in limited quantities, be disposed of down the sink, followed by a significant volume (e.g. 5 liters) of cold tap water. However, once they have come into contact with clinical material (i.e. gametes, embryos, semen or follicular fluid) they must be considered potentially infectious and disposed of in the same manner as other contaminated waste.

Contaminated waste disposal

All contaminated waste is placed in the appropriate designated CONTAMINATED WASTE bins or boxes, which should be sealed for collection by an authorized person or disposal company.

Do not over-fill the bins; no-one should ever have to force long items into the bin or have to try and break them in order to put the lids onto the bins.

Chemical materials – receiving, storing, and disposal

Upon receiving a chemical in the laboratory, locate local data safety sheets, e.g. COSHH assessments, and store the chemical according to the safety information that is provided. For disposal give all expired, unused or unwanted chemicals to the local Safety Officer for disposal.

Compressed gases

Safe handling of compressed gases includes not only the cylinders themselves, but also the regulators used to control the flow and/or pressure of the gas at delivery. Gas cylinders must only be transported using special dollies with safety straps around them. In the gas room or during use in the laboratory, cylinders must be stood upright and attached by safety straps to mounting brackets fixed securely to the bench or wall. Cylinders must be protected from mechanical shock and extremes of heat or cold.

Safe, proper use of regulators:

1. Regulators must be attached and removed using the correct wrench, spanner or key.
2. Ensure that the main (inlet) valve is tightly closed before attaching a regulator to a gas cylinder or removing a regulator from a cylinder.
3. Take great care not to damage the screw threads when attaching or removing a regulator.
4. When gas is not flowing, close the inlet valve from the cylinder to the regulator and open the outlet valve. Maintaining pressure inside the regulator when not in use will greatly shorten its life.
5. Always use appropriate tubing or piping for the gas being used and its purpose. For flammable gases use butyl rubber tubing, for high pressure gases use a tubing with a suitable pressure rating as well as any necessary security fittings (e.g. terry clips or worm-drive clamps where the tubing is attached to the regulator outlet).

Note that when using special gases (e.g. CO_2-in-air) suitable tubing must be used. Many materials are permeable to CO_2 and hence the carefully mixed gas could change greatly between leaving the cylinder and reaching its point-of-use.

Cryogenics

Because of its extremely cold temperature ($-196°C$), the handling and use of liquid nitrogen (LN_2) requires extreme care and attention. *Always wear appropriate protective clothing and equipment*, including long sleeves, suitable gloves and a whole-face visor or face shield.

Whenever possible, LN_2 should be transferred from its supply dewar vessel by transfer hose or other delivery device; open pouring should be discouraged.

Touching the inside of dewar vessels containing LN_2, or any object that has been in recent contact with LN_2, using bare fingers can cause severe cold burns. If frostbite does occur, warm the affected skin slowly against a warm part of your body (e.g. armpit). *Do not rub!* Keep the affected area immobile and cover with a sterile dressing.

Dewar vessels must be protected from mechanical insult. Glass dewar vessels must be treated with extreme caution, and it is worth considering the use of styrofoam boxes or stainless steel dewars for short-term uses involving small volumes of LN_2. Plastic-cased dewar vessels are perfectly suitable, except that spilling LN_2 over the plastic casing, especially at the vessel's open neck, often causes it to split. Remember, even steel or aluminum storage dewar tanks can be punctured, and the loss of vacuum between the outer and inner walls will result in rapid evaporative loss of the LN_2, and hence of the cryopreserved material.

Never seal or enclose a dewar vessel containing LN_2 as evaporation of the LN_2 will cause a substantial build-up of internal pressure that will certainly explode glass dewar vessels (e.g. thermos flasks or jugs). All lids or caps for LN_2 dewars must be loose fitting or include an emergency pressure release valve.

Be very careful when handling straws or vials that have been immersed in liquid nitrogen as there is a genuine risk of explosion. If a cryovial is not completely sealed LN_2 will enter it during its period of immersion; this liquid will rapidly turn to gas when returned to ambient temperature and the sudden huge increase in its volume can cause the vial to explode. This is an extremely serious concern with glass ampoules. With traditional straws, evaporation of the liquid that permeates the cotton plug at the top of the straw often causes violent expulsion of this plug the first time the straw is transferred, even for a few seconds, from the liquid phase to ambient temperature (e.g. while searching for a particular straw or batch of straws). This is not a risk if using High Security Straws. Protective goggles or visor must be worn when thawing straws or cryovials. Note that this does not equate to loss of the seal, which is internal to the outer cotton plug.

Although intended for an animal breeding audience, the double DVD *The Guide to Handling Frozen Semen and Embryos* (www.biotechproductions.com) is an excellent resource on safe handling of specimens in cryogenic storage.

Other hazards

All hazardous materials, whether in transit, storage or use, must be clearly labeled so as to alert handlers or users to the hazards and safe handling procedures of such materials. Material Safety Data Sheets and information must be kept on file for each chemical used in the laboratory.

Fire or explosion hazard

Relevant information includes the substance's conditions of flammability, including its flashpoint, and means of extinction. Sensitivity to mechanical impact and static discharge in relation to explosion hazards must also be identified. Information on any hazardous combustion products should also be available.

Reactivity data

This information includes a description of any conditions under which the substance is chemically unstable or any other substance (or class of substances) with which the substance is incompatible. Information on conditions of reactivity and any hazardous decomposition products is also relevant.

Toxicological properties

Information on possible routes of entry into the body including skin contact, skin absorption, eye contact, inhalation and ingestion, as well as the effects of both acute and chronic exposure to the substance should be available. Other relevant information includes the substance's irritant nature and the likelihood of sensitization to it. Specific information on general toxicity, carcinogenicity, teratogenicity, mutagenicity, and reproductive toxicological properties should be clearly identified.

Mercury

Laboratories should have a policy not to use mercury thermometers. However, in the event of breakage of a mercury thermometer, the spilt mercury must be dealt with as a hazardous material.

1. Wear gloves and avoid any skin contact with the mercury.
2. Clean up the spill using a specific cleaning kit, e.g. SPILFYTER Mercury Spill Kit.
3. Discard everything in the disposal box that is part of the kit.

Incident reports

An Incident Report form *must* be completed in any situation where an incident occurs that:

a. impacts the treatment of a patient; or

b. results in injury to a staff member; or

c. creates a safety risk; or

d. creates a security risk; or

e. compromises, or actually causes a failure of laboratory QC or QA.

This is a standard requirement of laboratory accreditation schemes, e.g. ISO 15189:2007 [7], as well as a common regulatory requirement [8]. In a number of countries it is also a legal responsibility of the employer and/or manager.

References

1. World Health Organization. *Laboratory Biosafety Manual 2004*. Geneva: WHO 2004: 186pp.
2. www.free-training.com; www.pp.okstate.edu/ehs/MODULES/index.htm
3. Schrader SM. Safety guidelines for the andrology laboratory. *Fertil Steril* 1989; **51**: 387–9.
4. World Health Organization. *WHO Laboratory Manual for the Examination of Human Semen and Sperm-Cervical Mucus Interaction*. 4th edn. Cambridge: Cambridge University Press 1999: 128pp.
5. Revised guidelines for human embryology and andrology laboratories. The Practice Committee for the American Society for Reproductive Medicine and the Practice Committee of the Society for Assisted Reproductive Technology. *Fertil Steril* 2006; **86** Suppl 4: S56-S72.
6. Magli MC, Vandne Abbeel E, Lundin K, *et al.*, Revised guidelines for good practice in

IVF laboratories. *Hum Reprod* 2008; **23**: 1253–62.

7. International Standard ISO 15189. *Medical Laboratories – Particular Requirements for Quality and Competence*. Geneva: International Organization for Standardization 2007.

8. European Union. Commission Directive 2006/86/EC implementing Directive 2004/ 23/EC of the European Parliament and of the Council as regards traceability requirements, notification of serious adverse reactions and events and certain technical requirements for the coding, processing, preservation, storage and distribution of human tissues and cells. *Official Journal of the European Union* 2006: L294/32, 24.10.2006.

Index

Note: Page numbers in *Italics* refer to figures and tables

A23187 calcium ionophore
121, 122
accident prevention
employees' responsibilities
315
supervisors' responsibilities
315
accreditation 229–232,
231, 232
definition 229
worldwide infrastructure
231–232
accumulative histogram 238
acrosin 26–27
acrosome(s)
defects 65
failure to develop 66
formation *8*
acrosome reaction (AR) 26–27
testing 121–124, *123*
calculations 123
equipment 121
interpretation guidelines
123–124
procedure 122–123
quality control 122
reagents 122
results 123
specimen 121
acrosome reaction following
ionophore challenge
(ARIC) testing 121
interpretation guidelines
123–124
procedure 122–123
reagent 122
response 122
standardized protocol 124
values 123
adrenoceptor alpha$_1$-receptors
17, 18
amplitude of lateral head
displacement
(ALH) 106
ampullae 17–18
analytical balance 279
analytical performance
evaluation 242–243

androgens 10
sperm transport 14
antisperm antibodies 1,
77–86
bacterial infections 86
biological effects 270
circulating 270
direct testing 78
forms 302
IgM 270
immobilizing 161
immunobead test *79*
direct 82–84
indirect 84–86
immunoglobulin
classes 77
indirect testing 78
mixed antiglobulin reaction
test 77–82
direct 78–80
primary screening test
77–78
reference values *264*, 270
sperm motility 48
sperm–mucus interaction
test (SMIT) 164
subfertility 77
Appraisal of Guidelines
Research and Evaluation
(AGREE) 232
asthenozoospermia 3
Australia, regulation 245
autocryopreservation 208
auxiliary sex glands,
secretion 1
average path velocity
(VAP) 106
azoospermia
factor
non-obstructive 219
obstructive 219
sample handling 46
semen sample
appearance 39
surgically retrieved
specimens 219
Wolffian duct system
agenesis 42

Baby Start™ Male Fertility
Test 295
bacteria, semen sample 45
bacterial infections
ejaculate examination
86–87
leukocytes 86, 87
semen microbiological
examination 86–87
see also named organisms
beat cross frequency (BCF),
CASA 106–107
biological materials, safety
317–319
bladder neck 18–19
Bland & Altman chart *235*
blood–testis barrier 10
bright-field microscopy,
TUNEL test 137–138
5-Br-PAPS 91, *92*
buffers 175
cryopreservation media
196, 197
see also sperm buffers
bulbocavernosus muscles 20

calcium ionophore 121, 122
cancer treatment,
autocryopreservation 208
capacitation, sperm 16, 26,
167, 179
seminal plasma
contamination *167*
sperm wash medium 175
CASA *see* computer-aided
sperm analysis (CASA)
cauda epididymis 16
CD45 pan-leukocyte antigen,
immunocytochemical
staining 88–91
calculation 90
calibration 89
equipment 88–89
interpretation guidelines 90
procedure 89–90
quality control 89
reagents 89
results 90

cell membrane, chilling
    effects 189
centrifuge 279
    see also density gradient
        centrifugation (DGC)
centrioles
    duplication 29
    male 28
centrosomes 28
    duplication 29
certification 231
    definition 230
cervical mucus
    cellularity 150
    ferning 150
    Insler score 149–150
        criteria for assigning
            component
            values 149
        crossed hostility
            testing
        Kremer sperm penetration
            test 160
        Kurzrok–Miller test 156
        post-coital test 154
    pH 150
        Kremer sperm penetration
            test 160
        Kurzrok–Miller test 156
        sperm–cervical mucus
            contact test 163
    post-coital test
        Insler score 154
        pH 154
    quantity assessment 150
    receptivity to sperm
        penetration 148
    sampling 148–150
        equipment 148
        estradiol pretreatment
            148
        procedure 148–149
        timing 148
    sperm passage 24
    sperm penetration 147
    spinnbarkeit 150
    storage 150
    substitutes 165
    see also sperm–mucus
        interaction tests
cervical os appearance 150
cervix, sperm reservoir 24
chelating agents 196
chemicals, safety 319
chemiluminescence, ROS
    measurement 114

children, maximum number
    from donor 213
chilling damage 189
Chlamydia trachomatis
    86, 317
    donor screening
        214–215
chorionic villi 29
chromatin, sperm 11–12, 20
    reference values 273–274
    stability 12, 21
    see also sperm chromatin
        structure assay (SCSA);
        sperm chromatin
        testing
chromosomes 5, 8
    balanced translocations/
        deletions 23
ciliary dyskinesia
    sperm motility 48
    sperm vitality 58
cilium, sperm 29
citrate 196
Creutzfeldt–Jakob disease
    (CJD) see variant
        Creutzfeldt–Jakob
        disease (vCJD)
Clinical Laboratory
    Improvement
    Amendments (CLIA)
    (1988, US) 245
clinical practice, evidence-
    based guidelines 232
clinical quality 232–233
    indicators 232
coefficient of variation
    (CV) 238
cold shock 189
College of American
    Pathologists (CAP)
colloidal silica 170–171, 180
Comet assay 259, 274
competence criteria,
    training 234
competitive (intact) zona-
    binding assay 125,
    128–131
    calculation 131
    equipment 126–129
    interpretation
        guidelines 131
    procedure 130–131
    quality control 130
    reagents 129
    results 131
    specimens 129–126

computer-aided sperm analysis
    (CASA) 1, 105
    amplitude of lateral head
        displacement 106
    average path velocity 106
    beat cross frequency
        106–107
    clinical applications
        293–294
    curvilinear velocity
        105, 106
    instrument 284
    instrumentation 291–292
    kinematic measures of sperm
        motility 105–107
    quality control 109
    recommendations 291
    reference values 269–270
    reproductive toxicology 294
    sperm concentration 107
        determination 292
    sperm functional potential
        assessment 107–108
    sperm hyperactivation 108,
        108, 117, 293
        procedure 120
    sperm morphology
        107, 293
    sperm motility 292–293
        percentage 107
        quality control 109
    sperm survival assay 140
    sperm–cervical mucus
        penetration 107–108
    straight line velocity 106
    technology applications
        291–294
confidence intervals 240
contaminated waste
    disposal 319
continuous variables 234
control charts 229
cooling
    mechanically-assisted vapor
        phase 198
    optimal range 191
    rate
        cell survival 190
        with packaging 200
    static vapor phase 198
counting chambers 279
crossed hostility testing (XHT)
    163–164, 163
    Insler score
    interpretation guidelines 164
    procedure 163–164

cryobanking 189–215, 252–255
  cryopreservation methods
    194–199
  donor screening 214–215
  equipment 282–284
  infection transmission
    253–254
  inventory control
    systems 212
  legal issues 212–213
  mistaken identity 253
  monitoring 254
  organization 209–210, *209*
  packaging 199–202, 254
  premature warming
    254–255
  sample storage 209–210
    dual 253
  samples 211
  sperm bank users *194*
  staff safety 253
  storage period 213
  tank types 211
  traceability 212
  transportation 213
  warning systems 254
cryobiology 189–193
cryogenic safety gear 283,
  319–320
cryogenic storage dewars 283
  safety 320
cryogenics, safety 319–320
cryopreservation 189–193
  autocryopreservation 208
  biological factors 195
  calibration 203
  cellular responses
    freezing 189–190
    thawing 190
  centrifuging before 209
  commercial *196*
  competence criteria 234
  cooling profile *201*
  cooling rate control 198
  cross-contamination risk
    200–202, 203
    storage systems 212
  cryodamage 190–192, *191*
  donor sperm 208
  equipment 202–203
  external quality
    assessment 204
  fecundity rates post-thaw 200
  freezing phase 205–207
  highly viscous samples
    208–209

identification of samples 212
intracellular ice formation
  189–190
intracervical insemination 208
intrauterine insemination 208
in-vitro fertilization 208
  methods 194–199, 205–207
  optimization *195*
  osmotic stress 190
  packaging 199–202, 254
    cross-contamination risk
      200–202
    fragility 200
    sealing 200
  post-thaw motility 207
  procedure 202–209
  quality control 203–205
  reagents 203, 204
  recrystallization 191–192
  refreezing of samples 209
  repeat freezing 208
  results 207–209
  samples
    identification 203
    traceability 212
    transportation 213
  second chance sperm
    donor 208
  specimens 205
  sperm
    fragility 209
    motility 207
  sperm preparation 184
    testicular 223–224
  storage
    period 213
    systems 212
  straws 205–206
    fragility 200
    homogeneity from same
      donor 204–205
    identification 212
    preparation 205–206
    semen storage 199–*201*
    thawing 207
    traceability of samples 212
  technical factors 195
  temperature 204
  testicular sperm preparation
    223–224
  thawing 199, 207
    suitability for use after 208
    traceability of samples 212
  transition zone 191
  transportation of samples 213
  very few sperm 209

vitrification 193–194, 198
warming profile *201*
warming rate control 199
water baths 204
cryopreservation media
  195–197
  addition 197
  agents interacting with
    plasma membrane
    195–196
  buffers 196, 197
  chelating agents 196
  formulation 196–197
  good manufacturing
    practice 197
  lipid peroxidation
    prevention 196
  quality control 204
  removal 197
cryoprotective agents
  (CPAs) 192–193
  benefits 192
  harmful effects 192–193
  nonpermeating 192
  osmosis 193
  permeating 192
  toxicity 192
cryosurvival factor (CSF) 207
cryovials, semen storage
  199–*201*
curvilinear velocity (VCL),
  CASA 105, *106*
cytomegalovirus (CMV)
  87, 317
  donor screening 214–215

decapacitation factors 167, 179
dehydration, cellular 190
Deming wheel *see* Plan-Do-
  Check-Act (PDCA) cycle
density gradient centrifugation
  (DGC) 170–174,
  179–182, 185
  buffers 175, 180
  calculations 182
  calibration 180
  centrifugation time/speed
    172–173
  colloidal silica 170–171, 180
  competence criteria 234
  discontinuous 174
  equipment 179–180
  gradient layer number/
    volume 172, *172*
  harvesting technique
    173, *173*

density gradient centrifugation (DGC) (cont.)
  interpretation guidelines 182
  post-gradient swim-up 174
  procedure 181–182
  products 170–171
  quality control 181
  reagents 180
  results 182
  rotors 171–172, *171*, *172*
  selective washing of sperm 170–174
  specimens 179
  tubes 171–172, *171*, *172*
  washing 174
diagnosis 255
Diff-Quik® stain 61
dihydrotestosterone 16
direct swim-up from semen (DSUS) 169, *169*, 174, 175–179
  buffers 178
  calculations 178
  calibration 176–177
  competence criteria 234
  equipment 176
  procedure 177
  quality control 177
  reagents 176
  results 178
  specimens 175
discrete variables 234
dithiothreitol (DTT) 157
DNA 5, 8, 11–12
  fragmentation 132–133, 258
  fragmentation index unique 10
DNA damage
  enzymatic tests 258
  iceberg effect 133, 134
  low sperm number 22
  ROS 132–133, 174
  sperm chromatin integrity tests 258
  sperm function tests 132–139
  sperm preparation 174
  during sperm storage 17
  see also TUNEL test
DNA tests
  enzymatic 258
  reference values 273–274
  sperm chromatin integrity 258
  see also TUNEL test

docosahexaenoic acid (DHA) 113–114
donors
  clinical history 214
  genetic screening 214
  maximum number for children 213
  microbiological testing 214–215
  physical screening 214
  psychological screening 214
  screening 214–215
  serological testing 214–215
dry bath 279
dry shipper 283

ejaculate
  composition 21
  sequence sample report form 303
  split *103*
  volume reference values 264–265
ejaculation 19, 20–21
  antegrade 19
  frequency 16–17
  zinc redistribution 21
  see also retrograde ejaculation
ejaculation sequence 20–21, 102–104
  abnormal 21
  calculations 104–*104*
  interpretation guidelines 104
  procedure 103–104
  results 104–*104*
ejaculatory ducts 17–18
  obstruction 102
ejaculatory flow speed 20
ejaculatory muscles 20
emission 18–19
  smooth muscle innervation 19
endometrium 29
endpoints of interest 261, 262
epididymal duct 13–14, *14*
epididymal spermatozoa preparation 219–221
  calibration 220
  equipment 220
  procedure 220–221
  reagents 220
  sperm buffers 220

epididymal transit time 15
epididymis
  biochemical tests 99–102
  sperm storage 16–17
  sperm transit 16
  sperm transport 15–16
epithelial cells, semen sample 45
Epstein–Barr virus (EBV) 87
equipment 277–*280*
  basic laboratory 277–282
  contaminated 314
  cryobanking 282–284
  inappropriate 250
  safety 315–316
  specialized assays 284–285
  sterilization 314
  supply companies 287–289
erythrocytes
  bacterial infections 86
  semen sample 45
Escherichia coli 86
estradiol 24
  pretreatment for cervical mucus sampling 148
ethylenediamine tetraacetic acid (EDTA) 196
European Union directives 244–245
evidence-based clinical practice guidelines 232
explosion hazard 320
external quality assurance (EQA) 242
  accuracy 237
  analytical performance evaluation 242–243
  cryopreservation 204
  functionality 243
  programmes 242
  schemes 242–243, *243*
extraordinary precautions 313
eye protection 315

face masks 316
failure modes and effects analysis (FMEA) 240–241, 249–250
Fallopian tubes, isthmus 25
fecundity rates post-thaw 200
female reproductive physiology 23–30
  cervical mucus 24
  fertilization 25–26

oocytes
  activation 28
  passage of competent
    sperm 27
  single 23
  sperm fusion 27–28
  sperm mitochondria
    destruction 30
oviductal ampulla 25
placental development
  initiation 29–30
sperm messages after fusion
  28–30
sperm responses to female
  genital tract signals
  26–27
uterotubal junction 25
ferning of cervical mucus 150
Fertell® 295
fertilization
  capacity of sperm 16
  passage of sperm through
    cervical mucus 24
  polyzoospermic
  reference values for sperm
    ability tests 273
  sperm reaching place for
    25–26
fire hazard 320
fire safety 316
flagella, sperm 29, 114
  high-amplitude waves 117
flash-freeze techniques 198
flavoproteins, semen
    sample 39
flow cytometry
  equipment 284
  TUNEL test 137, 138
fluorescence microscopy
  equipment 284
  TUNEL test 137, 138
follicle-stimulating hormone
  (FSH) 10
  estradiol production
    stimulation 24
freezer 279
  controlled rate 282–283
freezing
  cellular responses 189–190
  mechanically-assisted vapor
    phase cooling 198
  programmable systems 198
  static vapor phase
    cooling 198
  ultra-rapid 198
  vitrification 198

fructose, seminal fluid 18,
    94–97, 104
  qualitative assessment 97–98
  reference values 271
fume hood/adsorber 279, 316

gametes
  protection in laboratory 5
  protective role 5–6
  uniqueness 5
gases, compressed 319
genetic screening of donors 214
genital tract, male 15
germ cells 6
  immature in semen 90–91
glassware 280–281
globozoospermia 66
gloves, using 314
alpha-glucosidase
  neutral 99–102
  reference values 272
gonadotrophin-releasing
    hormone (GnRH) 10
good laboratory practice
  (GLP) 244
good manufacturing practice
  (GMP), cryopreservation
  media 197
Halo test 274
HAmax assay 117–118, 118
  interpretation guidelines 120
  procedure 120
  reagents 119
  results 120
hamster egg penetration test
    (HEPT) see zona-free
    hamster egg penetration
    test
hand protection 314, 315
Health Technology Assessment
    (HTA) 233
heated stirrer 279
Hemacolor® stain 61
hemizona assay (HZA) 125,
    126–128, 127
  calculations 127–128
  equipment 126
  interpretation guidelines 128
  procedure 127
  quality control 127
  reagents 126
  results 127–128
  specimens 126
hemizona index (HZI)
    127–128

hemocytometer 55, 279
  ejaculate dilution 52
hepatitis B virus (HBV) 87
  donor screening 214
  transmission 317
hepatitis C virus (HCV)
  donor screening 214
  transmission 317
herpes simplex virus
    (HSV) 87
high ion concentration
    hypothesis 190
highly viscous samples 183,
    208–209
HIV infection 87
  donor screening 214
  transmission 317
home testing 295
hot plate 280
human chorionic gonadotrophin
    (hCG) 10
human papillomavirus (HPV)
    87, 317
human resources,
    inadequate 251
human T cell lymphotropic
    virus (HTLV)
    214–215
humid chamber 280
hyaluronidase 26–27
hydrogen peroxide 114
hydroperoxyl radical 114
hyperactivation see sperm
    hyperactivation
hypogastric nerves 19
hypogastric plexus 19
hypothalamic hypogonadism 267

ice formation, intracellular
    189–190
  thawing 199
immotile cilia syndrome see
    Kartagener syndrome
antisperm antibodies 77–78
  direct 82–84
    calculations 84
    equipment 82
    immunobead preparation
      83
    interpretation guidelines
      84
    procedure 83–84
    quality control 83–84
    reagents 83
    results 84
    sperm preparation 83

immotile cilia syndrome (cont.)
  indirect 84–86
    calculations 86
    equipment 85
    interpretation guidelines 86
    procedure 85–86
    quality control 85
    reagents 85
    results 86
    specimens 84
immunoglobulin A (IgA)
  antisperm antibodies 77
  direct immunobead test 82–84
  mixed antiglobulin reaction
    test 78
immunoglobulin G (IgG)
  antisperm antibodies 77
  direct immunobead test
    82–84
  mixed antiglobulin reaction
    test 78
immunoglobulin M (IgM),
    antisperm antibodies 270
incident reports 321
incubators 280
infections
  bacterial 86–87
  protozoal 45, 45
  semen
    microbiological
      examination 86–88
    odor 40
  sperm motility 48
  transmission in cryobanking
    253–254
  viral 87
  see also named organisms
inflammation, bacterial
    infections 87
inflammatory cells
  peroxide-positive 70–72
  semen sample 39
information for patients 35
inhibin-B 10
Insler score for cervical mucus
  149–150
  criteria for assigning
    component values 149
  crossed hostility testing
  Kremer sperm penetration
    test 160
  Kurzrok–Miller test 156
  post-coital test 154
intact zona-binding assay see
    competitive (intact)
    zona-binding assay

internal quality control (IQC)
  236–237
International Laboratory
  Accreditation
  Corporation (ILAC)
  231–232
International Organization for
  Standardization (ISO)
  231–232
  see also ISO 15189:2007
inter-observer quality control
  237–238
intracervical insemination
  (ICI) 208
intracytoplasmic sperm
  injection (ICSI) 28
  epididymal sperm 221
  surgically retrieved
    sperm 219
  testicular sperm thawing 224
intra-urethral pressure 20
intrauterine insemination
  (IUI) 208
in-vitro fertilization (IVF) 208
ischiocavernosus muscles 20
ISO 231–232, 238, 244
  risk management 250
ISolate® 170–171

Kartagener syndrome
  sperm motility 48
  sperm vitality 58
kits, inappropriate 250
Kremer sperm penetration test
  156–161, 159
  calculations 160
  calibration 157–158
  equipment 157
  interpretation guidelines
    160–161
  procedure 158–160
  quality control 158
  reagents 157
  reference values 273
  results 160
  specimens 157
Kurzrok–Miller (K-M) test
  154–156, 155
  calculations 156
  disposable materials 155
  equipment 154–155
  interpretation guidelines 156
  procedure 155–156
  quality control 155
  reagents 155
  reference values 273

results 156
specimens 154

laboratory
  equipment 277–280
  gamete protection 5
  high-risk 250–251
  human resources 251
  inadequate resources 250
  supply companies 287–289
  systems 251
  work surface
    decontamination 314
  see also equipment
laboratory forms 297–303
laboratory methods
  bias 239
  comparing 241
  consistency 241
  controls 239
  error sources 239
  improvement 241–242
  inappropriate 250
  options 239
  practicality 240
  precision 239
  requirements of robust
    239–240
  review 241–242
  support 240
  training 240
  uncertainty 240–241
  see also quality; quality
    control
laboratory staff
  human resources 251
  vaccination 313
laboratory supplies
  disposal 314
  supply companies 287–289
legal issues, cryobanking
  212–213
leukocytes
  bacterial infections 86, 87
  CD45 pan-leukocyte antigen
    immunocytochemical
    staining 88–91
  destruction of sperm in
    uterus 24
  forms
  reference values 264
  ROS production 114
  semen 87–88
    cytology 69, 70
    sample 44–45
    staining 61, 69, 88, 88

leukocytospermia
Leydig cells 10
ligase chain reaction (LCR) 87
linearity (LIN)
lipid peroxidation, prevention 196
lipid phase transition 189
liquid nitrogen
    controlled cooling 198
    cryogenic storage dewars 283
    handling precautions 205, 253
    safety 319–320
    storage system 212
    supply vessels 283–284
    transport 253
lubricants, semen collection 35
luminol, ROS measurement 114, 115–116
luminometer 285
luteinizing hormone (LH) 10

Makler chamber 279
male pronucleus formation 28
measurement, uncertainty 240–241, 242, 255
mechanically-assisted vapor phase cooling 198
meiosis 7, 8
    evolution 5
    recombination 5
    spermatocytes 10
mercury, safety 321
messenger cells 11
microbiological testing, donors 214–215
micro-epididymal sperm aspiration (MESA) 219
    epididymal sperm preparation 219
micromanipulator 285
microorganisms, gamete protection against 5–6
microscopes 277–278, 278
    fluorescence 284
    inverted 285
minimum cellular volume hypothesis 190
mitochondria, destruction of sperm by oocytes 30
mitochondrial DNA (mtDNA), sperm 12–13
    destruction by oocytes 30
mitosis 7–8
    zygote 28

mixed antiglobulin reaction (MAR) test
    antisperm antibodies 77–82
    direct 78–80
        calculations 80
        interpretation guidelines 80
        procedure 79
        quality control 79
        results 80
    indirect 80–82
        calculations 81–82
        equipment 80
        interpretation guidelines 82
        procedure 81
        quality control 81
        reagents 81
        results 81–82
        specimens 80
Mycoplasma 317

National Association of Testing Authorities (NATA, Australia) 245
necrozoospermia
Neisseria gonorrhoeae 86, 317
    donor screening 214–215
Neubauer ruling 54
    hemocytometer 55
neutral alpha-glucosidase, seminal fluid 99–102
nick translation assays 258
nipple defect 65
nitrogen see liquid nitrogen
noradrenaline 17, 18, 25
normal range 261
nuclear chromatin decondensation (NCD)

oligozoospermia 3
    sample handling 46
    semen sample appearance 39
oocytes
    passage of competent sperm 27
    single 23
    sperm fusion 27–28
    sperm mitochondria destruction 30
osmotic stress 190
oviductal ampulla 25
ovulation, progesterone levels 25

packaging for cryopreservation 199–202
    cross-contamination risk 200–202

fragility 200
    sealing 200
Papanicolaou stain 61, 69
    leukocytes 88, 88
    procedure 62–63
parthenogenesis
pentoxifylline
    epididymal sperm preparation 221
    sperm hyperactivity testing 117–118, 118
Percoll® 170–171
percutaneous epididymal sperm aspiration (PESA) 219
    epididymal sperm preparation 219
pericentriolar material 28–29
peroxide-positive cell identification 70–72, 70
    calculations 72
    equipment 70–71
    interpretation 72
    materials 70–71
    procedure 71–72
    quality control 71
    reagents 71
    results 72
personal hygiene 314
physiology
    male reproduction 5–30
    see also female reproductive physiology
placental development initiation 29–30
Plan-Do-Check-Act (PDCA) cycle 228, 228, 241–242
polymerase chain reaction (PCR), viral infections 87
post-coital test (PCT) 147, 150–154, 153
    calculations 153–154
    calibration 152
    equipment 151
    interpretation guidelines 154
    procedure 153
    quality control 152
    reagents 151
    reference values 272–273
    results 153–154, 154
    specimens 151
    timing 150, 151
posthumous reproduction 213
post-synaptic short neurons 19
process analysis 228–229

process control 229
progesterone
  acrosome reaction testing 121
  levels after ovulation 25
  sperm hyperactivity testing
    117–118, *118*
prostaglandins, seminal
    vesicles 18
prostate 18
  biochemical tests 91–94
prostate-specific antigen
    (PSA) 21
prostatic fluid 18, 20
  delayed emptying 21
  urethral wall extension 20
  zinc assessment 91–94
protamines, sperm 12, *12*
protective clothing 314, 315–316
  cryogenic safety gear 283,
    319–320
protozoa, semen sample 45, *45*
PureSperm® 170–171

quality
  clinical 232–233
  concepts 227–228
  indicators *230*
  management 227–229
  training 233–236
quality assurance (QA) 1–2, 227
  accreditation 229–232
  see also external quality
    assurance (EQA);
    external quality
    assessment program
    (EQAP)
quality control (QC) 1–2, 227,
    236–242
  accumulative histogram 238
  coefficient of variation 238
  external 243, *243*
  internal 236–237
  inter-observer 237–238
  material 236–237
  method selection 238
  patient samples 237
  quality requirement
    definition 237
  requirements of robust
    method 239–240
  review of procedures 242
  rolling average 229, 238
  selection of levels 237
  Shewart control chart 237
  stability of method 237
  variation of method 237

quality improvement (QI)
    1–2, 228
quality management system
    (QMS) 228–229

reactive oxygen species (ROS)
  bacterial infections 87
  chemiluminescence
    methods 114
  DNA damage 132–133, 174
  measurement
    calculations 116
    equipment 114–115
    interpretation guidelines
      116
    procedure 115–116
    quality control 115
    reagents 115
    reference values 272
    results 116
    specimens 114
  production by sperm 66
  sperm function tests
    113–116
reactivity data 320–321
reagents, inappropriate 250
5-alpha-reductase
  type 1 16
  type 2 16
reference values 261–274
  antisperm antibodies *264*, 270
  CASA 269–270
  defined populations 262
  DNA tests 273–274
  ejaculate volume 264–265
  endpoints of interest 261, 262
  ethnicity 262
  fructose in seminal fluid 271
  geographical differences 262
  alpha-glucosidase in seminal
    fluid 272
  leukocytes *264*
  post-coital test 272–273
  semen analysis *264*
  semen volume 264–265, *264*
  seminal plasma biochemistry
    271–272
  sperm chromatin 273–274
  sperm chromatin structure
    assay 273–274
  sperm concentration
    264, 265
  sperm fertilizing ability
    tests 273
  sperm function tests
    272–273

sperm morphology assessment
    264, 268–269
sperm motility *264*,
    266–267
sperm progression
    grading 267
sperm vitality *264*, 267–268
sperm–mucus interaction
    tests 272–273
statistical techniques 262
technical methods 262
teratozoospermia index 269
total sperm count *264*,
    265–266
TUNEL test 274
zinc in seminal fluid 271
registration 231
  definition 230
regulation 244–245
  environment 244–245
  risk management 250
replicate counts 305–310
  acceptable differences 308
  uncertainty of results of
    sperm numbers
    306, 310
report forms 297–303
  computer-generated
    300, 302
reports 252
  incident 321
reproductive toxicology
    257–259
  CASA 294
  semen analysis 257–258
  sperm chromatin integrity
    tests 258–259
  training of technicians 258
respiratory protection 316
retrograde ejaculation 19
  semen collection 35
  urine specimens 184–185
risk management 249–255
  high-risk laboratories
    250–251
  proactive 249
  regulation 250
  retrospective 249
  tools 249–250
rolling averages 229, 238
root cause analysis (RCA)
    249–250
round cells
  forms
    semen sample 44–45, 46
  staining 61

safety 313–321
  accident prevention 315
  biological materials 317–319
  chemicals 319
  compressed gases 319
  contaminated waste
      disposal 319
  cryobanking 253
  cryogenic storage dewars 320
  cryogenics 319–320
  equipment 315–316
  explosion hazard 320
  fire hazard 316, 320
  incident reports 321
  liquid nitrogen 319–320
  mercury 321
  reactivity data 320–321
  recommendations 313–315
  responsibility 313
  semen handling 317–318
  spills 316–317
  staff 253
  straws 320
  toxicological 321
  see also protective clothing
safety cabinets 282
safety gear
  cryogenic 283, 319–320
  see also protective clothing
sample container handling
    36–37
secondary sex characteristics 10
secretory cells, innervation 19
seeding, ice formation 189–190
semen
  collection 317–318
  color 39
  disposal 318
  examination after vasectomy
      72–74
  handling 318
    safety 317–318
  immature germ cells 90–91
  leukocytes 87–88
  normal 44
  odor 39–40
  osmolarity 21–22
  packaging for cryopreservation
      199–202
  processing 318
  prognostic assessment 1–2
  specimen reception 317–318
  spills 318
  STD organisms 317
  viscous samples 60
  visual appearance 39

semen analysis 1–3, 33–74
  after vasectomy 72–74
    calculations 74
    interpretation guidelines
      74
    procedure 73
    quality control 73
    results 74
  analytical procedures 33
  biochemistry 271–272
  CASA technology 105,
      291–294
  characteristics variables 262
  competence criteria 234
  container labeling 36
  cytology 69–70
  diagnosis 255
  donor screening 215
  ejaculation sequence
      102–104
  extended 77–109
  home testing 295
  information for patients 35
  interpretation of results
      2–3, 255
  liquefaction 37–38
  microbiological examination
      86–88
  odor 39–40
  patient instructions 35
  peroxide-positive cell
      identification 70–72, 70
  pH 41–42
  prognostic information 2–3
  prostate biochemical tests
      91–94
  reference values 262–269, 264
  report form 301
  reproductive toxicology
      257–258
  sample
    collection 34–35
    container 34
    container handling
      36–37
    delivery 34–35
    depth 52
    dilution 41, 52, 52,
      53–54
    handling 46
    incubation 36
    numbers 2
    weighing 36
  sperm concentration 52–56
  sperm morphology 58–69,
      59–68

sperm motility assessment
    41, 44, 46–51, 49
  standardized methods 21,
      257–258
  terminology 3
  training of technicians 258
  treatment pathway 2–3
  variability 255
  viscosity 40–41
  visual appearance 39
  vitality 56–58, 58
  volume 36–37
  wet preparation
    investigation 43–46
    making 42–43
semen container labeling 36
semen liquefaction 37–38
  equipment/materials 38
  interpretation guidelines 38
  procedure 38
  results 38
semen pH 41–42
  equipment/materials 41
  interpretation guidelines 42
  procedure 42
semen sample
  debris 44–45
  incubation 36
  other cells 44–45
  weighing 36
semen viscosity 40–41
  equipment/materials 40
  highly viscous samples 183
  cryopreservation
      208–209
  interpretation guidelines 41
  procedure 40
  results 40
  viscous samples 60
semen volume 36–37
  calculations 37
  calibration 37
  equipment/materials 36
  high 37
  interpretation guidelines 37
  low 37
  procedure 37
  quality control 37
  reference values 264–265, 264
  results 37
seminal fluid
  biochemistry reference
      values 271–272
  fructose 18
    qualitative assessment
      97–98

seminal fluid (cont.)
  fructose quantitative
    assessment 94–97, *104*
    calculations 97
    calibration 95–96
    equipment 94–95
    interpretation guidelines 97
    quality control 96
    reagents 95
    results 97
  neutral alpha-glucosidase
    assessment 99–102
    calculations 101–102
    calibration 100–101
    equipment 99
    interpretation guidelines
      102
    procedure 101
    quality control 100–101
    reagents 100
    results 101–102
    specimen preparation 99
  sperm separation 179
  zinc assessment 91–94, *104*
    calculations 93
    calibration 92
    equipment 91
    interpretation
      guidelines 94
    procedure 92–93
    quality control 92
    reagents 92
    results 93
seminal vesicles 17–18
  biochemical tests 94–97
seminiferous cords 6
  Sertoli cells 10
seminiferous tubules *9, 14*
  germinal epithelium *9*
  Sertoli cells 10
  sperm transport 13
  spermatogenesis 9
serological testing, donors
  214–215
Sertoli cell-only syndrome 6
Sertoli cells 6, 8–9, 10
  seminiferous tubule
    germinal epithelium *9*
sexually transmissible diseases
  (STDs) 317
  viral 87
sharps accidents/disposal 313
Shewart control chart 237
short adrenergic neurons 19, 25
short tail syndrome 66
silica, colloidal 170–171, 180

single cell electrophoresis
  assay 259
small round-head defect 66
smooth muscle innervation 19
solution effect 190
specimens
  processing 252
  provenance 251–252
  results reporting 252
  storage 283
  witnessing 252
sperm/spermatozoa
  acrosome
    defects 65
    failure to develop 66
    formation *8*
  acrosome reaction 26–27
    testing 121–124
  agglutination 44
  aggregation 44
  aging 17
  anatomy *11*
  ATP production 114
  atypical 183–185
  axoneme 11
  cervical mucus penetration
    107–108, 147
  chromatin 11–12, 20
    reference values 273–274
    stability *12*, 21
  cilium 29
  clumping 44
  conservation 16
  cytoplasmic residues 66
  delayed expulsion 21
  diluents 53–54
  DNA 11–12
  donor for cryopreservation 208
    second chance 208
  fertilization
    capacity 16
    passage of through
      cervical mucus 24
    reaching place for 25–26
    reference values for ability
      tests 273
  flagella 29, 114
    high-amplitude waves 117
  fluorochrome labeling 130
  fragility of cryopreserved 209
  functional potential
    assessment 107–108
  head
    defects 65
    duplications 65
    loose 66

  human 11–13
  immaturity 66
  interpretation guidelines 58
  kinematic measures *105*,
    164, 269
  maturation 16
  messages after fusion 28–30
  midpiece defects 65
  mitochondria destruction by
    oocyte 30
  mtDNA 12–13
  neck defects 65
  number 22
    DNA damage risk 22
  oocytes
    activation 28
    barriers 27
    fusion 27–28
  in oviductal ampulla 25
  passage through cervical
    mucus 24
  penetration of cervical
    mucus 107–108, 147
  pinheads 66
  placental development
    initiation 29–30
  protamines 12, *12*
  rapid progressive 48
  reactive oxygen species 66,
    113–116
  replicate counts 305–310
  responses to female genital
    tract signals 26–27
  selection and semen osmolarity
    changes 21–22
  short tail syndrome 66
  small round-head defect 66
  specific gravity 170, 179
  standardized methods of
    handling 21
  sterilizing defects 66
  storage 16–17
    DNA damage 17
    size 16–17
  tail defects 65
  transit time 15–16
  transport 13–16
  uncertainty of results of
    numbers 306, 310
  unknown cells 66
  in uterotubal junction 25
  zinc 11–12, *12*, 20
    withdrawal 21
  see also capacitation;
    cryobanking
sperm aster formation 29

sperm bank users *194*
sperm buffers 175, 176, 178, 180
  epididymal spermatozoa
    preparation 220
  testicular sperm
    preparation 222
sperm chromatin structure
  assay (SCSA)
  133–134, 258
  reference values 273–274
sperm chromatin testing
  132–134, *133*
  dispersion test 259
  integrity tests 258–259
sperm concentration 52–56
  calculations 55, 56
  CASA 107, 269, 292
  ejaculate dilution *52*
  equipment 52–53
  forms
  home testing 295
  interpretation 56
  low 60
  materials 53
  procedure 53–55
  quality control 53
  reagents 53
  reference values *264*, 265
  results 55
sperm counting 22, 54–56
  reference values for total *264*,
    265–266
  wet preparation 43–44
sperm function tests 113–142
  acrosome reaction testing
    121–124, *123*
    calculations 123
    equipment 121
    interpretation guidelines
      123–124
    procedure 122–123
    quality control 122
    reagents 122
    results 123
    specimen 121
  chromatin assay 132–134, *133*
  DNA damage 132–139
  hyperactivation 117–120,
    117, *118*
    calculations 120
    calibration 119
    equipment 118–119
    interpretation
      guidelines 120
    procedure 120
    quality control 119

  reagents 119
  results 120
  specimens 118
  reactive oxygen species
    113–116
  reference values 272–273
  sperm survival assay 139–142
  sperm–zona binding
    124–128
  sperm–zona binding test
    competitive (intact) zona-
      binding assay 125,
      128–131
    hemizona assay 126–128
    materials 125
  TUNEL test 133, *133*,
    135–139
  zona-free hamster egg
    penetration test
    131–132
sperm hyperactivation 26,
  27, *117*
  CASA 108, *108*, 117, 293
  measurement 117–120, *118*
sperm immobilization (SIT)
  test, antisperm
  antibodies 78
sperm morphology 11, 58–69,
  59–74
  atypical 64–65
  calculations 68
  CASA 107, 293
  defects 65–66
  equipment 66–67
  evaluation 64–66
  fixation of smears 60–61
  forms
  interpretation of results 68
  materials 66–67
  microscopy 68–69
  mounting of stained smears
    63–64
  procedure 67
  quality control 67
  results 68
  smear preparation 59–60
  staining of smears 61–63, *62*
  Tygerberg strict criteria 64
  typical 64
sperm morphology assessment
  evaluation 236
  reference values *264*,
    268–269
  training 235–236
  typical forms 268
sperm motility 11, 24

  assessment 41, 44, 46–51
  calculation 47–48
  CASA 107, 109, 269, 292–293
  categories 46–48
  classification 239
  ejaculation sequence 104
  equipment 47
  home testing 295
  hyperactivation 26, 27
  index 141–142
  interpretation guidelines 48
  kinematic measures 105–107
  post-thaw in
    cryopreservation 207
  procedure 47
  progressive 266–267
  quality control 47
  rapid progressive 267
  reference values *264*,
    266–267
  results 47–48
  sperm survival assay 141–142
  testicular sperm
    incubation 221
  video monitoring 48–50
  video recording *49*, 50–51
  videomicrography system
    278–279
  wet preparation 42
  see also sperm
    hyperactivation
sperm penetration assay (SPA)
  see zona-free hamster
    egg penetration test
sperm penetration meter
  device 157
sperm preparation 167–187
  absolute yield 183
  adherence-based methods 170
  atypical specimens 183–185
  buffers 175, 178, 180
    epididymal sperm 220
    testicular sperm
      preparation 222
  competence criteria 234
  cryopreserved specimens 184
  density gradient
    centrifugation 170–174,
    179–182, 185
    buffers 175, 180
    competence criteria 234
  direct swim-up from
    semen 169, *169*, 174,
    175–179, 185
    competence criteria 234
  dirty specimens 184

sperm preparation (cont.)
  DNA damage 174
  epididymal 219–221
  evaluation of methods
    182–183
  highly viscous samples 183
  media 175, 178
  method selection 185
  migration-based techniques
    168–169
  migration-sedimentation
    technique 168–169
  poor quality specimens 184
  processing of multiple
    186–187, *186*
  relative yield 183
  retrograde ejaculation urine
    specimens 184–185
  safe methods 174–175
  selective washing using
    density gradient
    centrifugation 170–174
  separation from seminal
    plasma 179
  simple washing techniques
    168, 174
  surgically retrieved
    specimens 185, 219–225
    epididymal 219–221
  swim-up technique 168
    buffers 175, 178
    direct from semen 169,
      169, 174, 175–179,
      185, 234
    from washed pellet or
      sperm suspension 169
  testicular 221–225
sperm production 6–9
  genes controlling 6
sperm progression grading,
    reference values 267
sperm survival assay 139–142
  calculations 141–142
  calibration 140
  CASA 140
  equipment 139–140
  interpretation guidelines 142
  procedure 140–141
  quality control 140
  reagents 140
  results 141–142
  specimens 139
  sperm motility assessment 141
sperm vitality 56–58
  calculations 58
  equipment 57

preparation *58*
procedure 57–58
quality control 57–58
reagents 57
reference values *264,*
  267–268
results 58
Spermac® stain 61
spermarche 17
spermatids 7, 8, *8*
spermatocytes 8
  meiosis 10
spermatocytogenesis 7–8
spermatogenesis 6–9, *7*
  efficiency 13
  impaired 12–13
  pleiomorphism 13
  preparation in embryo 6
  processes 6–9
spermatogonia 6, 7–8, *7*
sperm–cervical mucus
    contact (SCMC) test
    161–164, *162*
  equipment 161
  procedure 161–162
  quality control 161
  reference values 273
  results *162*
  specimens 161
sperm–mucus interaction tests
    (SMITs) 82, 147–165
  antisperm antibody
    testing 164
  cervical mucus sampling
    148–150
  cervical mucus substitutes 165
  complementary tests
    164–165
  crossed hostility testing
    163–164
  Kremer sperm penetration
    test 156–161
  Kurzrok–Miller test
    154–156
  mucus sampling 147
  post-coital test 147,
    150–154, *154*
  reference values 272–273
  sperm kinematics 164
  sperm penetration assay *160*
  sperm–cervical mucus contact
    test 161–164, *162*
  timing 147
spermiation 7, 9
spermiogenesis *7*, 8
  steps *8*

sperm–zona binding test 124–128
  competitive (intact) zona-
    binding assay 125,
    128–131
  hemizona assay 125,
    126–128, *127*
  indirect 128
  materials 125
  standardization 128
spills
  dealing with 316–317
  semen 318
spinnbarkeit 150
staff safety, cryobanking 253
standard operating procedures
    (SOPs) 229, 251
static vapor phase cooling 198
stem cells, renewal 6
straight line velocity (VSL),
    CASA 106
straightness (STR)
straws 254
  fragility 200
  handling *555.30, 280,* 320
  homogeneity from same
    donor 204–205
  identification 212
  labeling 283
  preparation 205–206
  safety 320
  sealing devices 284
  semen storage 199–*201*
  thawing 207
  traceability 212
Streptococcus 317
subfertility 1–2
  antisperm antibodies 77
  home testing 295
  physical examination 3
  semen analysis 1–3
supercooling 189–190
superoxide anion 114
supply companies 287–289
swim-up techniques 168
  buffers 175, 176
  direct from semen 169, *169,*
    174, 175–179, 185
  competence criteria 234
  post-gradient 174
  from washed pellet or sperm
    suspension 169
syphilis, donor screening 214

tally counters 282
tanks, cryobanking 211
technicians, training 258

teratozoospermia index (TZI)
66, 68
reference values 269
testicular biopsy, surgically
retrieved sperm 219
testicular dysgenesis syndrome
262
testicular interstitium 10
testicular sperm aspiration
(TESA) 219, 221
testicular sperm extraction
(TESE) 219, 221
testicular sperm preparation
221–225
calibration 222
cryopreservation 224
equipment 222
freezing 223–224
incubation 221
procedure 223–224
reagents 222
specimen 222
thawing 224
testosterone 10
cauda epididymis 16
testosterone dehydrogenase
type 18
thawing
cellular responses 190
fecundity rates 200
post-thaw sperm motility 207
rate
control 199
with packaging 200
sample suitability for use
after 208
testicular sperm preparation
224
thermometers 282
total quality management
(TQM) 227–228
toxicology 257–259
see also reproductive
toxicology
training
comparing results of expert
and trainee 234, 235
competence criteria 234
laboratory methods 240
quality 233–236
sperm morphology
assessment 235–236
step-by-step 233
technicians 258
technique standardization
234

tray agglutination (TAT)
test, antisperm
antibodies 78
Trichomonas, semen sample
45, 45
TUNEL test 133, 133,
135–139, 258
bright-field microscopy
137–138
calculation 138
equipment 135
flow cytometry 137, 138
fluorescence microscopy
137, 138
interpretation guidelines 139
procedure 136–138
quality control 135–136
reagents 135
reference values 274
results 138
specimen 135
twin pregnancy, spontaneous 23
Tygerberg strict criteria for
sperm morphology 64

ultra-rapid freezing 198
uncertainty of measurement
240, 242, 255
controlling 240–241
determination 240–241
sources 240
United States regulation 245
universal precautions 313, 317
Ureaplasma urealyticum
86, 317
urethral wall, extension 20
uterotubal junction 25
uterus, leukocyte destruction of
sperm 24

vaccination, laboratory
staff 313
vagina 24
vapor phase cooling
mechanically-assisted 198
static 198
variables
continuous 241
discrete 241
vas deferens 14, 17
recanalization 74
sperm transport 14
vasectomy, semen examination
after 72–74
video monitors
calibration 49

sperm motility assessment
48–50
calibration 49–50
procedure 49–50
video recording, sperm
motility assessment
50–51
equipment 50
procedure 51
quality control 51
videomicrography system
278–279, 278
viral infections
semen microbiological
examination 87
see also hepatitis B virus;
hepatitis C virus; HIV
infection
viscosity see highly viscous
samples; semen
viscosity
vitrification 193–194, 198
vortex mixer 282

warming
premature 254–255
profile 201
rate
control 199
with packaging 200
see also thawing
waste disposal, contaminated
319
waterbath 282
wet preparation
air bubbles 43
debris 44–45
disposable materials 42
equipment 43
examination 43–45
forms
investigation 43–46
making 42–43
other cells 44–45
procedure 43
sperm aggregation/
agglutination 44
sperm counting 43–44
sperm motility
assessment 44
witnessing 252
wobble (WOB)
Wolffian duct system agenesis
18, 102
azoospermia 42
semen pH 41, 42

X-chromosomes 6

Y-chromosomes 6
  AZF region microdeletions
    219

zinc
  redistribution at ejaculation 21
  seminal fluid 91–94, *104*
    reference values 271

sperm 11–12, *12*, 20
  withdrawal 21
zona pellucida 27
  acrosome reaction
    26–27
  competitive (intact) zona-
    binding assay 126,
    130–131
  hemizona assay 126
  sperm binding 27

sperm–zona binding test
    124–128
zona-free hamster egg
    penetration test
    131–132, *132*, *160*
  seminal plasma
    contamination of sperm
    capacitation *167*
ZP3 glycoprotein 26–27, 121
zygote, mitosis 28